W9-AEJ-390

Acknowledgements

It takes a great deal of hard work, dedication, and persistence to transform a concept into a tangible reality. This book was no exception. Although the idea was conceived more than four years ago, it would not have progressed this far without the efforts and personal sacrifices of many individuals. This book was truly a team effort; here I will attempt to recognize those with the most direct roles.

A special thanks goes out to Meredith, my wife, for her unwavering support and guidance. Her editing, organizational skills, and overall perspective were absolutely essential. Next, I'd like to thank Lee, my mother, who meticulously collected, compiled, and interpreted the data necessary to rate over 600 foods. Amazingly, she remained enthusiastic even after I updated the system rules, essentially making her start over – twice! Although she declined to be listed as a co-author, her tremendous contribution to this endeavor merits recognition.

I'd like to thank Tim, my brother, whose computer savvy transformed the raw data into an easily understood format, which saved time and prevented headaches as we moved towards publication. I am grateful for the collaboration and advice of Drs. Michael McDaniel and Laurence Sperling, whose perspectives on cardiovascular disease prevention were truly enlightening. I look forward to continuing our collaboration in the future. My sincere appreciation goes out to Dr. Ai Mukai, one of the most multi-talented people I know. Her varied contributions included illustrations, cover and design ideas, and computer expertise.

I'd like to express my gratitude to Dr. B.R. Ashby, Fran Ashby, and Rick Ramsden, who took time out of their busy lives to make suggestions and help with the editing process. I also appreciate the keen insights of Dr. Hector Lopez, whose understanding of nutritional biochemistry never ceases to amaze me.

I'd like to thank Clarke Scott for designing a cover that is not only pleasing to the eye, but also reflects the contents of the book. I'm grateful for the hard work of Michael Navarro and Harold Graham from Commercial Graphics for making the publication process move as smoothly as possible.

Finally, I'd like to thank the many pioneering scientists and clinicians whose research has contributed to the impressive body of knowledge this book draws upon. While it is impossible to thank them all individually, their names appear in the reference lists at the end of each chapter.

Contents

PART ONE

INTRODUCTION

WHAT TO EXPECT FROM THIS GUIDE

Is Your Diet Making You Sick?

The United States is arguably the best place in the world to become *acutely* ill. Widespread availability of modern technologies, coupled with standardization of treatment protocols, has resulted in high survival rates for heart attacks, strokes, cancers, and other illnesses. Unfortunately, ***Americans are far more likely to be sick in the first place.***

Based on historical and scientific perspectives, it has become apparent that American dietary practices are a major contributor to the epidemic nature of the Big 7 U.S. diseases: heart disease, cancer, obesity, diabetes, Alzheimer's disease, arthritis, and depression. Over the last two decades, many of the actual molecular mechanisms responsible for these diseases have been identified. Simultaneously, we have witnessed the birth of ***nutritional biochemistry***, a new field that focuses on the predictable metabolic and health consequences of consuming individual dietary molecules. Scientists have identified nutrients that can aid in the prevention or attenuation of chronic diseases, and others that strongly promote disease. Although application of this knowledge has the potential to greatly improve health, the sheer complexity of nutritional biochemistry has proven a major obstacle to relaying these advances to the American public.

We created the ***nutritional quality index (NQI)*** as a tool to make the complex world of nutritional biochemistry accessible to everyone. The NQI assigns an all-inclusive health value to food items based on molecular content. Values range from -10 to 10, with -10 signifying a food that will contribute to disease if consumed regularly, 0 signifying neutral health effects, and +10 signifying profound health benefits (see Part 4 for details). The NQI can optimize your health by allowing you to simply choose foods based on the numbers, without even reading the rest of book. ***The work is done for you.***

Parts 2 through 4 of this book are dedicated to explaining the basics of nutritional biochemistry. Understanding this information allows you to make informed dietary decisions, even without the NQI ratings at your fingertips. This guide will teach you how to interpret food labels and ingredient lists efficiently and accurately in order to appreciate the molecular content of the foods you eat. Finally, Part 5 assigns ratings to over 600 commonly consumed food items to assist you in identifying and selecting the best possible foods.

Initially, you will need to refer to the book frequently before attaining a solid grasp of key concepts. We recommend that you first read Parts 1-4 in order to understand the basis of the NQI ratings. Alternatively, Part 5 can be utilized right away if desired, and you can refer back to previous chapters as needed.

- *Part 1* is the introduction to the book.
- *Part 2* introduces the 15 key dietary molecular categories.
- *Part 3* describes how these dietary molecules regulate the seven key metabolic processes and summarizes the relationships with the "Big 7" epidemic U.S. diseases.
- *Part 4* explains the basis for the NQI rating system.
- *Part 5* assigns NQI numerical ratings to more than *six hundred* breakfast cereals, breads, yogurts, fish, shellfish, poultry, red meats, eggs, cooking oils, fruits, vegetables, nuts and seeds, legumes, and other food items based on health attributes.

SCIENTIFIC AND HISTORICAL PERSPECTIVES

Scientific Perspective

The U.S. population is in the midst of an unprecedented explosion of chronic disease, with heart disease, cancer, obesity, diabetes, Alzheimer's disease, arthritis, and depression reaching epidemic proportions. These "Big 7" diseases negatively impact quality of life and longevity, and are draining healthcare resources. U.S. healthcare spending accounts for a staggering 16% of the gross domestic product (GDP), translating to well over $6,000 per person each year, easily the highest in the world [1, 2].

Despite the massive scale of healthcare spending, the U.S. population suffers from the highest rates of chronic illnesses amongst western countries, with roughly twice the prevalence of heart disease, diabetes, obesity, and cancer compared to Great Britain [1]. According to researchers, these disparities cannot be explained by smoking or other conventional risk factors. Another study of interest reported far higher rates of disease in the U.S. compared to neighboring Canada [3]. These differences are especially alarming when put into context - Great Britain and Canada have much higher rates of the "Big 7" diseases than countries in the Mediterranean, Asia, and other parts of the world!

Prevalence and Financial Burden of the "Big 7" U.S. Diseases

Disease	% of Population* (Prevalence)	Annual Indirect/Direct Cost
1) Cardiovascular Disease	32% [4]	>$400 billion [4]
Coronary Heart Disease	>6% [4]	>$140 billion [4]
2) Obesity (BMI>30)	33% [5]	>$150 billion [6]
Overweight (BMI>25)	66% [5]	**
3) Diabetes	>9% [7]	>$130 billion [7]
Pre-diabetes	>18% [7]	**
4) Depression	10% [8]	>$65 billion [9]
5) Alzheimer's Disease	13% above 65 years old [10] 42% above 85 years old [10]	>$100 billion [10, 11]
6) Arthritis	20% [12]	>$90 billion in 1997 [13]
Rheumatoid Arthritis	1% [14]	**

7) **Malignancy**	*Lifetime Risk*	**Annual Direct Cost**
Breast Cancer	1 in 8 [15]	>$7 billion [16]
Colon Cancer	Men - 1 in 17 [15] Women - 1 in 18 [15]	>$8 billion [17]
Prostate Cancer	1 in 6 [15]	>$5 billion [18]

*= Adult **= Unknown
BMI = Body Mass Index

Why are Americans so Sick?

A complex interaction between genetics and environmental factors determines which individuals will develop any given disease [19, 20]. Repetitive news stories of finding a "new gene responsible for" obesity, heart disease, diabetes, and cancer may lead some to conclude *genetics* are primarily responsible for the epidemic nature of these chronic diseases. However, three factors clearly demonstrate that *environmental* changes are largely to blame for the recent surge in the "Big 7" diseases [21]:

- rates have risen sharply over the last 50 years, despite insufficient time for major genetic changes to occur in the population [22-24]
- individuals with highly variable genetic susceptibilities suffer from many of the same epidemic diseases
- populations with low prevalence of disease in their native countries develop similar rates as Americans after relocating to the U.S. [25-30]

Could Diet be to Blame?

As the source of nearly all structural and functional molecules in the human body, diet is perhaps the most important environmental determinant of health. Mounting evidence suggests that a healthy diet is the common denominator amongst populations with very low incidence of chronic disease [31-38]. Simply put, populations with less "Americanized" dietary habits have dramatically lower rates of the Big 7 diseases and live longer, healthier lives.

Everything You Eat has Chemical Consequences

Any food or beverage, when reduced to the most fundamental level, is simply a unique combination of molecules. These bioactive molecules regulate high-leverage metabolic processes including (see Part 3):

- Inflammation
- Blood clotting
- Cholesterol metabolism
- Fat accumulation

- Sugar and insulin metabolism
- Antioxidant function
- Cell growth and replication

By regulating these crucial metabolic pathways, dietary molecules ultimately determine the overall impact of any given food on health and disease. Therefore, two foods that look and taste similar, but have different molecular contents, can have profoundly different health effects. By this reasoning, it is imperative to appreciate the precise molecular content of foods consumed.

Historical Perspective: The "Ancestral Human Diet"

Historically, human dietary patterns have varied to some extent by latitude, season, weather, culture, and other variables [39]. Thus, no universal ancestral human diet has ever existed. However, by necessity, the diets of our ancestors had several key features in common. Food sources were limited to unprocessed plant foods foraged from their own environment and unprocessed land and marine animal foods hunted from their own environment [40]. Importantly, these animals consumed *only* natural and unprocessed foods hunted or foraged from *their* own environments. With these limitations in mind, it becomes apparent that until recently, *all* human diets consisted of various combinations of lean wild meats (including brains, organs, and bone marrow), fish, shellfish, leafy vegetables, fruits, nuts, insects/larvae, and honey [41].

The human diet has remained relatively stable over millions of years of human evolution [42]. Historically, diet provided balance in the high-leverage metabolic functions listed above, favored health, and allowed our ancestors to thrive, reproduce, and pass their genes on to subsequent generations [40]. Modern humans are genetically adapted to the diets of our ancestors, which shaped our genetic makeup [43]. *In essence, the human body expects to be nourished by certain molecules within genetically determined ranges.*

However, modern U.S. dietary intake scarcely resembles that of our ancestors [40, 42, 44]. The first major change occurred between 3,000 and 8,000 B.C., roughly 200 - 400 generations ago, with the advent of the Agricultural Revolution and animal husbandry [39, 42]. More recently, the Industrial Revolution, approximately 150 - 200 years ago, heralded the onset of advances in food processing, crop manipulation, and intensive animal rearing practices, which boosted the speed and *quantity* of food production. These practices radically altered the qualitative and quantitative balance of nutrients in the food supply [45]. Ingestion of certain nutrients such as sugars, starches, saturated fats, sodium, and omega-6 fatty acids have risen to extreme levels. Meanwhile, other nutrients such as fibers and omega-3 fatty acids have nearly disappeared from the food supply In addition, food processing techniques, including hydrogenation of vegetable oils, have introduced novel toxins such as trans fats into our food supply with disastrous consequences [46, 47].

To put things into perspective, these radical changes occurred over less than 200 years, roughly 8 generations, which is not enough time to allow for genetic adaptation [48, 49]. Essentially, Americans are no longer consuming required nutrients within genetically determined ranges [50, 51]. Lack of harmony between our diet and genes (DNA) has disturbed the delicate balance in each of these crucial metabolic pathways. *Specifically, the "standard American diet" promotes excessive inflammation, blood clotting, and fat accumulation, distorts blood insulin and cholesterol metabolism, and favors oxidative stress and cancer (see Parts 2 and 3).* Each of these metabolic disturbances plays a major role in the rapid rise in the Big 7 epidemic U.S. diseases.

Evolution of Dietary Guidelines: From Nonspecific to Precise

For over 100 years, the U.S. government has developed and publicized "official" dietary guidelines for Americans [52]. Since the 1960s, an ever-increasing number of influential health promotion organizations including the American Heart Association, American Diabetes Association, National Cancer Society, and others have weighed in, publicizing their interpretations of how to eat a healthy diet. These dietary guidelines have shaped American ideas about nutrition and radically altered what we eat today [53]. Early U.S. guidelines were based on "proper" balances of the three macronutrient categories: *total* fats, *total* carbohydrates, and *total* proteins. Fats, carbohydrates, and proteins are broad classifications of dietary molecules grouped together based on having similar molecular makeup (though not necessarily similar metabolic or health properties).

Perhaps the most important policy shift in American dietary guidelines occurred in 1977 when a U.S. Senate Committee released a highly publicized report, known as the *Dietary Goals for the United States*, instructing Americans to drastically alter intake of the three major macronutrients [54]. Many of their recommendations were soon adopted and publicized by other governmental and private health promotion organizations [53].

Focus on Fat

Specifically, Americans were instructed to reduce *total* fat intake from 40% of energy to less than 30%, a recommendation based on the assumption that *total* fat played a key role in development of heart disease and other illnesses. Americans were further instructed to limit one subtype of fat, the saturated variety, from more than 16% to less than 10% of caloric intake, advice based on the association of saturated fats and heart disease. Saturated fats were to be replaced with "complex carbohydrates" and "unsaturated fats," a broad category of fatty acids with at least five different subsets of molecules [55]. These guidelines, which helped launch the "low-fat" craze, profoundly altered nutritional beliefs and dietary practices of the American people for decades to come.

If "You Are What You Eat" then "I Better Not Eat Fat"

Perceiving all fats as "bad" for their health, Americans reduced overall fat intake from 40 to 34% of caloric intake between 1977 and 1995 [53]. Simultaneously, saturated fat intake fell from more than 16% to 12% of caloric intake. Meanwhile, Americans boosted intake of unsaturated fats, especially from omega-6 rich vegetable oils in their hydrogenated and non-hydrogenated forms.

*Author's Note: Unfortunately, based on these guidelines, millions of Americans replaced butter with margarine and other foods rich in toxic, but unsaturated, trans fats, which accounted for more than 7% of all fats consumed in the 1990s! Many of these foods were labeled as "heart healthy," reflecting their lack of saturated fats. This situation illustrates the importance of **comprehensive** recommendations, including both beneficial and deleterious nutrients.*

In hindsight, guidelines instructing Americans to limit total fat to less than 30% seem arbitrary, particularly in light of the fact that populations with longer life expectancies and lower rates of chronic disease than the U.S. consume diets ranging from 10 to 40% of calories from fat [33, 34, 36, 38, 53]. Although they vary in *total* fat intake, dietary practices of these healthy populations have several features in common, namely low amounts of saturated fats, no artificial trans fats, a higher concentration of monounsaturated fats, and much higher ratios of omega-3 fatty acids to omega-6 fatty acids. Thus, populations consuming up to 40% of energy from high *quality* fats have much lower rates of disease than the U.S.

A large prospective U.S. study released in 2006 further supports the notion that *total* fat *quantity* has little, if any impact on the development of disease [56]. Expert groups are beginning to recognize that a wide range of *total* fat can be consumed as part of a healthy diet, as reflected in revamped dietary guidelines. Recently, the U.S. Department of Agriculture (USDA) and the American Heart Association (AHA) loosened recommendations from less than 30% to 20-35% of total caloric intake [57, 58]. It is quite likely that even wider ranges of total fat intakes are compatible with a healthy diet.

From "You Are What You Eat" to "Everything You Eat has Chemical Consequences"

It is now well established that not all fats are created equal. Subsets of fats have vastly different, even opposite, metabolic and health effects than others. Rather, it is the *quality* of dietary fat that determines the health properties [59-63]. Trans fats, despite being unsaturated, have a multitude of toxic effects [47]. Excessive consumption of saturated fats can also make a significant contribution to disease [63, 64]. Evidence is accumulating that over-consumption of omega-6 polyunsaturated fats, another subset of unsaturated fats, can contribute to certain diseases [65-73]. In contrast, other subsets of fats, especially monounsaturated fats and omega-3 polyunsaturated fats, have profoundly positive health effects [35, 60, 74-76].

Carbohydrates

Dietary guidelines have greatly influenced how Americans view carbohydrates. The same guidelines instructing Americans to reduce overall fat consumption recommended boosting intake of total carbohydrates to 50 – 60% or more of caloric intake [54, 58, 77]. Initial guidelines distinguished between undesirable "simple sugars" and desirable "complex carbohydrates" or starches based on the assumption that starches have superior health properties compared to sugars [54, 55, 78]. As instructed, Americans dramatically increased their consumption of starches, mostly in the form of refined grains. By 2000, total carbohydrates had increased to more than 50% of caloric intake [79]. However, advances in nutritional biochemistry have since demonstrated that starches, although more *complex* than sugars, are quickly digested and absorbed as sugars. *Metabolically speaking, pure starches are sugar equivalents* [78, 80-83]. Excessive intake of starches and sugars as part of the ensuing "low fat" craze actually fueled the epidemics of obesity and diabetes [53, 84-86]. Meanwhile, fibers, another category of carbohydrates, have essentially opposite metabolic effects as sugars and starches [87]. As a reflection of the improved understanding of properties of carbohydrates, dietary guidelines are transitioning from the inaccurate practice of grouping carbohydrates into *simple* and *complex* based on chain length to a more functional distinction of fibers and non-fiber carbohydrates [83].

Like fats, *quality* of carbohydrates consumed is far more important than *quantity* [83, 88-90]. Scientists are beginning to appreciate that a wide range of total carbohydrates can be consumed as part of a healthy diet. Although certain health promotion groups maintain more than 50% recommendations, others including the USDA have broadened total carbohydrate ranges to 40-65% of total caloric intake [57].

It is quite likely that an even wider range of *total* carbohydrate intakes are compatible with a healthy diet, as long as high fiber, high quality foods are consumed.

Proteins

Early studies suggested that animal protein consumption is associated with cardiovascular disease risk while vegetable protein (beans, nuts, etc) may be cardioprotective [91]. Ensuing guidelines suggested consumption of 15% of daily calories from protein [48, 77]. However, this advice was based on flawed preliminary studies which failed to account for the fact that most protein consumed in the U.S. comes from commercial meats and dairy, both highly concentrated sources of saturated fats [92-94]. Later studies demonstrated that both animal and vegetable proteins, when considered independently of saturated fat, have moderate *protective* effects against heart disease and diabetes [95-97]. Thus, unlike fats and carbohydrates, nutrition science has *yet* to demonstrate that certain subsets of proteins are of higher quality than others. Instead, *all* proteins appear to have modest health benefits, suggesting that protein sources should be selected based on the quality of accompanying fats and carbohydrates. Like fats and carbohydrates, a wide range of total protein can be consumed as part of a healthy diet, as reflected in 2005 USDA guidelines recommending consumption of between 10-35% of calories from protein [57].

Nutrient-based and Food-based Dietary Guidelines

The first nutrient-based guidelines were founded on the now obsolete assumption that intake of "proper" *ratios* of the broad classes of macronutrients (fats, carbohydrates, and proteins) is a key determinant of health. However, recent research clearly demonstrates that the *quality* of these macronutrients is more important than the ratio, and that wide ranges of *total* fats, carbohydrates, and proteins can be consumed as part of a healthy diet [56, 59, 60, 63, 68, 83].

It is now possible to predict the metabolic properties of specific subsets of dietary molecules, and in some cases, even individual dietary molecules. Studies strongly suggest that more specific dietary guidelines based on this understanding can dramatically improve outcomes [98-101].

Early nutrient-based dietary guidelines focused almost exclusively on reduction of serum cholesterol levels, an important but one-dimensional feature of health [48, 53, 77]. However, several other molecular parameters regulated by diet *also* play important roles in health and disease. In fact, diets that address these other metabolic parameters (inflammation, blood clotting, fat expansion, insulin regulation, oxidative stress, and cell growth) profoundly outperform simplistic "cholesterol-reducing" diets [98-101].

Reformulating dietary guidelines to reflect this new knowledge and relaying it to the public has proven challenging. Today, most Americans are admittedly confused about what constitutes a healthy diet. Part of this uncertainty stems from inconsistent and poorly defined dietary recommendations [53]. Advice to consume a certain percentage of daily calories from a particular nutrient subset is inherently difficult to apply to real world situations. For example, compliance with the recommendation to consume less than 10% of daily calories from saturated fat requires meticulous attention to detail regarding food labels, serving sizes, and servings consumed, as well as several complex mathematical calculations. Obviously, precise implementation of this recommendation is impractical for busy U.S. consumers. In reality, most Americans interpret advice to "consume less than 10% of calories from saturated fat" simply as "consume less saturated fat."

Furthermore, by simply listing a series of recommendations one after another, traditional nutrient-based guidelines do not provide adequate information to properly "weigh" the importance of suggestions. For example, advice to limit trans fats and *dietary* cholesterol is commonly listed together. While even small amounts of trans fatty acids pose serious health risks, consumption of relatively large quantities of *dietary* cholesterol has little or no effect on health [47, 102, 103]. Yet, Americans perceive *dietary* cholesterol to be one of the most important dietary factors [104]. Rather than leaving it up to the consumer to speculate, a more effective system would rank recommendations according to relative health impact.

In addition, nutrient-based guidelines may leave the consumer vulnerable to misleading product marketing. Buzzwords such as "low fat," "no trans fat," and "whole grain," which are designed to appeal to those with a superficial understanding of the latest nutrient-based guidelines, have permeated today's grocery stores. These buzzwords can be misleading because they do not take the *whole* food item into consideration. Health-conscious consumers may purchase these products unaware of potential health hazards. For example, a product labeled "low fat" may have added sugars and refined carbohydrates. Products labeled as "whole grain" may have very little fiber, with up to a 20 to 1 ratio of non-fiber carbohydrates (NFCs) to fiber (natural whole grains contain about a 5 to 1 ratio). Products labeled "zero grams of trans fat*" per serving* may have unrealistically small serving sizes. Consumption of a realistic serving size may result in significant intake of toxic trans fats. Despite health claims to the contrary, these supposedly wholesome foods may contribute to weight gain, diabetes, heart disease, and other epidemic U.S. diseases.

In the real world, an overall diet consists of a series of **isolated** food choices based on taste, texture, availability, cost, and perceived health attributes. On average, Americans make more than *fifty* decisions related to what foods they will eat each day [105]. A healthy diet results from **habitual** selection of food items with high concentrations of beneficial nutrients *and* low concentrations of detrimental nutrients and toxins. By focusing on a nebulous "percentage of daily caloric intake" from any given nutrient, traditional nutrient-based guidelines are not easily applied to determine the best **individual** food selections [106].

Toward Food-based Dietary Guidelines

These limitations of nutrient-based dietary guidelines have led some to suggest that food-based dietary guidelines may be more beneficial [53, 107]. Food-based guidelines, which recommend consumption of a certain number of servings per day of specific food groups, are user-friendly and are more easily applied to real life. Examples include recommendations to "choose" fruits and vegetables, whole grains, fish, lean meats, and low-fat dairy, and "limit" or "restrict" whole-fat dairy, soft drinks, and other foods with adverse health properties [107]. Advocates of food-based guidelines highlight the fact that people choose which **foods** to consume, rather than which **nutrients** to consume.

"People don't eat nutrition-They eat food."- Anthropologist Margaret Mead [53].

However, foods grouped within any particular category may have profoundly different molecular contents and health properties [53]. For example, certain fish contain high concentrations of beneficial omega-3 fatty acids and few toxins, while others contain little or no omega-3 fatty acids and relatively large amounts of mercury and PCBs [108, 109]. Likewise, although broccoli, onions, iceberg lettuce, and potatoes are all vegetables, each has markedly different health properties. The same situation applies to dairy products, cereals, breads, fruits, eggs, meats, vegetable oils, and to all other food groups!

In effect, current food-based guidelines sacrifice precision for the sake of simplicity. Because accompanying advice about choosing *within* a category is often superficial, consumers often fail to see the big picture [106]. For example, a consumer may select a "low-fat" yogurt or ice cream with massive amounts of added sugar while technically following dietary guidelines. Like nutrient-based guidelines, food-based guidelines *do not* prepare consumers to see through tricky advertising schemes.

The utility of both food-based and nutrient-based dietary guidelines are largely dependent on accurate representations of serving sizes. Unfortunately, serving sizes are far from uniform, and rarely match the actual amount of food consumed [110, 111]. In addition, water accounts for a large portion of many food items, a fact that further obscures the accuracy of serving sizes [112]. Dependence on the vagaries of serving sizes limits the precision of both food-based and nutrient-based dietary guidelines. In reality, few consumers know how to properly interpret serving size [113].

As nutrition science advances, it is becoming increasingly apparent that more specific and comprehensive dietary guidelines can dramatically improve health and reduce disease [37, 98-101]. In light of the current epidemics of obesity, diabetes, heart disease, cancers, and other illnesses, few would argue that U.S. dietary guidelines have succeeded in their goals [53]. Clearly, a new approach for selecting healthy foods is needed.

The Nutritional Quality Index (NQI)

The Nutritional Quality Index (NQI), which integrates the advantages of nutrient-based *and* food-based dietary guidelines, was designed to be this instrument. In fact, the NQI addresses *each* of the limitations of traditional guidelines. By taking advantage of the fact that wide ranges of *total* fats, carbohydrates, and proteins can be consumed as part of a healthy diet, the NQI is able to focus instead on *quality* of nutrients, a far more important determinant of health and disease. Like food-based guidelines, the NQI allows for selection of *individual* food items based on perceived health properties. However, because numerical rankings reflect precise molecular content rather than vague generalizations, the NQI is far more accurate. Individual food items are rated in terms of overall *quality* of nutrient content, which is expressed as an all-inclusive numerical ranking between -10 to +10, with -10 signifying a food that will contribute to disease if consumed regularly, 0 signifying neutral health effects, and +10 signifying profound health benefits. By focusing on all seven key metabolic processes (and the Big 7 epidemic U.S. diseases), rather than simply blood cholesterol reduction, the NQI takes a more holistic approach than traditional guidelines.

Thus, the NQI preserves the simplicity and ease of application of food-based guidelines without sacrificing the precision afforded by more complex nutrient-based guidelines. In addition, because numerical scores reflect content of each nutrient as a percentage of *water-free* weight, subjective serving sizes and water content cannot obscure the true *quality* of food consumed. Unlike traditional guidelines, which require speculation about the value of different recommendations, the NQI appropriately "weighs" both beneficial and deleterious nutrients according to relative importance. As such, the NQI exposes tricky advertising schemes intended to mislead consumers via use of trendy buzzwords.

Perhaps the simplest way to use the NQI is to identify food items within your current diet with the lowest NQI scores (the biggest "offenders"), and replace those items with higher quality choices. Alternatively, you may seek to consume more food items with outstanding health properties. For ease of application, the food items with the highest NQI ratings are listed at the beginning of each food category.

As a versatile tool that can be easily used to improve dietary choices, the NQI will empower Americans to apply recent advances in nutritional biochemistry to their everyday lives. Whatever your specific goals, our hope is that the NQI will serve as a useful tool to guide your food consumption and improve your health.

References:

1. Banks, J., et al., *Disease and disadvantage in the United States and in England.* Jama, 2006. **295**(17): p. 2037-45.
2. Catlin, A., et al., *National health spending in 2005: the slowdown continues.* Health Aff (Millwood), 2007. **26**(1): p. 142-53.
3. Lasser, K.E., D.U. Himmelstein, and S. Woolhandler, *Access to care, health status, and health disparities in the United States and Canada: results of a cross-national population-based survey.* Am J Public Health, 2006. **96**(7): p. 1300-7.
4. *American Heart Association & American Stroke Association: Heart Disease and Stroke Statistics - 2006 Update.* 2006 [cited 2006 July 12]; Available from: http://www.americanheart.org/downloadable/heart/1140534985281Statsupdate06book.pdf.
5. Ogden, C.L., et al., *Prevalence of overweight and obesity in the United States, 1999-2004.* Jama, 2006. **295**(13): p. 1549-55.
6. Herper, M. *The Hidden Cost of Obesity.* 2006 [cited 2006 July 31]; Available from: http://www.forbes.com/business/2006/07/19/obesity-fat-costs_cx_mh_0720obesity.html.
7. *National diabetes fact sheet: General information and national estimates on diabetes in the United States, 2005,* Atlanta, GA: U.S. Department of Health and Human Services, Centers for Disease Control and Prevention, 2005.
8. *National Institute of Mental Health - Depression: A treatable illness.* 2004 [cited 2006 July 14]; Available from: http://menanddepression.nimh.nih.gov/infopage.asp?ID=15.
9. *Quality Enhancement Research Initiative: Mental Health QUERI Fact Sheet.* 2006 [cited 2006 July 14]; Available from: http://www.hsrd.research.va.gov/publications/internal/mh_factsheet.pdf.
10. *Alzheimer's disease Facts and Figures 2007.* Alzheimer's Association 2007 [cited 2007 March 21]; Available from: http://www.alz.org/national/documents/Report_2007FactsAndFigures.pdf.
11. *Alzheimer's Association: Alzheimer's Disease Statistics.* 2006 [cited 2006 July 12]; Available from: http://www.alz.org/alzheimer_statistics.asp.
12. *National Center for Chronic Disease Prevention and Health Promotion: Arthritis Data and Statistics.* 2005 [cited 2006 July 14]; Available from: http://www.cdc.gov/arthritis/data_statistics/national_data.htm.
13. Yelin, E., et al., *Medical care expenditures and earnings losses of persons with arthritis and other rheumatic conditions in the United States in 1997: total and incremental estimates.* Arthritis Rheum, 2004. **50**(7): p. 2317-26.
14. Lawrence, R.C., et al., *Estimates of the prevalence of arthritis and selected musculoskeletal disorders in the United States.* Arthritis Rheum, 1998. **41**(5): p. 778-99.
15. *American Cancer Society: Cancer Statistics 2006.* [cited 2007 January 7]; Available from: http://www.cancer.org/downloads/STT/1.
16. Brown, M.L., J. Lipscomb, and C. Snyder, *The burden of illness of cancer: economic cost and quality of life.* Annu Rev Public Health, 2001. **22**: p. 91-113.
17. Brown, M.L., et al., *Estimating health care costs related to cancer treatment from SEER-Medicare data.* Med Care, 2002. **40**(8 Suppl): p. IV-104-17.
18. *National Prostate Cancer Coalition: Prostate Cancer Facts and Statistics.* 2006 [cited 2006 July 13]; Available from: http://70.84.59.4/~pcacoal/about_stats.htm.
19. Kaput, J. and R.L. Rodriguez, *Nutritional genomics: the next frontier in the postgenomic era.* Physiol Genomics, 2004. **16**(2): p. 166-77.
20. Simopoulos, A.P., *Genetics and nutrition: or what your genes can tell you about nutrition.* World Rev Nutr Diet, 1990. **63**: p. 25-34.
21. Hemminki, K., J. Lorenzo Bermejo, and A. Forsti, *The balance between heritable and environmental aetiology of human disease.* Nat Rev Genet, 2006. **7**(12): p. 958-65.
22. Fox, C.S., et al., *Trends in the incidence of type 2 diabetes mellitus from the 1970s to the 1990s: the Framingham Heart Study.* Circulation, 2006. **113**(25): p. 2914-8.
23. Morrill, A.C. and C.D. Chinn, *The obesity epidemic in the United States.* J Public Health Policy, 2004. **25**(3-4): p. 353-66.
24. Narayan, K.M., et al., *Impact of recent increase in incidence on future diabetes burden: U.S., 2005-2050.* Diabetes Care, 2006. **29**(9): p. 2114-6.

25. Kodama, M., T. Kodama, and M. Kodama, *Interrelation between western type cancers and non-western type cancers as regards their risk variations in time and space. III. A contrast between bladder cancer and stomach cancer.* Anticancer Res, 1991. **11**(5): p. 1895-904.

26. Wynder, E.L., et al., *Comparative epidemiology of cancer between the United States and Japan. A second look.* Cancer, 1991. **67**(3): p. 746-63.

27. Ziegler, R.G., et al., *Migration patterns and breast cancer risk in Asian-American women.* J Natl Cancer Inst, 1993. **85**(22): p. 1819-27.

28. Mooteri, S.N., et al., *Duration of residence in the United States as a new risk factor for coronary artery disease (The Konkani Heart Study).* Am J Cardiol, 2004. **93**(3): p. 359-61.

29. Goel, M.S., et al., *Obesity among US immigrant subgroups by duration of residence.* Jama, 2004. **292**(23): p. 2860-7.

30. Lauderdale, D.S. and P.J. Rathouz, *Body mass index in a US national sample of Asian Americans: effects of nativity, years since immigration and socioeconomic status.* Int J Obes Relat Metab Disord, 2000. **24**(9): p. 1188-94.

31. Sugano, M. and F. Hirahara, *Polyunsaturated fatty acids in the food chain in Japan.* Am J Clin Nutr, 2000. **71**(1 Suppl): p. 189S-96S.

32. McLaughlin, J., et al., *Adipose tissue triglyceride fatty acids and atherosclerosis in Alaska Natives and non-Natives.* Atherosclerosis, 2005. **181**(2): p. 353-62.

33. Fan, W.X., et al., *Erythrocyte fatty acids, plasma lipids, and cardiovascular disease in rural China.* Am J Clin Nutr, 1990. **52**(6): p. 1027-36.

34. Tao, S.C., et al., *CHD and its risk factors in the People's Republic of China.* Int J Epidemiol, 1989. **18**(3 Suppl 1): p. S159-63.

35. Siscovick, D.S., et al., *Dietary intake and cell membrane levels of long-chain n-3 polyunsaturated fatty acids and the risk of primary cardiac arrest.* Jama, 1995. **274**(17): p. 1363-7.

36. Kromhout, D., et al., *Food consumption patterns in the 1960s in seven countries.* Am J Clin Nutr, 1989. **49**(5): p. 889-94.

37. Scarmeas, N., et al., *Mediterranean diet and risk for Alzheimer's disease.* Ann Neurol, 2006. **59**(6): p. 912-21.

38. Trichopoulou, A., et al., *Diet and survival of elderly Greeks: a link to the past.* Am J Clin Nutr, 1995. **61**(6 Suppl): p. 1346S-1350S.

39. Gowlett, J., *What actually was the Stone Age diet?* J Nutr Environ Med 2003. **13**: p. 143-7.

40. O'Keefe, J.H., Jr. and L. Cordain, *Cardiovascular disease resulting from a diet and lifestyle at odds with our Paleolithic genome: how to become a 21st-century hunter-gatherer.* Mayo Clin Proc, 2004. **79**(1): p. 101-8.

41. Lindeberg, S.e., *Biological and Clinical Potential of a Paleolithic Diet.* J Nutr Environ med 2003, 2003. **13**: p. 149-60.

42. Cordain, L., et al., *Origins and evolution of the Western diet: health implications for the 21st century.* Am J Clin Nutr, 2005. **81**(2): p. 341-54.

43. Cordain, L., *The Nutritional Characteristics of a Contemporary Diet.* JANA, 2002. **5**(3): p. 15-25.

44. Muskiet, F.A., et al., *Is docosahexaenoic acid (DHA) essential? Lessons from DHA status regulation, our ancient diet, epidemiology and randomized controlled trials.* J Nutr, 2004. **134**(1): p. 183-6.

45. Ghebremeskel, K. and M.A. Crawford, *Nutrition and health in relation to food production and processing.* Nutr Health, 1994. **9**(4): p. 237-53.

46. Emken, E.A., *Nutrition and biochemistry of trans and positional fatty acid isomers in hydrogenated oils.* Annu Rev Nutr, 1984. **4**: p. 339-76.

47. Willett, W.C., *Trans fatty acids and cardiovascular disease-epidemiological data.* Atheroscler Suppl, 2006. **7**(2): p. 5-8.

48. Eaton, S.B., M. Konner, and M. Shostak, *Stone agers in the fast lane: chronic degenerative diseases in evolutionary perspective.* Am J Med, 1988. **84**(4): p. 739-49.

49. Goldsmith, M.F., *Ancestors may provide clinical answers, say 'Darwinian' medical evolutionists.* Jama, 1993. **269**(12): p. 1477-80.

50. Ridker, P.M., *On evolutionary biology, inflammation, infection, and the causes of atherosclerosis.* Circulation, 2002. **105**(1): p. 2-4.

51. Eaton, S.B. and M. Konner, *Paleolithic nutrition. A consideration of its nature and current implications.* N Engl J Med, 1985. **312**(5): p. 283-9.

52. Atwater, W.O., *Foods: Nutritive Value and Cost.* Washington, D.C.: U.S. Department of Agriculture, 1894. Farmer's Bulletin 23.

53. Gifford, K.D., *Dietary fats, eating guides, and public policy: history, critique, and recommendations.* Am J Med, 2002. **113 Suppl 9B**: p. 89S-106S.

54. *Dietary Goals for the United States.* February, 1977, Washington, D.C.: U.S. Senate Select Committee on Nutrition and Human Needs.

55. Grundy, S.M., et al., *Rationale of the diet-heart statement of the American Heart Association. Report of Nutrition Committee.* Circulation, 1982. **65**(4): p. 839A-854A.

56. Howard, B.V., et al., *Low-fat dietary pattern and risk of cardiovascular disease: the Women's Health Initiative Randomized Controlled Dietary Modification Trial.* Jama, 2006. **295**(6): p. 655-66.

57. U.S. Department of Health and Human Services, *U.S. Department of Agriculture: Dietary Guidelines for Americans,* 6th ed., Washington, D.C. 2005 [cited 2006 August 15]; Available from: http://healthierus.gov/dietaryguidelines/

58. Krauss, R.M., et al., *Dietary guidelines for healthy American adults. A statement for health professionals from the Nutrition Committee, American Heart Association.* Circulation, 1996. **94**(7): p. 1795-800.

59. Hu, F.B., J.E. Manson, and W.C. Willett, *Types of dietary fat and risk of coronary heart disease: a critical review.* J Am Coll Nutr, 2001. **20**(1): p. 5-19.

60.   de Lorgeril, M. and P. Salen, *The Mediterranean diet in secondary prevention of coronary heart disease.* Clin Invest Med, 2006. **29**(3): p. 154-8.
61.   *Dietary Fat-how much? What type? Consensus Statement from the Scientific Exchange.* Nutrition Today, 1998. **33-34**(173).
62.   Khor, G.L., *Dietary fat quality: a nutritional epidemiologist's view.* Asia Pac J Clin Nutr, 2004. **13**(Suppl): p. S22.
63.   Hu, F.B., et al., *Dietary saturated fats and their food sources in relation to the risk of coronary heart disease in women.* Am J Clin Nutr, 1999. **70**(6): p. 1001-8.
64.   Kromhout, D., *Serum cholesterol in cross-cultural perspective. The Seven Countries Study.* Acta Cardiol, 1999. **54**(3): p. 155-8.
65.   Yam, D., A. Eliraz, and E.M. Berry, *Diet and disease--the Israeli paradox: possible dangers of a high omega-6 polyunsaturated fatty acid diet.* Isr J Med Sci, 1996. **32**(11): p. 1134-43.
66.   Berry, E.M., *Who's afraid of n-6 polyunsaturated fatty acids? Methodological considerations for assessing whether they are harmful.* Nutr Metab Cardiovasc Dis, 2001. **11**(3): p. 181-8.
67.   Hodgson, J.M., et al., *Can linoleic acid contribute to coronary artery disease?* Am J Clin Nutr, 1993. **58**(2): p. 228-34.
68.   de Lorgeril, M. and P. Salen, *Dietary prevention of coronary heart disease: focus on omega-6/omega-3 essential fatty acid balance.* World Rev Nutr Diet, 2003. **92**: p. 57-73.
69.   Rose, G.A., W.B. Thomson, and R.T. Williams, *Corn Oil in Treatment of Ischaemic Heart Disease.* Br Med J, 1965. **1**(5449): p. 1531-3.
70.   Lands, W.E., *Primary prevention in cardiovascular disease: moving out of the shadows of the truth about death.* Nutr Metab Cardiovasc Dis, 2003. **13**(3): p. 154-64.
71.   Lands, W.E., *Dietary fat and health: the evidence and the politics of prevention: careful use of dietary fats can improve life and prevent disease.* Ann N Y Acad Sci, 2005. **1055**: p. 179-92.
72.   Ritch, C.R., et al., *Dietary fatty acids correlate with prostate cancer biopsy grade and volume in Jamaican men.* J Urol, 2007. **177**(1): p. 97-101; discussion 101.
73.   Takase, B., et al., *Arachidonic acid metabolites in acute myocardial infarction.* Angiology, 1996. **47**(7): p. 649-61.
74.   Iso, H., et al., *Intake of fish and n3 fatty acids and risk of coronary heart disease among Japanese: the Japan Public Health Center-Based (JPHC) Study Cohort I.* Circulation, 2006. **113**(2): p. 195-202.
75.   Stark, A.H. and Z. Madar, *Olive oil as a functional food: epidemiology and nutritional approaches.* Nutr Rev, 2002. **60**(6): p. 170-6.
76.   Erkkila, A.T., et al., *n-3 Fatty acids and 5-y risks of death and cardiovascular disease events in patients with coronary artery disease.* Am J Clin Nutr, 2003. **78**(1): p. 65-71.
77.   *Dietary guidelines for healthy American adults. A statement for physicians and health professionals by the Nutrition Committee, American Heart Association.* Circulation, 1986. **74**(6): p. 1465A-1468A.
78.   Pereira, M.A. and S. Liu, *Types of carbohydrates and risk of cardiovascular disease.* J Womens Health (Larchmt), 2003. **12**(2): p. 115-22.
79.   Gerrior, S., L. Bente, and H. Hiza, *Nutrient Content of the U.S. Food Supply, 1909-2000.* 2004, Home Economics Research Report No. 56. U.S. Department of Agriculture, Center for Nutrition Policy and Promotion.
80.   Wahlqvist, M.L., E.G. Wilmshurst, and E.N. Richardson, *The effect of chain length on glucose absorption and the related metabolic response.* Am J Clin Nutr, 1978. **31**(11): p. 1998-2001.
81.   Bantle, J.P., et al., *Postprandial glucose and insulin responses to meals containing different carbohydrates in normal and diabetic subjects.* N Engl J Med, 1983. **309**(1): p. 7-12.
82.   Dahlqvist, A. and B. Borgstrom, *Digestion and absorption of disaccharides in man.* Biochem J, 1961. **81**: p. 411-8.
83.   Liu, S., et al., *A prospective study of dietary glycemic load, carbohydrate intake, and risk of coronary heart disease in US women.* Am J Clin Nutr, 2000. **71**(6): p. 1455-61.
84.   Gross, L.S., et al., *Increased consumption of refined carbohydrates and the epidemic of type 2 diabetes in the United States: an ecologic assessment.* Am J Clin Nutr, 2004. **79**(5): p. 774-9.
85.   Bray, G.A., S.J. Nielsen, and B.M. Popkin, *Consumption of high-fructose corn syrup in beverages may play a role in the epidemic of obesity.* Am J Clin Nutr, 2004. **79**(4): p. 537-43.
86.   Schulze, M.B., et al., *Glycemic index, glycemic load, and dietary fiber intake and incidence of type 2 diabetes in younger and middle-aged women.* Am J Clin Nutr, 2004. **80**(2): p. 348-56.
87.   Asp, N.G., *Classification and methodology of food carbohydrates as related to nutritional effects.* Am J Clin Nutr, 1995. **61**(4 Suppl): p. 930S-937S.
88.   Griel, A.E., E.H. Ruder, and P.M. Kris-Etherton, *The changing roles of dietary carbohydrates: from simple to complex.* Arterioscler Thromb Vasc Biol, 2006. **26**(9): p. 1958-65.
89.   Ludwig, D.S., *Symposium 2: Nutrition and Chronic Disease. Diet and development of the insulin resustence syndrome.* Proceedings of the Nutrition Society of Australia, 2003. **27**: p. S4.
90.   Suter, P.M., *Carbohydrates and dietary fiber.* Handb Exp Pharmacol, 2005(170): p. 231-61.
91.   Carroll, K.K., *Dietary protein in relation to plasma cholesterol levels and atherosclerosis.* Nutr Rev, 1978. **36**(1): p. 1-5.
92.   Laugesen, M., *Decreased red meat fat consumption in New Zealand: 1995-2002.* N Z Med J, 2005. **118**(1226): p. U1751.
93.   Ferlay, A., et al., *Influence of grass-based diets on milk fatty acid composition and milk lipolytic system in Tarentaise and Montbeliarde cow breeds.* J Dairy Sci, 2006. **89**(10): p. 4026-41.
94.   Dannenberger, D., et al., *Diet alters the fatty acid composition of individual phospholipid classes in beef muscle.* J Agric Food Chem, 2007. **55**(2): p. 452-60.
95.   Hu, F.B., et al., *Dietary protein and risk of ischemic heart disease in women.* Am J Clin Nutr, 1999. **70**(2): p. 221-7.

96. Li, D., et al., *Lean meat and heart health*. Asia Pac J Clin Nutr, 2005. **14**(2): p. 113-9.
97. Cordain, L., et al., *The paradoxical nature of hunter-gatherer diets: meat-based, yet non-atherogenic*. Eur J Clin Nutr, 2002. **56 Suppl 1**: p. S42-52.
98. McCullough, M.L., et al., *Diet quality and major chronic disease risk in men and women: moving toward improved dietary guidance*. Am J Clin Nutr, 2002. **76**(6): p. 1261-71.
99. de Lorgeril, M., et al., *Mediterranean dietary pattern in a randomized trial: prolonged survival and possible reduced cancer rate*. Arch Intern Med, 1998. **158**(11): p. 1181-7.
100. de Lorgeril, M., et al., *Mediterranean diet, traditional risk factors, and the rate of cardiovascular complications after myocardial infarction: final report of the Lyon Diet Heart Study*. Circulation, 1999. **99**(6): p. 779-85.
101. Fung, T.T., et al., *Diet-quality scores and plasma concentrations of markers of inflammation and endothelial dysfunction*. Am J Clin Nutr, 2005. **82**(1): p. 163-73.
102. McDonald, B.E., *The Canadian experience: why Canada decided against an upper limit for cholesterol*. J Am Coll Nutr, 2004. **23**(6 Suppl): p. 616S-620S.
103. *Dietary Guidelines Advisory Committee: Nutrition and your health - dietary guidelines for Americans*. 2005 Dietary Guidelines Advisory Committee Report. Washington, D.C.: Department of Agriculture [cited 2006 July 15]; Available from: http://health.gov/dietaryguidelines/dga2005/report/
104. *U.S. Department of Agricultural Research Service. 1997. Data Tables: Results from USDA's 1996 Continuing Survey of Food Intakes by Individuals and 1996 Diet and Health Knowledge Survey.* [cited 2006 August 10]; Available from: http:barc.usda.gov/bhnrc/foodsurvey/home.htm.
105. Wansink, B.e., *Mindless Eating: The 200 Daily Food Choices We Overlook*. Environment and Behavior, 2007. **39**: p. 106-23.
106. Scheidt, D.M. and E. Daniel, *Composite index for aggregating nutrient density using food labels: ratio of recommended to restricted food components*. J Nutr Educ Behav, 2004. **36**(1): p. 35-9.
107. Schneeman, B.O., *Evolution of dietary guidelines*. J Am Diet Assoc, 2003. **103**(12 Suppl 2): p. S5-9.
108. Mozaffarian, D. and E.B. Rimm, *Fish intake, contaminants, and human health: evaluating the risks and the benefits*. Jama, 2006. **296**(15): p. 1885-99.
109. *US Department of Health and Human Services and Environmental Protection Agency. Mercury Levels in Commercial Fish and Shellfish.* [cited December 12, 2005]; Available from: http://www.cfsan.fda.gov/~frf/sea-mehg.html.
110. *Food labeling: Serving sizes of products that can reasonably be consumed at one eating occasion; Udating of reference amounts customarily consumed; Approaches for recommending smaller portion sizes*. 2005 [cited 2006 December 19]; Federal register]. Available from: http://www.cfsan.fda.gov/~lrd/fr05404c.html.
111. *Food portions and servings: How do they differ?*, in *Nutrition Insights*. 1999, Center for Nutrition Policy and Promotion, USDA: Washington, DC.
112. Drewnowski, A., *The role of energy density*. Lipids, 2003. **38**(2): p. 109-15.
113. Rothman, R.L., et al., *Patient Understanding of Food Labels The Role of Literacy and Numeracy*. Am J Prev Med, 2006. **31**(5): p. 391-398.

PART TWO

MEET THE 15 KEY DIETARY MOLECULAR PLAYERS

THE 15 KEY DIETARY MOLECULAR PLAYERS

The NQI recognizes fifteen dietary molecular categories including nutrients, toxins, and artificial sweeteners.

15 Molecular Categories
1 - Saturated fatty acids
2 - Monounsaturated fats
3 - ω-6 Linoleic acid
4 - ω-6 Arachidonic acid
5 - ω-3 Alpha-linolenic acid
6 - ω-3 EPA and DHA
7 - Trans fats
8 - Dietary Cholesterol
9 - Non-fiber carbohydrates
10 - Fiber
11 - Protein
12 - Sodium
13 - Antioxidants
14 - Toxins
15 - Artificial sweeteners

ω = Omega

These fifteen categories were selected because they regulate inflammation, blood clotting, cholesterol metabolism, fat accumulation, insulin metabolism, oxidative stress, and cellular replication. Basic understanding of the properties of these molecules will help you predict the health consequences of consuming any food item simply by examining the product label and ingredients. The ensuing information will allow you to make sound dietary choices, even without the NQI numerical ratings at your fingertips.

Eight of the thirteen nutrient categories fall under the broad classification of fats: saturated fats, monounsaturated fats, four subsets of polyunsaturated fats, trans fats, and cholesterol.

BACKGROUND OF FATS

Fatty acids, commonly known as fats, are a group of molecular compounds with a carbon (-C) backbone attached to hydrogen (-H) atoms. Fatty acids are broadly classified into three types, saturated, monounsaturated, and polyunsaturated, according to the number of double bonds [1].

Saturated fatty acids, which have the maximum number of hydrogen atoms attached to every carbon atom, are said to be "saturated" with hydrogen atoms. All of the carbon atoms of a saturated fatty acid are attached to one another by *single* bonds.

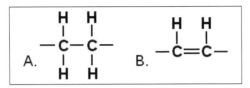

Figure 1: A. Carbon single bond. B. Carbon double bond.

Unlike saturated fatty acids, the carbon backbones of *un*saturated fatty acids are *not* fully saturated by hydrogen atoms. Each missing pair of hydrogen atoms creates a gap that leaves two carbon atoms connected by a *double* bond rather than a single bond.

Unsaturated fats are further classified into "*mono*unsaturated" and "*poly*unsaturated" fatty acids, depending on the total number of gaps, or double bonds. A fatty acid with one double bond, or gap, is called *mono*unsaturated. Fatty acids with more than one gap are called *poly*unsaturated [1, 2].

Classification of Fatty Acids by Number of Double Bonds

Saturated fatty acid	No double bonds	"Saturated" with hydrogens
Monounsaturated fatty acid	One double bond	Mono = one gap
Polyunsaturated fatty acid	> One double bond	Poly = many gaps

Fatty acids are further classified by length of the carbon chain, which can range from four to twenty-four carbons.

Each fatty acid has a name and a corresponding number. For example, the sixteen carbon saturated fatty acid, palmitic acid, can be expressed as 16:0. The first number, 16, refers to the chain length while the second number, 0, refers to the number of double bonds. Since palmitic acid is saturated, it has no double bonds.

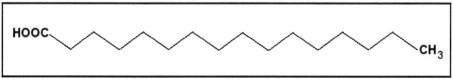

Figure 2: Palmitic Acid (16:0). The sixteen carbon saturated fatty acid has no double bonds. Each point represents a carbon atom attached to two hydrogen atoms.

The primary monounsaturated fat (MUFA) in the diet is oleic acid, which can be expressed as 18:1. The first number, 18, refers to the number of carbon atoms in the fatty acid chain. The second number, 1, refers to the number of double bonds between carbon atoms. Since oleic acid (18:1) is monounsaturated, it has one double bond [2].

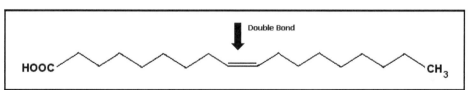

Figure 3: Oleic acid (18:1). The eighteen carbon mono-unsaturated fatty acid has one double bond (arrow).

*Poly*unsaturated fatty acids (PUFA), which have multiple double bonds, are further divided into two main types based on position of the *first* double bond. Omega-6 fatty acids, abbreviated ω-6, are PUFAs with their first double bond located *six* carbons from the (ω) end. Omega-3 fatty acids, abbreviated ω-3, have their first double bond located *three* carbons from the (ω) end.

The primary polyunsaturated fatty acid in the U.S. diet is linoleic acid, which can be expressed as 18:2 ω-6. The first number in this formula indicates that linoleic acid has eighteen carbons. The second number, 2, signifies two double bonds, making linoleic acid a polyunsaturated fatty acid. The last part of the formula, ω-6, signifies that the first double bond is located six carbons from the "ω" end, making linoleic an ω-6 or omega-6 polyunsaturated fatty acid.

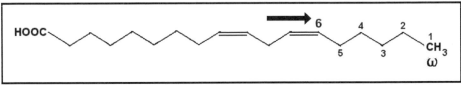

Figure 4: Linoleic acid (18:2 ω-6). Linoleic acid has two double bonds, the first (arrow) of which is six carbons from the CH3 or ω end.

The chain length, position, and number of double bonds determine the unique molecular signature and specific metabolic actions of each different fatty acid [2, 3].

Thus, identification of the precise fatty acid composition of any item helps one predict the consequences of its consumption.

TOTAL FAT

Total fat intake, which accounts for 33-34% of U.S. caloric intake, varies widely across populations, and is poorly correlated with any disease [4]. Despite previous U.S. recommendations to limit total fat intake to <30% of calories based on perceived cardiac benefit, it is now known that subtypes of fatty acids have distinct health attributes: some good and some bad. For this reason, *quality* of fat intake is far more important than total *quantity* consumed [5-10].

SATURATED FATTY ACIDS (SFAs)

The carbon atoms forming the backbone of saturated fats are fully *saturated* with hydrogen atoms, meaning they contain no double bonds. The resulting straight structure allows them to pack tightly together, making them solid at room temperature.

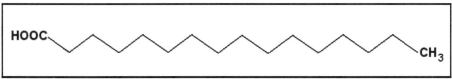

Figure 5: Palmitic acid (16:0).

Saturated fatty acids are concentrated in whole-fat dairy products, grain-fed beef and poultry, and palm, palm kernel, and coconut oils [11].

Total saturated fatty acids supply about 11.6% caloric intake of the average American adult, roughly 27 grams per day [12-14]. Two molecules, palmitic acid (16:0) and stearic acid (18:0), account for the bulk of U.S. intake [14].

Daily Consumption of Saturated Fatty Acids

Name	Molecule	Grams	% Calories
Stearic acid	18:0	7.0	3.0
Palmitic acid	16:0	15.0	6.4
Myristic acid	14:0	2.3	1.0
Lauric acid	12:0	0.9	0.4
Short Chain	4-10:0	1.9	0.8
Total SFAs	**4-18:0**	**27.1**	**11.6**

[12-14]

SFAs accounted for an estimated 6% of caloric intake of pre-agricultural humans [15]. Wild game, like that consumed in abundance by our ancestors, contains a much lower concentration of saturated fats than commercial meats widely available today [15-17]. Modern corn-fed cattle, which account for over 95% of U.S. beef consumption, contain 2-4 times as much saturated fat as animals raised naturally [15, 18]. Dairy, the other major source of SFAs, was not available for human intake until after the Agricultural Revolution, about 10,000 years ago [18]. Overall, modern humans consume nearly twice the saturated fat as our ancestors.

Excessive consumption of long-chain SFAs: stearic (18:0), palmitic (16:0), myristic (14:0), and lauric acid (12:0), which account for 93% of total SFA intake, has several adverse metabolic consequences [8, 19, 20]. Although these four long-chain SFAs have distinct *metabolic* properties, there is insufficient evidence to make any distinctions in their *overall health* properties at this time. For example, stearic acid (18:0) has comparatively little effect on blood cholesterol levels, but may predispose to excessive blood clotting [21, 22]. Collective adverse effects on cholesterol metabolism, insulin regulation, and blood clotting help explain the association between *total* saturated fatty acid consumption and cardiovascular disease [23].

Several U.S. expert groups, including the USDA, recommend Americans consume less than 10% of calories from saturated fats [2]. In 2006, the American Heart Association amended guidelines to further reduce SFA to less than 7% of caloric intake [24].

NQI Analysis: The NQI does not currently differentiate between individual saturated fatty acids, which are considered one molecular category. All saturated fats are rated as moderately negative.

MONOUNSATURATED FATTY ACIDS (MUFAs)

*Mono*unsaturated fatty acids (MUFAs) have one double bond, or gap without hydrogens on the carbon atoms. This double bond, which gives MUFAs a "kinked" structure, results in higher fluidity than saturated fats, making MUFAs liquid at room temperature.

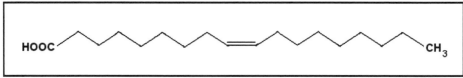

Figure 6: Oleic acid (18:1). Oleic acid, the primary dietary mono-unsaturated fat, has one double bond.

MUFAs account for approximately 13% of U.S. caloric intake, representing about 30 grams per person daily [14, 25-27]. Oleic acid, the major dietary MUFA, accounts for well-over 90% of total U.S. MUFA consumption and 12% of overall U.S. caloric intake [14].

Daily Consumption of Monounsaturated Fatty Acids

Name	Molecule	Grams/day	% Calories
Oleic acid	18:1	28.5	12.2
Palmitoleic acid	16:1*	1.9	0.8
Total MUFA	**16-18:1**	**30.4**	**13.0%**

[14, 25, 26] *Palmitoleic acid includes 0.1% calories from 20:1 and 22:1

Concentrated sources of oleic acid include olive oil, whole olives, avocados, and many nuts, especially macadamias, almonds, and cashews. Seed oils vary widely in oleic acid content, reflecting the fatty acid properties of the whole seeds from which they were obtained.

Oleic Acid-rich Nuts, Seeds, and Fruits

Nut, seed, or fruit	Oleic Acid (as % of total fat)*
Macadamia	80
Olive	75
Avocado	70
Almond	70
Cashew	65
Pecan	60
Pistachio	58

[28, 29] *Somewhat variable by season, climate, latitude, etc.

Throughout human history, MUFAs are believed to have accounted for about half of total dietary fat and 16-25% of total caloric intake [30, 31]. Nuts, wild animal meats, and bone marrow provided concentrated sources of oleic acid. MUFAs account for well over half of the *total* fat of wild and grass-fed animals consumed by pre-industrial humans [30-32].

The diets of wild ruminant animals (deer, sheep, goats) consist of a variety of grasses supplemented by flowers, low hanging branches, moss, seeds, and clovers [33]. In nature, these animals migrate long distances to find adequate pasture and food sources.The lean meats of these animals reflect their grass-based diet and ample physical activity [15, 17]. However, modern animal rearing practices have profoundly altered the composition of beef, poultry, and other meats consumed today, resulting in the replacement of MUFAs with saturated fats [15, 17, 18, 31].

Although MUFAs are widely recognized as beneficial for health, no specific
recommendations have been made for healthy adults [2, 34, 35]. However, according to
one U.S. health promotion agency, consumption of up to 20% of total calories from
MUFAs may be beneficial for those with cholesterol abnormalities [36].

NQI Analysis: The NQI rates MUFAs as modestly to moderately positive.

POLYUNSATURATED FATTY ACIDS (PUFAs)

*Poly*unsaturated fatty acids, or PUFAs, are fatty acids with two or more double bonds.
These double bonds account for the highly fluid nature of PUFAs, which like MUFAs,
are liquid at room temperature.

Polyunsaturated fatty acids are divided into two principal types based on position of the
first double bond. Omega-*6* fatty acids, abbreviated ω-6, are PUFAs with their first
double bond located *six* carbons from the (ω) end. Omega-3, or ω-3 fatty acids, have
their first double bond located *three* carbons from the (ω) end.

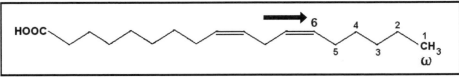

Figure 7: Linoleic acid (LA; 18:2 ω-6) has two double bonds. The first double bond is located six
carbons from the omega (ω) end, making LA an omega-6 fatty acid.

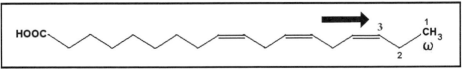

Figure 8: Alpha-linolenic acid (ALA; 18:3 ω-3) has three double bonds. The first double bond is
located three carbons from the omega (ω) end, making ALA an omega-3 fatty acid.

Omega-6 and ω-3 fatty acids serve vital, yet often opposite, functions in the human body.
In general, ω-6 fatty acids promote and ω-3 fatty acids inhibit inflammation, blood
clotting, and cell growth and replication. Both absolute and relative intakes of short *and*

long-chain ω-6 and ω-3 PUFAs have profound and widespread metabolic implications [37-40]. Accumulating evidence suggests that *balanced* intake of all major ω-6 and ω-3 fatty acids is required for optimal health [41-47]. Unfortunately, the modern U.S. food supply provides massive amounts of ω-6 fats and minimal ω-3 fats, a situation strongly linked to the current epidemics of the Big 7 U.S. diseases [44, 48-52].

The most important ω-6 PUFAs are linoleic acid (LA) and arachidonic acid (ArA). Key ω-3 PUFAs include alpha-linolenic acid (ALA), eicosapentaenoic acid (EPA), and docosahexaenoic acid (DHA). Together, these five PUFAs account for an estimated 7.2% of caloric intake or 16.7 grams per day [14, 27, 53].

The NQI breaks these five key molecules into four distinct categories based on health properties: two categories of ω-6 PUFAs, LA and ArA, and two categories of ω-3 PUFAs, ALA and EPA/DHA.

Omega-6 Polyunsaturated fatty acids (PUFAs)

	Short Chain	Chain length	Formula
1	**Linoleic acid (LA)**	18 Carbons	18:2ω-6
	Long Chain		
2	**Arachidonic acid (ArA)**	20 Carbons	20:4ω-6

The two major omega-6 fatty acids are the short-chain, 18 carbon linoleic acid, abbreviated LA, and the long-chain, 20 carbon arachidonic acid, abbreviated ArA.

Omega-6 and ω-3 PUFAs come in short chain and long chain varieties. Short chain PUFAs have 18-carbon backbones and long chain PUFAs have 20 or 22 carbons.

Omega-3 Polyunsaturated fatty acids (PUFAs)

	Short Chain	Chain Length	Formula
3	**Alpha linolenic acid (ALA)**	18 Carbons	18:3ω-3
	Long Chain		
4	**Eicosapentaenoic acid (EPA)**	20 Carbons	20:5ω-3
	Docosahexaenoic acid (DHA)	22 Carbons	22:6ω-3

The chief categories of omega-3 fatty acids are the short-chain, 18 carbon alpha linolenic acid, abbreviated ALA, and the long chain, 20 and 22 carbon EPA and DHA, respectively.

The short chain versions of ω-6 and ω-3 fatty acids, ω-6 LA and ω-3 ALA, are considered "essential fatty acids," meaning that *small amounts* of these molecules are required in the diet, and that humans cannot make them from scratch [54]. Nuts, beans, fruits, vegetables, and other plant foods supply *only* these short-chain ω-6 and ω-3 fatty acids. After human or animal consumption, ω-6 LA and ω-3 ALA compete with one another for liver enzymes which convert some LA and ALA to their **long chain** ω-6 and ω-3 counterparts: the 20 carbon ω-6 fatty acid Arachidonic acid (ArA) and the 20 and 22 carbon ω-3 fatty acids EPA and DHA.

Omega-6 LA ⟹ ArA	**Figure 9: Conversion of short chain ω-6 and ω-3 fatty acids to their long chain counterparts.**
Omega-3 ALA ⟹ EPA ⟹ DHA	

Thus, fish, meats, eggs, and other animal products supply **long-chain** ω-6 ArA and ω-3 EPA/DHA, in addition to their short chain counterparts.

Plant Foods	Animal Foods		
Short chain	**Long chain**	**AND**	**Short Chain**
ω-6 LA	ω-6 ArA		ω-6 LA
ω-3 ALA	ω-3 EPA + DHA		ω-3 ALA

Dietary ω-6 (LA, ArA) and ω-3 (ALA, EPA, and DHA) fatty acids interact with one another in a complex network [37-40, 54-57]. Tissue accumulation and activity of both short and long chain ω-6 and ω-3 fatty acids are dependent upon both relative and absolute intake of *all five* of these molecules [44, 50, 56-59]. Therefore, it is imperative to consider dietary intakes of these five PUFAs in context of one another.

OMEGA – 6 POLYUNSATURATED FATS

ω-6 LINOLEIC ACID (LA; 18:2ω-6)

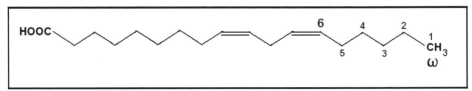

Figure 10: Linoleic acid (18:2 ω-6).

The 18 carbon, short-chain ω-6 polyunsaturated fatty acid linoleic acid (LA) is highly concentrated in most vegetable and seed oils consumed in the U.S., especially safflower, sunflower, corn, cottonseed, soybean, peanut, and canola oils.

Omega-6 Linoleic acid - rich Vegetable Oils

Vegetable oil	ω-6 LA (as % of fatty acids)
Safflower	78
Sunflower	70
Corn	60
Cottonseed	54
Soybean	53
Peanut	33
Canola	24

[28, 29, 60]

On average, Americans consume 15 grams of linoleic acid each day [14, 53]. Therefore, this single molecule accounts for 6.4% of total caloric intake and nearly 90% of polyunsaturated fatty acid intake in the U.S.!

Historically, pre-agricultural humans *may* have consumed *as many as* 8 grams of LA per day, mostly from nuts and wild animal meats [32]. As cereal grains replaced nuts and wild game during the Agricultural Revolution, consumption of linoleic acid intake declined until the turn of the 20th century, when technological advances allowed for solvent extraction of seed and vegetable oils [55]. Over the last 100 years, as solvent extraction of oils has expanded, intake of LA-rich seed and vegetable oils has soared and continues to escalate. Today, the average American consumes about three times as much LA as in 1909, at least twice as much as any population in human history [11]!

U.S. dietary guidelines do not differentiate between specific polyunsaturated fatty acids; instead, they cite beneficial effects of the broad classifications of either "unsaturated" or "polyunsaturated" fats as a whole [61]. In the 1950s, it was demonstrated that "high LA" diets can reduce serum cholesterol, especially when replacing saturated and trans fats [62]. Several, but not all, ensuing studies in the 1960s through 1980s suggested that replacement of *typical* fats with LA-rich vegetable oils reduced the risk of heart disease [63-67]. However, interpretations of these studies failed to account for the fact that the *typical* fats replaced by LA-rich oils consisted of moderate to massive amounts of trans fatty acid-rich shortenings and margarines, which are *now* known to have overwhelmingly negative health consequences [63, 65, 66]. Other studies showed no benefit, increased coronary events, and/or higher cancer incidence which negated any overall mortality benefit [65, 67-70]. Nevertheless, subsequent recommendations to replace saturated fats with "unsaturated" or "polyunsaturated" fats, coupled with widespread availability of LA-rich vegetable oils, has boosted the intake of LA to unprecedented levels.

Once consumed, a significant portion of dietary ω-6 linoleic acid is converted to its long-chain ω-6 counterpart, arachidonic acid (ArA), in the human liver and other tissues [37, 55]. Excessive accumulation of arachidonic acid and ArA metabolites in blood and tissues, a situation termed "ArA Overload," is associated with fat tissue expansion, inflammation, and a host of other metabolic disturbances [42, 71-75]. *Resulting unrestrained ArA metabolism plays a major role in the epidemic nature of the Big 7 U.S. diseases* [42, 43, 45, 46, 50, 56, 76-78].

Growing recognition of adverse health consequences of excessive LA intake has motivated a number of individual experts and international bodies to propose reducing ω-6 LA intake with the goal of achieving more balanced ω-6 to ω-3 ratios [41, 43-47, 50, 79-81]. Generally speaking, overall ω-6 intake should be no more than 4-5 times that of ω-3 intake, although intake of closer to the 1 to 1 or 2 to 1 ratio consumed by our ancestors is considered ideal [79-82].

In 1999, a panel of experts associated with the International Society for the Study of Fatty Acids and Lipids (ISSFAL) and the National Institutes of Health (NIH) suggested that LA should account for no more than 3% of daily calories, or 6.7 grams per day, in order to "reduce adverse effects of excesses of arachidonic acid and its eicosanoid products" [51]. This ceiling of 3% of calories places virtually the entire U.S. population well above the upper limit of LA intake! A July 2004 statement of the ISSFAL board reiterated that "a healthy upper limit to the intake of LA" exists, but failed to reach a numerical consensus [83].

The Lyon Diet Heart study, a secondary prevention study which pitted an ALA-rich, LA-poor Mediterranean diet against a prudent diet similar to the National Cholesterol Education Program Step I diet recommended at the time, strongly supports the potential of limiting LA and balancing ω-6 to ω-3 ratios. The ALA-rich, LA-poor diet resulted in a remarkable 50-70% reduction of cardiac events, cancers, and overall mortality despite similar blood cholesterol levels [6, 45-47]!

However, despite growing evidence and international recognition that excessive ω-6 LA intake may predispose to certain diseases, U.S. health advocacy groups continue to advocate high intakes of "unsaturated" or "polyunsaturated" fatty acids. In fact, in March of 2007, the U.S. Food and Drug Administration voted to allow "heart healthy" labeling claims on products containing 80% or more of "unsaturated" fats, including spreads, shortenings, potato chips, corn chips, pretzels, popcorn, cookies, and other snacks containing ω-6 LA-rich vegetable and seed oils.

NQI Analysis: The NQI rates ω-6 LA as modestly negative.

ω-6 ARACHIDONIC ACID (ArA; 20:4ω-6)

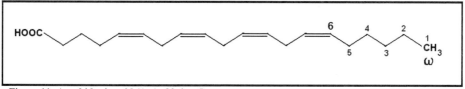

Figure 11: Arachidonic acid (ArA; 20:4 ω-6).

The 20 carbon ω-6 polyunsaturated fatty acid, arachidonic acid (ArA), is found in most animal fats: especially red meat, poultry, eggs, and tropical and certain farm-raised fish [28, 84, 85].

While estimated non-vegetarian ArA intake can range from 100 to 1000 milligrams (mg) per day, most Americans consume between 200-300 mg [57, 69, 76, 86]. Although intake is modest in comparison to other PUFAs, dietary ArA has several profound metabolic effects [42, 59, 71-73, 76, 87, 88].

Historical intake of ArA is a matter of controversy. Adequate intakes of both ω-6 ArA and ω-3 DHA were required for the rapid brain growth during evolution of modern humans [89, 90]. However, quantitative estimates are highly dependent upon whether early humans lived at the land-water interface, which allowed for consumption of ω-3 rich fish and shellfish, or the African grassland, which required hunting and scavenging of ω-6 ArA-rich mammals. In brief, early humans would have consumed far less ω-6 ArA if they lived at the land-water interface rather than the grassland [32, 89, 91].

Regardless of precise historical intakes, modern agribusiness practices have radically altered the relative amounts of ω-6 ArA and ω-3 EPA/DHA in domesticated animal meats. Corn-fed livestock maintain moderate amounts of ω-6 ArA, but only a tiny fraction of EPA/DHA levels of pasture-fed and wild counterparts [15, 17, 18, 92-98]. Similar changes have occurred in poultry, eggs, and other animal products [99-101]. Farm-raised fatty fish, including salmon, have undergone even more extreme changes. Farmed fish, often fed ω-6 LA enriched vegetable oils, accumulate large quantities of ArA. For instance, farm-raised Atlantic salmon contain 4 to 15 times as much ArA as wild salmon. These farm-raised salmon, which account for over 50% of U.S. salmon intake, are the most concentrated source of ArA in the U.S. food supply [28, 102]!

There is growing evidence that dietary ArA, even with modest to moderate intake, can have a significant impact on several key molecular processes including: inflammation, fat accumulation, blood clotting, and cell replication [42, 56, 59, 71-73, 75, 76, 87, 88]. Tissue and blood levels of ArA reflect direct consumption of ArA *and* conversion of dietary LA to ArA in the liver [37, 55, 57-59, 84, 103]. Even in the context of massive background intake of ω-6 LA and *pre-existing* blood and tissue ArA accumulation, nearly all *dietary* ω-6 ArA enters the eicosanoid precursor pool, further magnifying "ArA Overload" [59, 87, 103]. Accumulating evidence suggests that excessive ArA and ArA-derived metabolic mediators play key roles in the development and progression of many epidemic U.S. diseases including heart disease, stroke, obesity, depression, Alzheimer's dementia, arthritis, and certain cancers [42, 44, 49, 50, 52, 76-78, 104-107].

While individual experts have suggested that patients with inflammatory diseases such as rheumatoid arthritis should limit ω-6 ArA intake (to <90 mg per day), national or international expert groups have yet to make specific recommendations for ArA intake [56].

NQI Analysis: The NQI rates ω-6 ArA as profoundly negative.

OMEGA – 3 POLYUNSATURATED FATS

ALPHA-LINOLENIC ACID (ALA; 18:3ω-3)

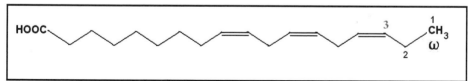

Figure 12: Alpha-linolenic acid (ALA; 18:3 ω-3).

The most concentrated dietary source of the short-chain (18 carbon) ω-3 alpha linolenic acid (ALA) is flaxseed. However, less concentrated sources, especially soybean oil-based mayonnaises and salad dressings, provide the bulk of U.S. ALA intake [108]. Although certain vegetable and seed oils provide modest amounts of ω-3 ALA, their intake is generally accompanied by massive amounts of ω-6 LA.

ω-6 LA and ω-3 ALA in Vegetable and Seed Oils

Type	ω-6 LA	ω-3 ALA	LA:ALA ratio
Safflower	78%	0%	>100:1
Sunflower	69%	0%	>100:1
Corn	60%	1%	60:1
Cottonseed	54%	0%	>100:1
Soybean	53%	7%	7.5:1
Sesame	43%	0%	>100:1
Peanut	33%	0%	>100:1
Canola	24%	8%	3:1

[28, 29, 60] **LA and ALA expressed as percentages of total fatty acids.**

Walnuts, and to a lesser extent certain vegetables and fruits, also provide small amounts of ALA.

ω-6 LA to ω-3 ALA Ratios of Vegetables, Fruits, Walnuts, and Grains

Food	ω-6:ω-3 ratio
Vegetables (average)	1.5:1
Fruit (average)	2:1
English walnuts*	4.2:1
Grains (average)	20:1
Wheat	11:1
Corn	60:1

[28] * **California supplies the majority of "English" or "Persian" walnuts, which account for more than 90% of U.S. walnut intake. "English" walnuts have a higher ω-3 ALA concentration than "black" walnuts.**

On average, Americans consume approximately 1.35 grams of ω-3 ALA per day, representing about 0.6% of caloric intake [13, 27, 53, 69, 108, 109]

Pre-agricultural humans, with a natural diet rich in fruits, vegetables, nuts, and wild game, *may* have consumed up to 10 times as much ALA as modern Americans [32]. In fact, prior to the agricultural revolution, humans may have consumed more ω-3 ALA than ω-6 LA [32]! However, over the last 5,000 to 10,000 years, humans began consuming less ω-3 ALA as nuts, seeds, vegetables, and fruits were replaced with cultivated grains. More recently, agribusiness, selective plant breeding, and food processing have removed much of the remaining ω-3 ALA from the U.S. food supply [29, 44]. Simultaneously, massive consumption of ω-6 LA-rich vegetable oils has raised the ω-6 LA to ω-3 ALA ratio 12-20 fold since pre-agricultural times [32, 41, 43, 44, 110].

Like their human counterparts, U.S. livestock consume far fewer ω-3 fatty acids than their wild ancestors. Unlike the ω-3 ALA-rich grasses, leaves, herbs, clovers, flowers, seeds, and moss consumed by wild ruminants, ω-6 LA-rich, ω-3 ALA-poor corn-based diets produce U.S. meat and dairy products deficient in ALA [33, 100, 101, 111, 112]. Importantly, the high ALA content of meat and dairy from naturally-raised Alpine cattle has been linked to the low levels of heart disease despite high dairy fat intake, a situation known as the "Alpine Paradox" [101].

Accumulating evidence suggests that dietary ω-3 ALA may have a host of beneficial health effects including reduction of coronary heart disease mortality, prevention of certain cancers, and lower overall mortality [45-47, 69, 78, 108, 113-115]. However, enthusiasm for increasing ALA intake has been tempered by the inconsistent association with prostate cancer seen in some but not all epidemiological studies [116]. Of three *prospective* studies estimating *dietary* ALA intake, one reported a modest protective effect, another a modest increased incidence of high-grade prostate cancer risk (but no overall increased risk), and the most recent no relationship with prostate cancer of any grade [117-119]. In contrast, molecular, animal, and even some experimental studies *suggest* that a high LA/ALA ratio may predispose to several cancers and increasing ω-3 ALA intake may actually *prevent* various cancers including prostate cancer [46, 69, 78, 120]. Likewise, a 2007 Duke University study found that a high ω-3 ALA flaxseed diet slowed tumor growth in patients with established prostate cancer [115, 121]. Clearly, more research is needed to evaluate this controversial subject [109, 122].

Several international and U.S. health promotion agencies suggest that the *minimum* requirement for ALA is around 0.6% of calories, and ideal intake somewhat higher, perhaps 1% of calories or 2 grams/day [28, 51, 83, 123, 124]. Evidence supports the notion that intake at about this level "reduces all-cause mortality and various cardiovascular disease states" [2]. Most health advocacy groups specify no upper limit for ALA intake, citing insufficient evidence of risk at any amount of intake [2].

Overall, Americans consume even less ALA than these conservative guidelines advocate. In fact, it may be difficult to consume even 1% of calories from ω-3 ALA-depleted American foods without supplementing with flaxseed or canola oil. For now, a conservative recommendation to boost intake to 2 to 3 grams per day (0.9 to 1.3% caloric intake) seems reasonable.

Author's Note: In the author's opinion, the supposed link between ALA and elevated risk of prostate cancer will eventually be refuted [78, 115, 119, 122]. When this occurs, Americans may further take advantage of the beneficial health properties of ω-3 ALA at considerably higher levels than the current 10-20% of historical intake.

NQI Analysis: The NQI rates ω-3 ALA as moderately positive. Due to the current controversy surrounding ALA and prostate cancer, a limit is placed on positive points attributable to ALA.

ω-3 EPA (20:5ω-3) + DHA (22:6ω-3)

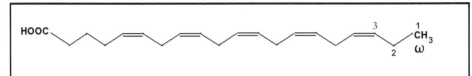

Figure 13: Eicosapentaenoic acid (EPA; 20:5 ω-3).

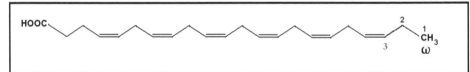

Figure 14: Docosahexaenoic acid (DHA; 22:6 ω-3).

The richest dietary sources of the 20 and 22-carbon long-chain ω-3 PUFAs, EPA and DHA, in the U.S. food supply are cold water fatty fish including salmon, mackerel, anchovies, herring, halibut, sardines, and tuna. Less concentrated sources include mussels, shrimp, squid (calamari), octopus, and scallops [28]. Marine ω-3 EPA and DHA are ultimately derived from microscopic plants known as phytoplankton which accumulate up the food chain in crustaceans, fish, and other marine organisms [125]. Meat from *wild* and *pasture-fed* mammals also contains modest to moderate amounts of EPA and DHA, reflecting intake of ω-3 ALA-rich grasses and other plants [33, 95, 96, 98].

On average, Americans consume only about 45 mg and 75 mg of EPA and DHA, respectively, a tiny fraction of the amount consumed throughout human history [53, 70]. Importantly, approximately 25% of the U.S. population consumes no detectable EPA or DHA [70]!

Although the idea that our ancestors consumed plentiful ω-3 EPA and DHA-rich marine foods has gained momentum, some evolutionary biologists maintain that brain, organ, and muscle tissue of *land* mammals may have provided adequate ω-3 DHA [32, 89-91]. Regardless of source, scientists agree that adequate dietary DHA was essential for the rapid brain growth which allowed prehistoric humans to develop and use tools, create complex cultures, and develop innovative means of communicating with one another [89]. Humans subsisting on a natural diet of our ancestors likely consumed *at least* 660 mg of EPA and DHA, roughly 6 times that of modern Americans [32]. Other estimates which place our ancestors at the land-water interface are considerably higher [89, 90].

Modern domesticated cattle, poultry, fish, dairy, and egg yolks all contain much lower concentrations of EPA and DHA and higher ω-6 to ω-3 ratios than their more naturally reared counterparts and the wild animals consumed by our ancestors [18, 31, 82, 92, 93, 98, 99, 111, 126]. For instance, the pasture-fed cattle consumed by our recent ancestors were low in total and saturated fats, and relatively high in ω-3 fatty acids, reflecting their intake of ω-3 ALA-rich grasses [18]. Over the last 100 years, however, ALA–rich grasses have been largely replaced with ω-6 LA-rich corn-based feed. Therefore, historically speaking, lack of ω-3 EPA and DHA and high ω-6 to ω-3 ratios in meats consumed by humans is an unprecedented situation.

Studies have repeatedly demonstrated that consumption of long chain ω-3 fatty acids can prevent or attenuate several of the Big 7 U.S. epidemic diseases. The strongest evidence of beneficial effects relates to protection against heart disease, stroke and other cardiovascular diseases, and reduction of overall mortality [127-129]. Accumulating evidence suggests that increased intake of ω-3 EPA and DHA may reduce the risk of developing depression and other psychiatric illnesses, Alzheimer's dementia and cognitive decline, excessive weight gain and obesity, certain cancers, arthritis, macular degeneration, and a host of other illnesses [42, 52, 56, 130-140].

Omega-3 EPA and DHA exert their beneficial effects via a wide variety of molecular mechanisms. Interestingly, ω-3 EPA and DHA regulate several high-leverage metabolic processes at the DNA level by modulating gene expression [141-143]. Importantly, ω-3 EPA and DHA antagonize "ArA Overload" syndrome. By inhibiting conversion of dietary ω-6 LA and by directly competing with ω-6 ArA throughout the body, ω-3 EPA and DHA block excessive inflammation and blood clotting, inhibit fat cell accumulation, and block unrestrained cell growth and replication [42, 53, 57, 113, 136, 137, 144-148].

Several national and international agencies advocate increased dietary ω-3 EPA and DHA intake. Americans consume nowhere near even the most modest of these guidelines [53]. The USDA suggests that Americans should consume a bare minimum of 200 mg, nearly double the average U.S. intake [2]. Several other bodies recommend at least 500 mg [83]. The American Heart Association suggests that those with documented coronary heart disease should consume approximately 1000 mg per day of EPA and DHA, more than eight-times the average amount consumed by Americans [53, 149].

Intriguingly, a recent study in Japan reported that the risk of developing coronary heart disease, cardiac mortality, and overall mortality may *continue* to decrease with *very high* fish consumption, corresponding to 15 to 20 times average U.S. intake of EPA and DHA [128]. These results are consistent with the strong inverse association between ω-3 EPA and DHA intake and heart disease mortality seen across multiple diverse populations (see pages 110-112, Part 3: Diet and Blood Clotting) [50, 73, 74, 79, 150-154].

NQI Analysis: The NQI rates ω-3 EPA and DHA as profoundly positive.

TRANS FATS

Trans fatty acids are *un*saturated fatty acids that contain at least one double bond in the "trans" configuration instead of the natural "cis" configuration.

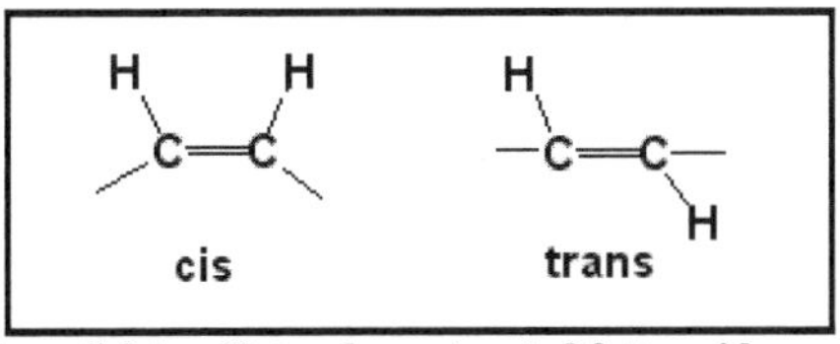

Figure 15: "cis" and "trans" fats. Natural unsaturated fatty acids contain hydrogen atoms on the same side, known as the "cis" configuration. However, by moving hydrogen atoms around to an unnatural "trans" configuration, the hydrogenation process alters the biochemical attributes of fatty acids.

Artificial trans fatty acids are created by partial hydrogenation of liquid vegetable oils. Hydrogenation, which straightens the "kinks" caused by natural double bonds, hardens the oils giving them a semisolid consistency similar to saturated fatty acids [155]. Trans fats are desirable for food manufacturers because they greatly extend the shelf-life of foods, remain stable during deep-frying, and enhance the palatability and texture of some baked goods and sweets [156].

Two molecules account for the bulk of U.S. trans fat intake, trans-oleic (t18:1), the *trans* isomer of oleic acid (18:1), and trans-linoleic (t18:2), the *trans* isomer of linoleic acid (18:2ω-6).

Trans Fatty Acids in U.S. Food Supply

Name	Molecular formula(s)	Grams/day	% caloric intake
Trans Oleic* (Elaidic)	t18:1	3.5	1.5%
Trans Linoleic	t18:2	0.6	0.3%
Total Trans	t18:1 + t18:2	4.1	1.8%

[27, 53]*Trans oleic includes trans palmitoleic (0.08g/day)
Estimates based on 25-35% reduction in TFA intake since 2001-2002.

The majority of artificial trans fats consumed in the U.S. are supplied by three categories of food items: household shortenings and margarines, foods fried in partially hydrogenated oils (french fries, fried chicken), and baked goods (cakes, cookies, pies, donuts). Other processed foods, including certain breakfast cereals, salad dressings, crackers, chips, and candies supply modest amounts of trans fats [157].

Author's Note: Beef and dairy products naturally contain small amounts of trans fatty acids (<0.5% caloric intake), mostly in the form of trans-vaccenic acid. However, because naturally occurring trans fatty acids found in beef and dairy products do not appear to have substantial adverse health effects, this section will focus on artificial trans fatty acids formed during partial hydrogenation of vegetable oils [156].

Aside from naturally occurring trans fats in the meat and dairy products of grazing animals, trans fatty acids were absent from human diet prior to the invention of hydrogenation around 1900. However, in 1911 with the widespread commercialization of Crisco™ (made of partially hydrogenated cottonseed oil), significant amounts of trans fatty acids began to enter the U.S. food supply. The low cost of partially hydrogenated vegetable oils made them an attractive alternative to saturated animal fats, and their use slowly climbed over the ensuing decades. In the 1970s and 1980s, several studies firmly established a link between *saturated* fats and coronary heart disease [23]. Subsequent guidelines from health promotion agencies focused on reducing consumption of saturated fats, which were to be replaced with "unsaturated fats" and "complex carbohydrates." Perhaps because trans fats fit into the broad category of *un*saturated fats, their use continued to increase. Throughout the 1980s and 1990s, trans fatty acid-rich margarines were widely recommended as a supposedly "heart healthy" alternative to butters rich in saturated fat and cholesterol [158]. By the late 1990s, U.S. trans fat intake peaked at around 7-8% of total fat intake and roughly 3% of total caloric intake [13, 159].

Despite the widespread addition of trans fats to the U.S. food supply for over 75 years, essentially nothing was known about the health consequences of their consumption until studies in the 1990s suggested they may have a multitude of toxic effects [156, 160]. Since then, evidence has accumulated that trans fatty acid consumption promotes cholesterol and insulin dysregulation, contributes to excessive inflammation and blood clotting, alters function of cell membranes, and may disrupt normal neurotransmitter turnover and neuronal function [145, 161-163]. Substantial evidence suggests that trans fatty acids, even in relatively small amounts (1-3% of calories), *greatly* increase the risk of developing heart disease [9]. Chillingly, on a *per gram* basis, trans fats increase the risk of disease more than any other macronutrient. In fact, the adverse effects of trans fats appear to be many magnitudes greater than even saturated fats [164, 165]. Near elimination of partially hydrogenated oils from the U.S. food supply would prevent an estimated 72,000 to 228,000 coronary events per year [156]. In addition, emerging research suggests that trans fat intake *may* also predispose to a wide variety of epidemic U.S. diseases including diabetes, obesity, Alzheimer's dementia and cognitive decline, mood disorders, and certain cancers [161, 166-169]. Disturbingly, consuming even small quantities of trans fats appears to increase the risk of ovulatory infertility [170].

As evidence belatedly accumulated that trans fats predispose to chronic disease in the 1990s, health advocacy groups began trying to curb their consumption. However, early suggestions to limit intake were generally overshadowed by standard guidelines to reduce *total* fat, saturated fat, and cholesterol [61]. In 2003, Denmark passed legislation effectively banning the use of hydrogenated oils [171, 172]. Later in 2003, the U.S. FDA issued a regulation requiring manufacturers to list trans fatty acids on the Nutrition Facts panel, effective January 1, 2006 [1]. Thus, prior to 2006, only U.S. consumers who knew how to recognize the presence of trans fatty acids in ingredient lists had any idea whether or not foods consumed contained them, and had no way of quantifying the amount of trans fatty acids in any food item.

---

*Author's Note: **Identifying Trans Fats** - Oils labeled "partially hydrogenated" generally contain significant amounts of trans fatty acids. Although "fully hydrogenated", or simply "hydrogenated," oils contain smaller amounts, the hydrogenation process does not achieve 100% efficiency, so at least traces of trans fats are present. In addition, partial hydrogenation of oils produces countless other altered fatty acids with unknown health consequences, and both partially or fully hydrogenated oils often contain nickel, aluminum or other potentially toxic heavy metals used in the hydrogenation process.*

Recent guidelines require manufacturers to list the amount of trans fats in the Nutrition Facts panel of most food items [1]. While these guidelines are a major improvement, a "trans fat loophole" exists which allows manufacturers to continue discretely adding trans fats to processed foods. Under current guidelines, food items containing up to 500 milligrams of trans fatty acids *per serving* can legally label and market foods as "trans fat free," "no trans fat," and "0 grams of trans fat" [1, 173]. In some instances, by manipulating listed serving sizes and rounding down manufacturers have been able to list food items fairly concentrated in trans fats as "trans fat free" with *per serving* in small print. Because many "servings" may be consumed at one sitting, total trans fat intake may add up to several grams. By expressing trans fats as a percentage of weight (using *true* grams) rather than rounding off to the nearest gram, the NQI eliminates the trans fat loophole.

Despite this loophole, intake of unnatural trans fatty acids has declined as manufacturers scrambled to reformulate products by either replacing trans fats with other ingredients, or by reducing them to less than 500 mg per serving. While it is difficult to say for sure, the author estimates that trans fat intake dropped by 30-35% percent over the last few years, to about 1.8% of total caloric intake. Pending legislation and voluntary substitution of fast food cooking oils may further reduce intake.

Given the strong link between trans fat intake and coronary events (estimated 72,000 –
228,000 events per year), and likely role in other common causes of death, even a modest
population-wide decline would be expected to significantly reduce overall mortality
[156]. Intriguingly, as manufacturers began reformulating products to reduce trans fats in
anticipation of January 2006 labeling requirements, a sharp drop in overall U.S. mortality
was observed, the first such drop in decades, and the largest single-year drop since the
1940s [174].

Unlike other fats and nutrients, trans fatty acids are not required and have *no* known
beneficial effects. Health advocacy groups now universally recommend that unnatural
trans fats should be sharply limited "as much as possible" [2]. Given the profoundly
deleterious health properties of unnatural trans fatty acids, the optimal level of intake is
zero [156].

NQI Analysis: The NQI assigns trans fatty acids a strongly negative rating.

DIETARY CHOLESTEROL

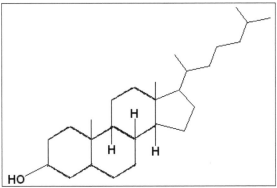

Figure 16: Cholesterol. A simplified schematic of the molecular structure of cholesterol.

Dietary cholesterol is derived entirely from animal products. Eggs, red meat, poultry, and fish are the principal sources of *dietary* cholesterol in the U.S. food supply [11]. Nuts, fruits, vegetables, beans, and other plant foods do *not* contain cholesterol. On average, American adults consume about 290 mg of *dietary* cholesterol per day [27, 53].

Historically, our ancestors are believed to have consumed closer to 500 mg of cholesterol each day, reflecting their higher intake of animal products [175-177]. However, despite higher intake of *dietary* cholesterol, preagricultural humans likely had much lower *blood* cholesterol levels than modern Americans [30].

DIETARY CHOLESTEROL VERSUS BLOOD CHOLESTEROL: A HISTORY OF CONFUSION

Over the last half-century the role of elevated *blood* cholesterol in heart disease has become well established [178]. However, a key distinction must be made between *dietary* cholesterol and *blood (or serum)* cholesterol. Importantly, *dietary* cholesterol has only a modest effect on *blood* cholesterol levels [2, 179-183]. By comparison, trans fatty acids, saturated fatty acids, and nonfiber carbohydrates play a much larger role in the regulation of *blood* cholesterol levels than does *dietary* cholesterol [2].

These facts likely explain why studies have failed to demonstrate a significant relationship between *dietary* cholesterol and heart disease or any other disease [2, 184]. Yet many Americans erroneously believe reduction of *dietary* cholesterol is the single most important dietary change necessary to reduce the risk of coronary heart disease [185].

Rather than specifying an upper limit for *dietary* cholesterol intake, Canadian health advocacy groups emphasize the importance of choosing the right kinds of fats [186]. However, U.S. health promotion agencies uniformly recommend reducing intake of "saturated fats and cholesterol," along with an upper limit of 300 mg of cholesterol intake per day [2]. The argument that many foods rich in cholesterol are also rich in saturated fat is often used to justify the inclusion of cholesterol in guidelines, despite lack of solid evidence that *dietary* cholesterol promotes disease. Two notable examples of high cholesterol foods with little saturated fat are fish and eggs [28]. Thus, guidelines to limit cholesterol intake may inadvertently reduce consumption of foods with beneficial health effects [128, 187].

Regardless of whether *dietary* cholesterol has a minimal impact on the development of coronary disease (as the fine print of U.S. guidelines suggest) or no impact at all as some studies suggest, recognition that the importance of *dietary* cholesterol is minuscule in comparison to that of trans fats, saturated fats, and other macronutrients will allow Americans to make more informed food choices.

NQI Analysis: The NQI assigns dietary cholesterol a minimally negative rating reflecting its minimal impact on health and disease.

CATEGORIES OF CARBOHYDRATES

BACKGROUND

Carbohydrates are *carbo*n-based compounds that contain large quantities of *hydr*oxyl (-OH) groups [188].

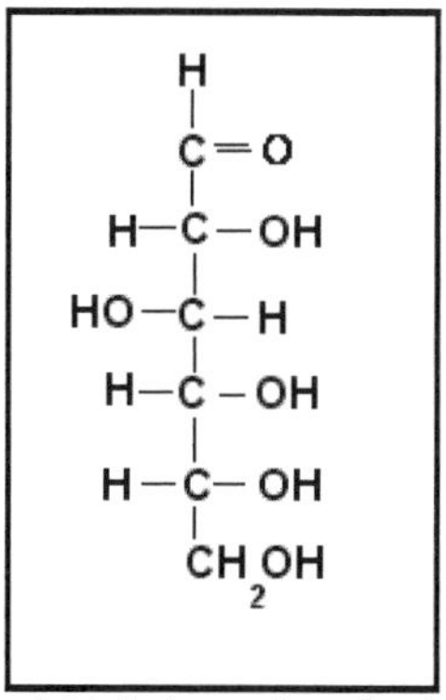

Figure 17: Glucose. Simplified straight chain version of a glucose molecule consisting of carbon (-C), oxygen (-O), and hydrogen (-H) atoms. A single oxygen attached to a single hydrogen is known as a hydroxyl (-OH) group.

Total dietary carbohydrates can be divided into two groups: fibers and non-fiber carbohydrates (NFC).

Dietary fibers are edible parts of plants which are resistant to digestion in the small intestine, and therefore are not absorbed into the bloodstream. Fibers are classified as either soluble or insoluble, based on their behavior in water [189]. *In*soluble fibers pass through the small and large intestines without being digested or absorbed before being passed out in the stool [190]. Soluble fibers, however, are converted into short chain fatty acids which supply energy to colonic cells [190].

Unlike fibers, which account for only a modest amount of caloric intake, non-fiber carbohydrates (NFC) supply about *half* of all calories consumed in the U.S. NFCs can be subdivided into two groups, sugars and starches, based on the number of single sugar units per molecule. Dietary sugars contain either one or two sugar units.

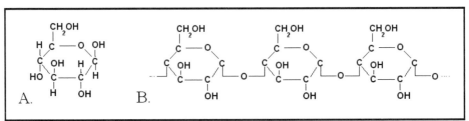

Figure 18: Examples of carbohydrates: A. Glucose, a single unit sugar.   B. Amylose, a starch.

Starches, or *poly*saccharides, are simply hundreds to thousands of sugar molecules linked together into long chains [188]. Like sugars, *poly*saccharides are readily digested in the human small intestine into one-unit sugar molecules which are then absorbed into the bloodstream [191-193].

Author's Note: The digestion of starches to single unit sugar molecules begins in the mouth, where salivary amylase dissolves the bonds between glucose molecules . Amylases in the small intestine generally complete the job within minutes [194].

Thus, both dietary sugars and starches are transported by the human bloodstream and presented to various tissues in the form of simple sugars.

FIBERS

Major sources of fiber in the U.S. diet include unrefined cereal grains, vegetables, fruits, nuts, and legumes [11]. Low intake of high-fiber fruits, vegetables and nuts, combined with high intake of refined cereal grains stripped of fiber, has profoundly reduced the fiber content of the American food supply [185].

In fact, the average American consumes only 16 grams of total fiber per day, a small fraction of the estimated 60-120 grams consumed by our ancestors [27, 53, 176, 195]. Roughly two-thirds, or 10 grams, of this fiber is of the insoluble variety; the remaining one-third is soluble fiber [27]. Although they account for only a trivial amount of caloric intake, dietary fibers play important and beneficial roles in several key metabolic processes [189, 190].

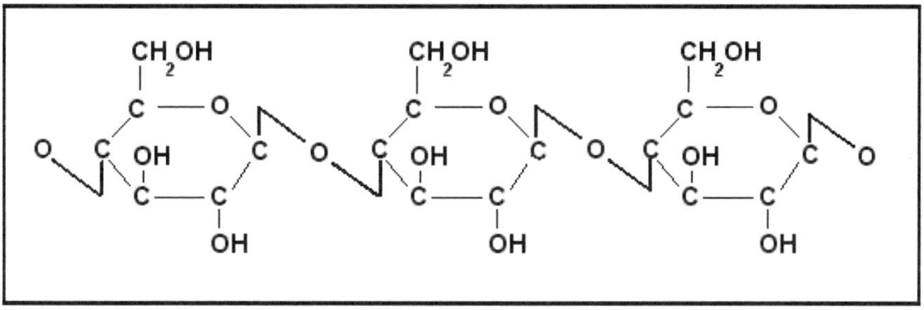

Figure 19: Cellulose, an example of a dietary fiber.

Both soluble and insoluble fibers improve insulin sensitivity, reduce excessive inflammation and blood clotting, and reduce the risk of developing diabetes, heart disease, and obesity [196-200]. However, soluble and insoluble fibers do *not* have identical metabolic properties. For instance, soluble fibers reduce LDL cholesterol more than insoluble fibers [201]. Despite metabolic differences, studies suggest that *all* fibers have significant beneficial health properties, and currently no *overall* health distinctions can be made amongst them [189, 202]. Despite the many well-recognized beneficial health properties of fiber, most Americans consume nowhere near the modest current recommendations of 25 to 40 grams per day [2, 203].

NQI Analysis: The NQI does not distinguish between soluble and insoluble fibers; both are grouped together into a single category of total fiber which is given a moderately positive rating.

NON-FIBER CARBOHYDRATES (NFCs): SUGARS AND STARCHES

Non-fiber carbohydrates (NFCs) include both sugars *and* starches. Unlike dietary fiber which provides little or no calories, NFCs account for approximately 50% of caloric intake of U.S. adults [27, 204]. Sugars and starches have similar molecular compositions and share many metabolic properties [191, 205].

SUGARS

The simplest sugars, known as *mono*saccharides, consist of a single sugar molecule. The most important dietary monosaccharides are glucose and fructose [188].

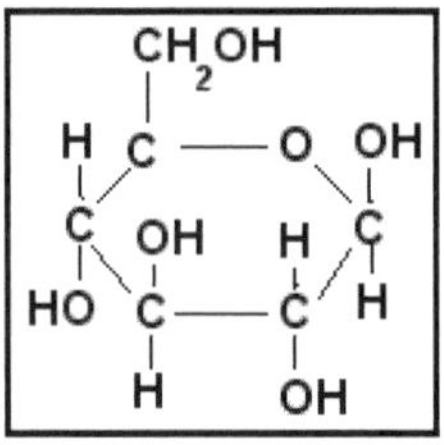

Figure 20: Glucose. Glucose is one of the two major dietary monosaccharides.

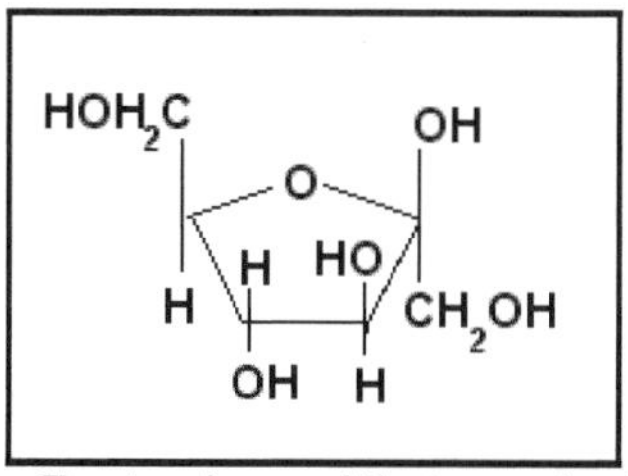

HOH2C
OH
O
H
HO
H
CH2OH
OH
H

Figure 21: Fructose. Fructose is one of the two major dietary monosaccharides.

Another monosaccharide, galactose, is quickly metabolized to glucose, and can be considered a glucose equivalent [188]. More complex sugars, known as *di*saccharides, consist of two monosaccharides attached end-to-end. The most important dietary disaccharide, known as sucrose, consists of one glucose molecule and one fructose molecule attached end-to-end.

CH2OH
H
C
O
H
HOH2C
OH
O
C
OH
H
C
H
HO
HO
C
C
α
O
β
CH2OH
H
OH
OH
H

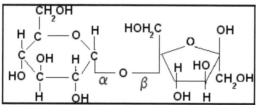

Figure 22: Sucrose. Sucrose, a dissacharide, consists of a glucose molecule and a fructose molecule attached end-to-end.

Other *di*saccharides include lactose (milk sugar) and maltose, both of which are quickly metabolized into two glucose molecules [188]. Therefore, all mono and disaccharides can be expressed as glucose or fructose equivalents.

Sugars Expressed as Glucose and Fructose Equivalents		
Monosaccharides	**Content**	**Equivalents**
Glucose	Glucose	1 Glucose
Fructose	Fructose	1 Fructose
Galactose	Glucose isomer	1 Glucose
Disaccharides		
Sucrose	Glucose-Fructose	1 Glucose+ 1 Fructose
Lactose	Glucose-Galactose	2 Glucose
Maltose	Glucose-Glucose	2 Glucose

Although glucose and fructose share many similar metabolic effects, they do have some important differences. For instance, glucose has a higher glycemic index and load than fructose, meaning that dietary glucose raises blood sugar (glucose) more than dietary fructose. However, fructose raises blood fats known as triglycerides more than glucose, and may be less satiating than glucose [206, 207]. Despite their differences, ultimately glucose and fructose appear to have similar effects on fat accumulation and insulin resistance, and excessive consumption of each is associated with increased risk of developing several of the Big 7 epidemic U.S. diseases [208-210]. For this reason, the NQI does not make a numerical distinction between them, and all sugars are grouped together.

Unrefined foods, including fruits, honey and some vegetables, naturally contain sugars. Throughout millions of years of human history, before processed foods became available, these natural foods were the only sources of sugars available for human consumption [18, 195]. Today, however, the major U.S. sources of sugars are processed foods including soft drinks, juices and other beverages, baked goods, snacks, jams, candies, yogurts, and ice creams [11].

Currently an estimated 18-19% of American calories, roughly 150 pounds per person each year, are supplied by highly concentrated *added* sugars in the form of high-fructose corn syrup (HFCS), sucrose, glucose, fruit juice concentrate, honey, and syrups [11, 211]. HFCS, a mixture of free fructose and glucose, alone accounts for over 40% of U.S. added sugar consumption, which works out to more than 70 pounds per American every year [206]! U.S. intake of HFCS, the major added sugar in sodas, sports drinks, and some juices, increased over 1000% between 1970-1990, and continues to climb [206]. Another estimated 7-8% of calories are supplied by *intrinsic* sugars *naturally* present in fruits, vegetables, and dairy products. Overall, sugars account for slightly more than one-quarter of all calories consumed in the U.S. [11].

U.S. Per Capita Sugar Intake (natural *and* added sugars)

Monosaccharide	Grams consumed/day	% caloric intake
Glucose	30	5.7
Fructose	31	5.9
Disaccharides		
Sucrose (glucose-fructose)	56	10.7
Lactose (glucose-galactose)	17	3.2
Maltose (glucose-glucose)	3	0.6
Total mono and disaccharides	137	26

[11, 27, 53, 204, 212, 213] Based on 2100 calorie diet.

Per Capita Daily Intake of Glucose and Fructose *Equivalents*

Equivalents	Grams per day	% caloric intake
Glucose	78	15
Fructose	59	11
Total sugar	137	26

[11, 27, 53, 204, 212, 213] Based on 2100 calorie diet.

Throughout the vast majority of human history, pre-agricultural humans consumed an estimated 30-40% of *total* caloric intake from non-fiber carbohydrates (NFCs), mostly from fiber-rich fruits, vegetables, and other plant-derived foods [175, 195, 214-216]. Based on this, many of our ancestors may have consumed between 15 and 20% of total calories from naturally present sugars. Thus, *total* sugar accounts for a far larger percentage of U.S. caloric intake than ever before in human history [18, 195].

Excessive sugar consumption contributes to cholesterol and insulin dysregulation and has been linked to obesity, diabetes, heart disease, and other epidemic U.S. diseases [217-219]. U.S. dietary guidelines uniformly recommend reduction of added sugars [2, 24].

STARCHES

Dietary starches, or *poly*saccharides, are essentially just large chains of glucose molecules attached end-to-end [188]. The simplest dietary starch molecule, amylose, consists of 500-20,000 glucose molecules with very few branches. The other major dietary starch, known as amylopectin, consists of up to one million glucose molecules, with a new branch every 20-30 molecules [188].

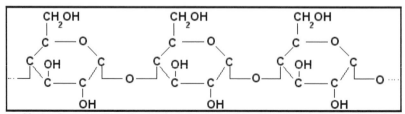

Figure 23: Amylose. Amylose, the simplest starch, consists of hundreds to thousands of glucose molecules, attached end-to-end, with few branches.

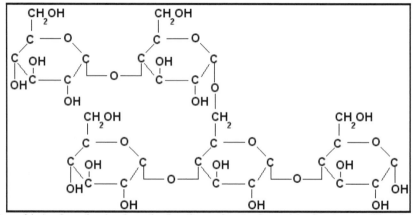

Figure 24: Amylopectin. Amylopectin, the other major starch, consists of up to one million glucose molecules, with more branches than amylose.

Starches are naturally abundant in whole-grain, unprocessed cereal grains including corn, wheat, and rice. They can be further concentrated through processing or refining, which removes most of the fiber, fatty acids, vitamins, and phytochemicals, leaving almost pure starch [220]. In fact, 85% of U.S. grain-products, already rich in starches, are highly refined before being sold as breads, cereals, crackers, corn chips, pretzels, and other snack foods [185]. Although potatoes are a naturally concentrated source of starch, most unprocessed vegetables, legumes, and nuts contain much lower concentrations.

Highly concentrated *refined* starches account for approximately 20% of total U.S. caloric intake [18]. Less concentrated sources of starch, including potatoes, unrefined whole grains, and certain vegetables provide another 4-5% of caloric intake. Together, starches supply an average of 122 glucose equivalents per day, or slightly less than one quarter of all calories consumed in the U.S. [11].

Glucose and Fructose Equivalents Consumed from Sugars _and_ Starches (NFCs)

	Grams (g) per day 2100 kcal diet	% caloric intake
Glucose equivalents from sugars	78	15
Glucose equivalents from starches	122	23
Total Glucose equivalents	200	38
Total Fructose equivalents	59	11
NFC total	259	49

Calculation of glucose equivalents = [Glucose+Amylose+Amylopectin+Galactose+½(Sucrose and HFCS)]
Calculation of fructose equivalents = [Fructose+½(Sucrose and HFCS)]   [11, 27, 53, 204, 212, 213]

Throughout the vast majority of human evolution, our ancestors consumed fewer _total_ non-fiber carbohydrates, which accounted for an estimated 30-40% of total caloric intake, mostly from fiber-rich fruits, vegetables, nuts, and other plant-derived foods [175, 195, 214, 215]. These natural foods contain much lower concentrations of starches (and higher concentrations of fiber) than refined carbohydrates and even whole grain cereals. Beginning with the Agricultural Revolution 10,000 years ago, many populations began consuming larger amounts of unprocessed "whole" grains with higher starch to fiber ratios than the fruits, nuts, and vegetables historically consumed [18]. Since the Industrial Revolution 100-150 years ago, widespread refining of cereal grains has radically increased the concentration of starches and further reduced the fiber which naturally accompanies these starches [18, 196].

In the past, U.S. guidelines differentiated between "simple sugars" and "complex carbohydrates" (starches), based solely on carbohydrate chain length [196, 221]. Expert bodies, who assumed that sugars are more rapidly digested and absorbed in the small intestine than starches, recommended Americans increase "complex carbohydrate" intake at the expense of simple sugars [222]. However, metabolic studies suggest that *pure* starches, which are quickly digested to and absorbed as glucose, have virtually the same glycemic and insulin responses as glucose when given in the same amounts [191-193].

Excessive consumption of pure starches, like sugars, reduces HDL or "good cholesterol," raises triglycerides (VLDL), promotes inflammation (CRP) and oxidative stress, and favors insulin resistance and weight gain [223-229]. Studies demonstrating similar or equivalent metabolic and health effects of consuming purified starches and sugars question the rationale of grouping carbohydrates based on chain lengths, and suggest that a functional classification of fiber and non-fiber carbohydrates may be more appropriate [196, 219, 226, 229, 230].

The distinct effects of foods containing sugars and starches are primarily due to accompanying fiber, protein, fats, minerals, and phytochemicals [219, 220, 231]. For this reason, the NQI weighs sugars and *pure* starch molecules equally and groups all sugars and starches into the single category of "non-fiber carbohydrates" (NFCs). Thus, grain-based food items rate higher than sugars solely based on accompanying protein, fiber, fatty acids, minerals, and antioxidants.

HISTORICAL PERSPECTIVE

Fibers and non-fiber carbohydrates have opposite effects on several key metabolic processes, and balanced intake is a crucial component of a healthy diet. The fruits, vegetables, and nuts consumed by our ancestors for over 99% of human evolution, even when combined with a small amount of seasonal honey, naturally provided *at least* one gram of fiber for every four grams of non-fiber carbohydrates [18, 28]. The switch to cereal grains in the last 5-10,000 years boosted the non-fiber carbohydrates to dietary fiber ratio to approximately 5 to 1. Today, however, massive consumption of added sugars and refining of cereal grains has distorted this important ratio to more than 16 to 1 with disastrous metabolic consequences! This radical shift plays a major role in the current explosion of obesity, diabetes, heart disease, and other U.S. epidemic diseases.

Historical Human NFC to Fiber Ratio

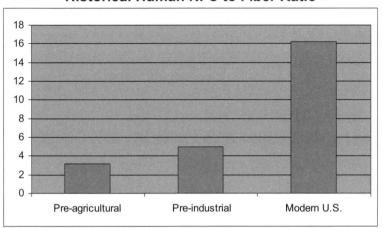

Cumulative Per Capita U.S. Carbohydrate Intake

	Grams (g) per day 2100 kcal diet	% caloric intake
Glucose equivalents	200	38
Fructose equivalents	59	11
Total NFC	259	49
Soluble fiber	5.5	1
Insoluble fiber	10.5	0
Total Fiber	16	1
Total Carbohydrate	275	>50
NFC:Fiber ratio	259:16 = 16:1	

[11, 27, 53, 204, 212, 213]

NQI Analysis: As a reflection of the role of the NFC to fiber ratio in health and disease, the NQI rates NFCs as modestly negative, and fibers as moderately positive.

PROTEINS

Proteins are a group of complex molecules consisting of amino acids attached by peptide bonds.

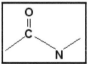

Figure 25: Peptide bond. Proteins consist of amino acids attached by nitrogen (-N) containing peptide bonds.

Twenty distinct dietary amino acid building blocks are relevant to the makeup of human proteins, nine of which are considered "essential," meaning they must be consumed in the diet for proper function [232]. The remaining eleven "non-essential" amino acids can be synthesized by the human body and are not required in the diet.

Essential and Non-Essential Amino acids

Essential	Non-Essential
Histidine	Alanine
Isoleucine	Arginine*
Leucine	Asparagine
Lysine	Aspartate
Methionine	Cysteine
Phenylalanine	Glutamate
Threonine	Glutamine
Tryptophan	Glycine
Valine	Proline
	Serine
	Tyrosine

[232] *Additional arginine must be obtained by growing children.

The unique amino acid sequences of proteins determine their diverse three-dimensional structures and functions [232]. Examples of important proteins include hemoglobin, which delivers oxygen to tissues, collagen, which provides structural integrity to tissue, and HMG-CoA reductase, an enzyme which synthesizes cholesterol. In addition, amino acids serve as precursors for the neurotransmitters serotonin, norepinephrine, and dopamine which regulate mood, pain, and a variety of other important metabolic processes [233]. Although interesting, the potential roles of specific dietary amino acids in human health and disease is beyond the scope of this book. Instead, the NQI will focus on the health consequences of consuming proteins as a whole.

The primary U.S. sources of protein include poultry, red meats, dairy, eggs, fish, shellfish, nuts, and beans [11]. Total protein, from both plant and animal sources, currently accounts for 16% of U.S. caloric intake, roughly half of the estimated 30% caloric intake throughout the last 50,000 years of human evolution [17, 175, 177, 195, 204]

Average U.S. Protein Intake

Protein Source	Grams/day	% Caloric intake
Animal protein	60	11.5
Vegetable protein	24	4.5
Total	84	16

[11, 18, 27, 53, 204]

In the late 1970s, after studies suggested a link between animal protein and cardiovascular disease, U.S. health promotion agencies advocated limiting protein to around 15% of caloric intake [234, 235]. However, modern American animal protein sources have radically different fat concentrations than those consumed throughout human history. For example, domesticated, grain-fed cattle contain two to four times as much saturated fat as their wild or grass-fed counterparts [17, 195]. More recent studies which accounted for this difference, suggest that saturated fat, rather than the animal protein itself, was primarily responsible for the association with cardiovascular disease [236]. When considered independently of saturated fat, both animal protein and vegetable protein have several beneficial metabolic effects, and may moderately reduce the risk of heart disease, diabetes, obesity, and other epidemic U.S. diseases [17, 231, 237-240]. More recently, a large U.S. study failed to reveal any safety concerns of high protein diets [241]. Current USDA guidelines advocate that protein should account for 10-35% of total calories, suggesting that a wide range of protein can be consumed as part of a healthy diet.

Unlike fats and carbohydrates, evidence that specific subsets of protein have distinct effects on health is lacking. Instead, both animal and vegetable proteins appear to have similar, but modest, health benefits [236]. Thus, when selecting high-protein food items, it is most important to consider the quality of accompanying fats, carbohydrates, other nutrients, and toxins.

NQI Analysis: The NQI rates all protein as modestly positive.

SODIUM (and OTHER MINERALS)

Sodium, a mineral supplied in the diet, serves a variety of important functions in the human body. The term "salt" refers to the combination of two minerals, sodium and chloride. Sodium accounts for about 40% of the *total* weight of salt, and chloride accounts for the other 60%.

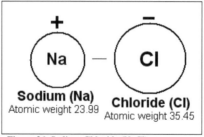

Figure 26: Sodium Chloride (NaCl).

Americans consume an average of about 3600 to 4000 mg of sodium per day [14, 27, 53]. Salt added to processed foods accounts for 75% of this sodium, with another 15% added during cooking or at the table [242]. Thus, sodium naturally present in foods is responsible for only 10% of sodium intake [243]! Throughout over 99% of human history, before the widespread availability of processed foods, humans consumed 500 to 800 mg per day of sodium from natural foods [244, 245]. *Thus, modern Americans consume at least five times as much sodium as our ancestors!*

U.S. health promotion agencies including the USDA and American Heart Association recommend consumption of less than 2300 mg of sodium per day, and less than 1500 mg/day for individuals with high blood pressure, African Americans, and anyone middle aged or older [2, 24].

Multiple studies have established the connection between excessive sodium consumption and elevated blood pressure, and high salt intake is a major contributor to hypertension, an epidemic affecting over a third of U.S. adults [246-248]. Not surprisingly given the link between high blood pressure and cardiovascular disease, a prospective experimental study demonstrated that high sodium intake predisposes to heart attack, stroke, and higher overall mortality [249, 250]. However, the fact that epidemiological studies have shown inconsistent or even opposite results, has motivated some experts to question the rationale of sodium restriction guidelines [251]. Emerging research suggests that excessive sodium intake is only part of the story, and that balanced intake of several other minerals may be a key to healthy blood pressure.

MINERAL BALANCE

Potassium, magnesium, and calcium have anti-hypertensive effects which counteract the hypertensive effects of sodium [244, 252-255]. Increased dietary intake of these three minerals lowers blood pressure significantly more than sodium restriction alone. Because processed foods contain only a small fraction of the potassium, magnesium, and calcium as their natural counterparts, modern Americans consume only a tiny fraction of the historical and current recommended intakes of these minerals [244, 245].

Mineral Imbalance in the U.S.

Mineral	% of Historical Intake
Sodium	500%
Potassium	25%
Magnesium	25%
Calcium	55%

[244, 245]

In light of the many complex interactions between these four minerals in human biochemical processes, optimal effects can be expected to occur with balanced intake similar to that consumed in a natural diet. Increased intake of potassium, magnesium, and calcium, alongside sodium restriction, can significantly reduce blood pressure. In addition, a more balanced intake of these minerals may reduce the risk of osteoporosis and a variety of other diseases [244].

Modified salts, which replace some of the sodium with potassium and magnesium, are available to season foods and have been shown to reduce blood pressure [256]. However, because processed foods account for 75% of U.S. sodium intake, the only way to effectively reduce intake is to choose more foods in their natural, unprocessed state. A combination of using a modified table salt and eating more natural foods has the potential to reduce blood pressure towards more natural levels and reduce the risk of cardiovascular and other diseases.

NQI Analysis: Currently potassium and magnesium are not listed on Nutrition Facts labels. Thus, for consistency, the NQI in its current form rates only sodium, which is assigned a moderately negative rating. Foods with high concentrations of beneficial potassium, calcium, and magnesium, receive a modest positive adjustment.

ANTIOXIDANTS

Antioxidants are a diverse group of molecules grouped together because they neutralize oxygen-derived free radicals, thereby preventing tissue damage [257, 258]. In addition, some antioxidants have potent effects on inflammation, blood coagulation, cell growth, and other important metabolic processes [259-261]. Antioxidants can be classified according to solubility: hydro*philic* antioxidants, such as vitamin C, are water soluble and hydro*phobic* antioxidants, including vitamin E, are fat soluble.

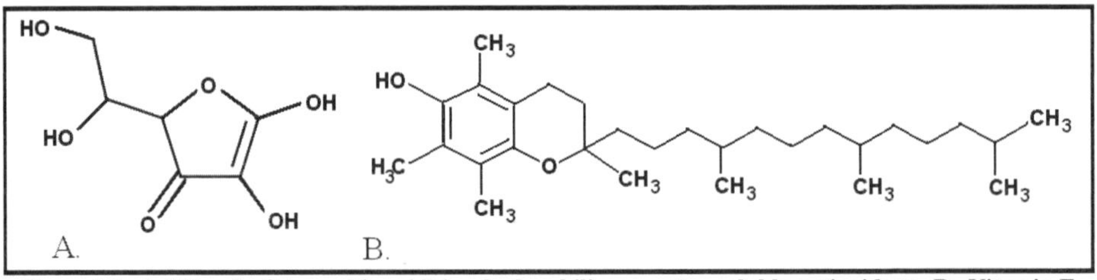

Figure 27: A. Vitamin C (ascorbic acid) is a hydrophilic, or water-soluble antioxidant. B. Vitamin E (tocopherol) is a hydrophobic, or fat-soluble antioxidant.

Although vitamins C, E, and other vitamin antioxidants traditionally receive much of the attention, non-vitamin molecules known as polyphenolic antioxidants may have even more potent biological and health effects [262-264]. *Poly*phenolic antioxidants, also known as flavonoids, are compounds with multiple phenol groups.

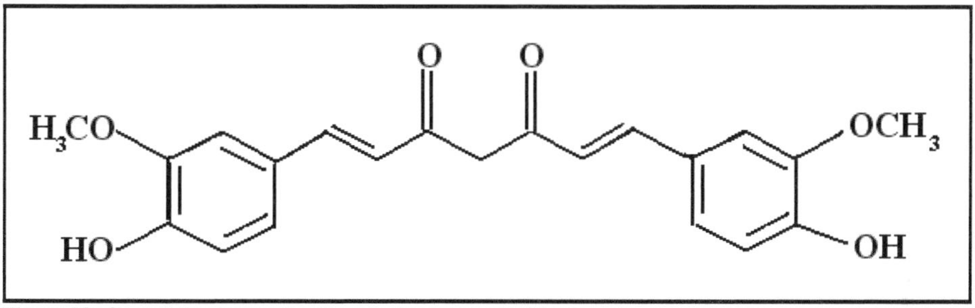

Figure 28: Curcumin. Example of a polyphenolic antioxidant.

Classes of polyphenolic antioxidants include anthocyanidins, catechins, flavonols, flavones, flavanones, and isoflavones [265]. Each of these can be further classified into individual molecules based on their precise molecular makeup [266]. Concentrated sources of antioxidants in the U.S. food supply include fruits and vegetables, spices, extra virgin olive oil, nuts, whole grains, dark chocolate, teas, red wines, and ales [220, 259, 262-264, 267].

Total antioxidant intake is difficult to quantify and appears to vary markedly amongst different populations [268]. *Average* U.S. *total* polyphenolic antioxidant intake may fall somewhere between 400 mg to over one gram per day, with wide variations depending on individual dietary practices [269, 270]. A recent study estimated that Americans, on average, consume over 420 mg of polyphenolic antioxidants per day from fruits and vegetables alone [263].

Compared to plant-based foods in their natural forms, refined foods preserve only a tiny fraction of antioxidants. For example, nearly all the antioxidant content of whole grains is found in the bran and germ, components generally removed during processing [220].

Therefore, refined grains provide only a tiny fraction of the antioxidants naturally present in unprocessed whole grains [185, 220]. Historically, humans consumed much larger quantities of antioxidants, reflecting higher intake of fruits, vegetables, nuts, whole grains, and other unprocessed plant-based foods [18, 214].

As the beneficial metabolic and health promoting properties of polyphenolic and other antioxidants have become more recognized, U.S. and international health promotion agencies have begun stressing the importance of high intake of antioxidant-rich plant-based foods and beverages [24]. However, aside from a select few antioxidant vitamins, namely vitamin C, vitamin E, and beta-carotene, no specific guidelines have been made for antioxidant intake. Although studies have shown that individuals with higher *blood* levels of antioxidants have a lower risk for many of the Big 7 epidemic U.S. diseases, supplementation of high doses of one or a few antioxidant vitamins has failed to show benefit, and in some cases may actually increase the risk of disease [271-273]. Rather than simply taking mega-doses of single antioxidants in pill form, it appears that optimization of a complex antioxidant network is required to get the most benefit from antioxidant intake [257, 273]. This can best be accomplished through *habitual* consumption of foods and beverages rich in a wide *variety* of antioxidants, as discussed in detail in Part 3: Diet and Oxidative Stress, pages 151-158.

NQI Analysis: The NQI rates total antioxidants as modestly to moderately positive.

TOXINS

The modern U.S. food supply contains several established toxins and thousands of other *potential* toxins. Established toxins in uncooked foods include mercury and polychlorinated biphenyls (PCBs), both of which are concentrated in certain fish sources, and nitrates (converted to nitrosamines) which are present in processed meats. Other established toxins, including heterocyclic amines (HCAs), are introduced by cooking (essentially burning) meats at high temperatures [274]. A variety of other *potential* toxins include pesticides and fertilizers used to improve crop yields, and artificial colors, flavors, sweeteners, and other food additives used in food processing, as well as various chemicals used in cookware and food packaging.

The NQI focuses on two of the more established toxins, mercury and PCBs, because reasonably reliable data is available in which to base fish recommendations. Nitrates, which have been linked to various cancers, will also be taken into consideration. However, because the amounts of cancer-causing HCAs are dependent upon cooking method and temperature rather than inherent properties of foods, they will not be included in the NQI ratings for overall quality of food items. Steps which can be taken to reduce HCA exposure will be briefly discussed. While it is probable that *some* of the more than 40,000 chemicals entering the U.S. food supply from pesticides, fertilizers, food additives, and packaging may have toxic effects, there is not enough information available to quantify their presence, nor enough evidence of specific adverse consequences to include them in the NQI rating system [275].

MERCURY

Although a small amount of mercury is *naturally* present in the environment, the chief source is industrial pollution [276, 277]. Bacteria present in water sources convert mercury to highly toxic, fat-soluble methylmercury, which accumulates in certain fish species, especially large, fatty fish at the top of the food chain. Methylmercury is especially toxic to the developing human brain, and exposure should be limited by pregnant women and young children [278]. In addition, mercury appears to have adverse effects on the cardiovascular system, and may partially negate some of the beneficial effects of ω-3 fatty acids [279]. Fish and shellfish contain highly variable amounts of methylmercury, ranging from essentially zero to potentially dangerous amounts. Given the vast and growing evidence that consumption of long chain ω-3 fatty acids EPA and DHA have a variety of beneficial effects on the heart, brain, joints, eyes, and mood, it is important for consumers to identify and select fish and shellfish rich in ω-3 fatty acids with little or no mercury [42, 127-131, 134, 135, 137, 280-282].

Mercury in U.S. Fish and Shellfish in Parts Per Million (ppm)

Fish	Mercury (ppm)	Fish	Mercury (ppm)
Tilefish (Gulf of Mexico)	**1.45**	Flounder	0.09
Swordfish	**1.31**	Cod	0.08
Shark	**0.99**	Whitefish	0.07
Mackerel (King)	**0.73**	Mackerel (Atl/Pacific)	0.07
Tuna (Big eye)	**0.62**	Mussels	0.07
Grouper	**0.55**	Squid/calamari	0.07
Orange roughy	**0.54**	Crab	0.06
Marlin	**0.49**	Scallop	0.05
Chilean sea bass	**0.38**	Catfish	0.05
Tuna (Canned Albacore)	**0.38**	Anchovies	0.04
Bluefish	**0.35**	Crawfish/crayfish	0.04
Tuna (Yellowfin)	0.34	Herring	0.04
Lobster (Atlantic-Maine)	0.31	Haddock	0.03
Halibut	0.23	Octopus	0.03
Red snapper	0.19	Sardine	0.02
Tilefish (Atlantic)	0.15	Perch (Ocean)	0.01
Carp	0.14	Tilapia	0.01
Perch (Freshwater)	0.14	Salmon	0.01
Tuna (Canned Light)	0.12	Clam	0.01
Freshwater trout	0.11	Oysters	0.01
Spiny (Rock) Lobster Warm water	0.09	Shrimp	0.01

[283-286]

Prior to the Industrial Revolution, humans were only exposed to the comparatively small amounts of mercury naturally present in the environment. As a result of industrial pollution, modern Americans are exposed to far higher amounts of mercury [276, 277].

The FDA provides warnings about fish with mercury concentrations of 0.35 parts per million (ppm) or higher. However, the legal limit for mercury levels in fish sold in the United States is 1.0 ppm, twice as high as the legal limit in Canada. The EPA specifies that pregnant women and children should eat *no more* than 12 ounces of *low* mercury fish per week, and that shark, swordfish, king mackerel, and tilefish should be avoided [287]. Guidelines to limit fish intake may explain the reduction of blood mercury levels in women of childbearing age in recent years [288]. However, given the crucial role of ω-3 DHA in the developing brain and retina and widespread U.S. DHA deficiency, suggestions to limit fish intake may have negative consequences [289-291]. By identifying fish with the highest concentrations of ω-3 DHA and lowest mercury and PCBs, the NQI can help solve this problem.

NQI Analysis: The NQI rates mercury as strongly negative.

POLYCHLORINATED BIPHENYLS (PCBs)

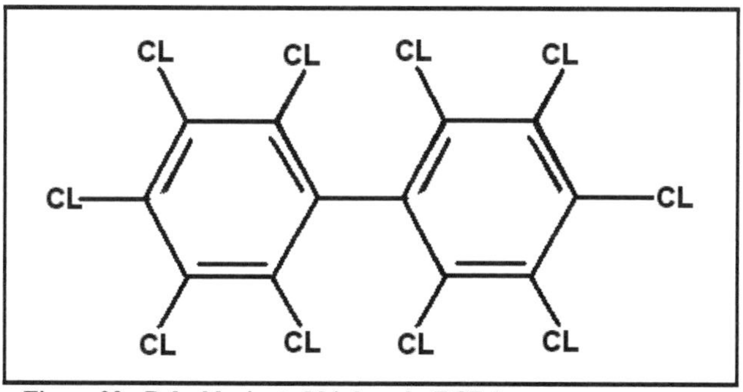

Figure 29: Polychlorinated biphenyls (PCBs).

Polychlorinated biphenyls (PCBs) are unnatural chlorinated byproducts of industrialization [292]. Although the manufacturing of PCBs was banned by the United States in 1977, PCBs are still found throughout the environment in soil, water, and contaminated food sources. Like methylmercury, fat-soluble PCBs accumulate in animals at the top of the food chain, especially certain fatty fish. After human consumption, PCBs accumulate in the liver, skin, fat, and breast milk. Exposure to PCBs has been linked to several cancers, prediabetes and diabetes mellitus, decreased immunity, impaired learning and memory, and a host of other adverse effects [293-295]. Children appear especially susceptible to PCB induced neurotoxicity, highlighting the importance of limiting exposure during pregnancy and childhood [292, 296, 297].

Dietary intake is the main source of exposure to PCBs, and concentrations vary widely across and within food groups. Although the highest concentrations of dietary PCBs are found in farm-raised fish, Americans may actually be exposed to more PCBs from cattle and dairy products, reflecting much higher overall U.S. intake of beef and dairy than fish [102, 298]. Farm-raised salmon appear to be the most concentrated source of PCBs in the U.S. food supply, with some samples exceeding the EPA's health-based limits for weekly consumption [299, 300]. In contrast, wild-caught salmon have a much lower concentration of PCBs than most farm-raised sources [102].

Because PCBs do not occur naturally and all PCB exposure is a result of industrial pollution, our ancestors were not exposed to *any* amount of PCBs. Fortunately, dietary intake has declined dramatically since PCBs were effectively banned in the late 1970s [301]. The federal government has set an upper limit for 0.2-3 ppm of PCBs for fish, dairy, poultry, and red meat [301].

NQI Analysis: The NQI rates PCBs as moderately negative.

NITRATES/NITRITES

The consumption of processed meats is associated with increased risk of certain cancers [302]. Compounds present in hot dogs, bacon, sausages, salami and hams known as nitrates/nitrites, which are converted to carcinogenic nitrosamines, may be responsible for this association [302, 303].

NQI Analysis: The NQI makes a modest negative adjustment to food items containing nitrates/nitrites.

HETEROCYCLIC AMINES

Heterocyclic amines (HCAs) are a group of compounds formed in meats cooked at high temperatures, especially during grilling, pan frying, and deep frying [274]. Individuals consume widely variable amounts of HCAs: those who regularly pan-fry or grill meats may consume more than twenty times as much as those who cook via other methods [274]. Dietary exposure to HCAs *may* account for an estimated 28,000 cases of breast, colon, and other U.S. cancers each year [304, 305]. Because the concentration of HCAs increases with "doneness," meats should be cooked at moderate temperatures and not overcooked or charred [306].

ARTIFICIAL SWEETENERS

As the epidemic of overweight and obesity has accelerated over the past several decades, U.S. consumers have increased consumption of low and no-calorie artificial sweeteners in the hopes of losing weight [307]. Popular artificial sweeteners include aspartame, acesulfame, saccharin, and sucralose. Despite studies suggesting that *long-term* consumption of reasonable doses of the older sweeteners aspartame and saccharin are safe for most people, questions persist about the increased risk of certain cancers seen in animal studies [210, 308]. Long-term effects of human consumption of newer sweeteners, such as sucralose, are largely unknown [309]. Perhaps more importantly, the role of low-calorie, artificially sweetened foods in weight loss has recently come into question. For instance, in the San Antonio Heart Study, consumption of artificially sweetened "diet" beverages paradoxically predicted future weight gain even more than regular soda consumption [310]! Later analysis demonstrated a dose-response association between artificial sweetener intake and weight gain (Fowler, S. personal communication 2007). Similarly, in the Framimgton Heart Study, long-term consumption of diet soft drinks was closely associated with a variety of metabolic abnormalities, weight gain, and obesity [311]. While the mechanism responsible for this long-term weight gain is poorly understood and controversial, animal studies suggest that artificial sweeteners may contribute to weight gain via appetite dysregulation, later overeating, and increased *future* caloric intake [312, 313].

NQI Analysis: This association, coupled with the lack of any established health benefits, suggests that consumers may benefit from restricting intake of artificial sweeteners. The NQI automatically assigns a modestly negative rating to all foods and beverages containing artificial sweeteners.

DEFINING THE "STANDARD" AMERICAN DIET

Various surveys and collection data have allowed for the description and statistical characterization of the average U.S. dietary intakes of macronutrients. Because dietary intakes vary to some extent by region, culture, educational level, and personal preference, there is no "standard American diet." *However, Americans share many key dietary features.* Analysis of the molecular and health consequences of these common features strongly suggests that the "American diet" is a major driving force behind the Big 7 U.S. epidemic diseases.

Per Capita U.S. Daily Macronutrient Intake: The "Standard American Diet"

Macronutrient	Molecular name(s)	Grams(g)	Calories	%Calories
Total	Fats, Carbohydrates, Protein	437 g	2100	100%
Total Fat		78.3 g	705	33.6%
Total Saturated Fats		27.1 g	244	11.6%
18:0	Stearic	7.0 g	63	3.0%
16:0	Palmitic	15.0 g	135	6.4%
14:0	Myristic	2.3 g	20.7	1.0%
12:0	Lauric	0.9 g	8.1	0.4%
10:0-4:0	Capric, Caprylic, Caproic, Butyric	1.9 g	17.1	0.8%
Total Monounsaturated		30.4 g	273.6	13.0%
18:1	Oleic	28.5 g	12.2	12.2%
16:1	Palmitoleic* (and other)	1.9 g	17.1	0.8%
Total Polyunsaturated		16.7 g	150.3	7.2%
Total ω-6				6.55%
20:4 ω-6	ω-6 Arachidonate (ArA)	250 mg	2.25	0.11%
18:2 ω-6	ω-6 Linoleate (LA)	15.0 g	135	6.4%
Total ω-3				0.6%
22:6 ω-3	ω-3 Docosahexaenoate (DHA)	75 mg	0.68	0.03%
20:5 ω-3	ω-3 Eicosapentaenoate (EPA)	45 mg	0.41	0.02%
18:3 ω-3	ω-3 Alpha-linolenic (ALA)	1.35 g	12.2	0.58%
Total Trans Fats		4.1 g	36.9	1.8%
t18:1, t16:1	Trans Oleic (Elaidic) + Trans Palmitoleic	3.5 g	31.5	1.5%
t18:2	Trans Linoleic	0.6 g	5.4	0.3%
Cholesterol		290 mg	0	<<<1%
Total Carbohydrates		275 g	1059	50.4%
Non-fiber Carbohydrates	Sugars + Starches	259 g	1036	49.3%
Total Sugars	Glucose, Fructose, Sucrose, Lactose, Maltose	137 g	548	26.1%
Total Starches	Amylose + Amylopectin	122 g	488	23.2%
Total Fibers		16 g	22	1.0%
Soluble		5.5 g	22	1.0%
Insoluble		10.5 g	0	0%
Total Protein		84 g	336	16.0%

[11-14, 18, 25-27, 53, 108, 159, 185, 212, 213] Other references throughout text. Based on 2100 calorie diet. Not including alcohol consumption which accounts for up to 3% of caloric intake.
*Palmitoleic includes 0.1% of calories from 20:1 and 22:1.

References

1. *Questions and Answers about Trans Fat Nutrition Labeling. U.S. Food and Drug Administration.* . CFSAN Office of Nutritional Products, Labeling and Dietary Supplements 2003, July 9 [cited 2006 September 15]; Available from: http://www.cfsan.fda.gov/~dms/qatrans2.html.
2. 2005, D.o.A. *Dietary Guidelines Advisory Committee. Nutrition and your health: dietary guidelines for Americans.* Dietary Guidelines Advisory Committee report [cited 2006 July 15]; Available from: http://health.gov/dietaryguidelines/dga2005/report/.
3. Madsen, L., R.K. Petersen, and K. Kristiansen, *Regulation of adipocyte differentiation and function by polyunsaturated fatty acids.* Biochim Biophys Acta, 2005. **1740**(2): p. 266-86.
4. Howard, B.V., et al., *Low-fat dietary pattern and risk of cardiovascular disease: the Women's Health Initiative Randomized Controlled Dietary Modification Trial.* Jama, 2006. **295**(6): p. 655-66.
5. Khor, G.L., *Dietary fat quality: a nutritional epidemiologist's view.* Asia Pac J Clin Nutr, 2004. **13**(Suppl): p. S22.
6. de Lorgeril, M. and P. Salen, *The Mediterranean diet in secondary prevention of coronary heart disease.* Clin Invest Med, 2006. **29**(3): p. 154-8.
7. Hu, F.B., J.E. Manson, and W.C. Willett, *Types of dietary fat and risk of coronary heart disease: a critical review.* J Am Coll Nutr, 2001. **20**(1): p. 5-19.
8. Ludwig, D.S., *Symposium 2: Nutrition and Chronic Disease. Diet and development of the insulin resustence syndrome.* Proceedings of the Nutrition Society of Australia, 2003. **27**: p. S4.
9. Ascherio, A., *Epidemiologic studies on dietary fats and coronary heart disease.* Am J Med, 2002. **113 Suppl 9B**: p. 9S-12S.
10. *Dietary Fat-how much? What type? Consensus Statement from the Scientific Exchange.* Nutrition Today, 1998. **33-34**(173).
11. Gerrior, S., Bente, L, & Hiza, H, *Nutrient Content of the U.S. Food Supply, 1909-2000 (Home Economics Research Report No. 56).* 2004, U.S. Department of Agriculture, Center for Nutrition Policy and Promotion.
12. Briefel, R.R. and C.L. Johnson, *Secular trends in dietary intake in the United States.* Annu Rev Nutr, 2004. **24**: p. 401-31.
13. Allison, D.B., et al., *Estimated intakes of trans fatty and other fatty acids in the US population.* J Am Diet Assoc, 1999. **99**(2): p. 166-74; quiz 175-6.
14. Ahuja, J., J. Exler & N. Raper. *Data Tables: Individual Fatty Acid Intakes: Results from 1995 Continuing Survey of food Intakes by Individuals.* ARS Food Surveys Research Group. 1997 [cited 2006 July 14]; Available from: http://www.barc.usda.gov/bhnrc/foodsurvey/home.htm.
15. Eaton, S.B., *Humans, lipids and evolution.* Lipids, 1992. **27**(10): p. 814-20.
16. Sinclair, A.J., et al., *Effects on plasma lipids and fatty acid composition of very low fat diets enriched with fish or kangaroo meat.* Lipids, 1987. **22**(7): p. 523-9.
17. Mann, N., *Dietary lean red meat and human evolution.* Eur J Nutr, 2000. **39**(2): p. 71-9.
18. Cordain, L., et al., *Origins and evolution of the Western diet: health implications for the 21st century.* Am J Clin Nutr, 2005. **81**(2): p. 341-54.
19. Mensink, R.P., et al., *Effects of dietary fatty acids and carbohydrates on the ratio of serum total to HDL cholesterol and on serum lipids and apolipoproteins: a meta-analysis of 60 controlled trials.* Am J Clin Nutr, 2003. **77**(5): p. 1146-55.
20. Das, U.N., *A defect in the activity of Delta6 and Delta5 desaturases may be a factor predisposing to the development of insulin resistance syndrome.* Prostaglandins Leukot Essent Fatty Acids, 2005. **72**(5): p. 343-50.
21. Yu, S., et al., *Plasma cholesterol-predictive equations demonstrate that stearic acid is neutral and monounsaturated fatty acids are hypocholesterolemic.* Am J Clin Nutr, 1995. **61**(5): p. 1129-39.
22. Renaud, S.C., *What is the epidemiologic evidence for the thrombogenic potential of dietary long-chain fatty acids?* Am J Clin Nutr, 1992. **56**(4 Suppl): p. 823S-824S.
23. Keys, A., *Seven Countries: a multivariate analysis of death and coronary heart disease.*, Cambridge, Mass: Harvard University Press, 1980.
24. Lichtenstein, A.H., et al., *Diet and lifestyle recommendations revision 2006: a scientific statement from the American Heart Association Nutrition Committee.* Circulation, 2006. **114**(1): p. 82-96.
25. Ganji, V. and N. Betts, *Fat, cholesterol, fiber and sodium intakes of US population: evaluation of diets reported in 1987-88 Nationwide Food Consumption Survey.* Eur J Clin Nutr, 1995. **49**(12): p. 915-20.
26. Troiano, R.P., et al., *Energy and fat intakes of children and adolescents in the united states: data from the national health and nutrition examination surveys.* Am J Clin Nutr, 2000. **72**(5 Suppl): p. 1343S-1353S.
27. Bialostosky, K.e., *Dietary intake of macronutrients, micronutrients, and other dietary constituents:United States 1988-94.* National Center for Health Statistics. Vital Health Stat, 2002. **11**(245).
28. U.S. Department of Agriculture, A.R.S. *USDA Nutrient Database for Standard Reference. Release 18, Nutrient Data Laboratory Home Page.* [cited Jan 1, 2006 Available from: http://www.nal.usda.gov/fnic/foodcomp
29. Hu, X., et al., *Mapping of the loci controlling oleic and linolenic acid contents and development of fad2 and fad3 allele-specific markers in canola (Brassica napus L.).* Theor Appl Genet, 2006. **113**(3): p. 497-507.
30. Cordain, L., et al., *The paradoxical nature of hunter-gatherer diets: meat-based, yet non-atherogenic.* Eur J Clin Nutr, 2002. **56 Suppl 1**: p. S42-52.
31. Cordain, L., et al., *Fatty acid analysis of wild ruminant tissues: evolutionary implications for reducing diet-related chronic disease.* Eur J Clin Nutr, 2002. **56**(3): p. 181-91.
32. Eaton, S.B., et al., *Dietary intake of long-chain polyunsaturated fatty acids during the paleolithic.* World Rev Nutr Diet, 1998. **83**: p. 12-23.
33. Dannenberger, D., et al., *Effect of diet on the deposition of n-3 fatty acids, conjugated linoleic and C18:1trans fatty acid isomers in muscle lipids of German Holstein bulls.* J Agric Food Chem, 2004. **52**(21): p. 6607-15.

34.   Brynes, A.E., et al., *A randomised four-intervention crossover study investigating the effect of carbohydrates on daytime profiles of insulin, glucose, non-esterified fatty acids and triacylglycerols in middle-aged men.* Br J Nutr, 2003. **89**(2): p. 207-18.
35.   Heilbronn, L.K., M. Noakes, and P.M. Clifton, *Effect of energy restriction, weight loss, and diet composition on plasma lipids and glucose in patients with type 2 diabetes.* Diabetes Care, 1999. **22**(6): p. 889-95.
36.   *Third Report of the National Cholesterol Education Program (NCEP) Expert Panel on Detection, Evaluation, and Treatment of High Blood Cholesterol in Adults (Adult Treatment Panel III) final report.* Circulation, 2002. **106**(25): p. 3143-421.
37.   Hussein, N., et al., *Long-chain conversion of [13C]linoleic acid and alpha-linolenic acid in response to marked changes in their dietary intake in men.* J Lipid Res, 2005. **46**(2): p. 269-80.
38.   Goyens, P.L., et al., *Conversion of alpha-linolenic acid in humans is influenced by the absolute amounts of alpha-linolenic acid and linoleic acid in the diet and not by their ratio.* Am J Clin Nutr, 2006. **84**(1): p. 44-53.
39.   Schwab, U.S., et al., *Effects of hempseed and flaxseed oils on the profile of serum lipids, serum total and lipoprotein lipid concentrations and haemostatic factors.* Eur J Nutr, 2006. **45**(8): p. 470-7.
40.   Emken, E.A., et al., *Effect of dietary docosahexaenoic acid on desaturation and uptake in vivo of isotope-labeled oleic, linoleic, and linolenic acids by male subjects.* Lipids, 1999. **34**(8): p. 785-91.
41.   Okuyama, H., T. Kobayashi, and S. Watanabe, *Dietary fatty acids--the N-6/N-3 balance and chronic elderly diseases. Excess linoleic acid and relative N-3 deficiency syndrome seen in Japan.* Prog Lipid Res, 1996. **35**(4): p. 409-57.
42.   Ailhaud, G., et al., *Temporal changes in dietary fats: role of n-6 polyunsaturated fatty acids in excessive adipose tissue development and relationship to obesity.* Prog Lipid Res, 2006. **45**(3): p. 203-36.
43.   Simopoulos, A.P., *Evolutionary aspects of diet, the omega-6/omega-3 ratio and genetic variation: nutritional implications for chronic diseases.* Biomed Pharmacother, 2006. **60**(9): p. 502-7.
44.   Simopoulos, A.P., *The importance of the ratio of omega-6/omega-3 essential fatty acids.* Biomed Pharmacother, 2002. **56**(8): p. 365-79.
45.   de Lorgeril, M., et al., *Mediterranean diet, traditional risk factors, and the rate of cardiovascular complications after myocardial infarction: final report of the Lyon Diet Heart Study.* Circulation, 1999. **99**(6): p. 779-85.
46.   de Lorgeril, M., et al., *Mediterranean dietary pattern in a randomized trial: prolonged survival and possible reduced cancer rate.* Arch Intern Med, 1998. **158**(11): p. 1181-7.
47.   de Lorgeril, M. and P. Salen, *Modified cretan mediterranean diet in the prevention of coronary heart disease and cancer: an update.* World Rev Nutr Diet, 2007. **97**: p. 1-32.
48.   Dwyer, J.H., et al., *Arachidonate 5-lipoxygenase promoter genotype, dietary arachidonic acid, and atherosclerosis.* N Engl J Med, 2004. **350**(1): p. 29-37.
49.   Spanbroek, R., et al., *Expanding expression of the 5-lipoxygenase pathway within the arterial wall during human atherogenesis.* Proc Natl Acad Sci U S A, 2003. **100**(3): p. 1238-43.
50.   Lands, W.E., *Dietary fat and health: the evidence and the politics of prevention: careful use of dietary fats can improve life and prevent disease.* Ann N Y Acad Sci, 2005. **1055**: p. 179-92.
51.   Simopoulos, A.P., A. Leaf, and N. Salem, Jr., *Workshop on the Essentiality of and Recommended Dietary Intakes for Omega-6 and Omega-3 Fatty Acids.* J Am Coll Nutr, 1999. **18**(5): p. 487-9.
52.   Kiecolt-Glaser, J.K., et al., *Depressive symptoms, omega-6:omega-3 fatty acids, and inflammation in older adults.* Psychosom Med, 2007. **69**(3): p. 217-24.
53.   Moshfegh, A.G., Joseph; and Cleveland, Linda, *What We Eat in America, NHANES 2001-2002: Usual Nutrient Intakes from Food Compared to Dietary Reference Intakes.* , A.R.S. U.S. Department of Agriculture, Editor. 2005.
54.   Cunnane, S.C., *Problems with essential fatty acids: time for a new paradigm?* Prog Lipid Res, 2003. **42**(6): p. 544-68.
55.   Budowski, P. and M.A. Crawford, *a-Linolenic acid as a regulator of the metabolism of arachidonic acid: dietary implications of the ratio, n-6:n-3 fatty acids.* Proc Nutr Soc, 1985. **44**(2): p. 221-9.
56.   Adam, O., et al., *Anti-inflammatory effects of a low arachidonic acid diet and fish oil in patients with rheumatoid arthritis.* Rheumatol Int, 2003. **23**(1): p. 27-36.
57.   Kinsella, J.E., K.S. Broughton, and J.W. Whelan, *Dietary unsaturated fatty acids: interactions and possible needs in relation to eicosanoid synthesis.* J Nutr Biochem, 1990. **1**(3): p. 123-41.
58.   Chan, J.K., et al., *Effect of dietary alpha-linolenic acid and its ratio to linoleic acid on platelet and plasma fatty acids and thrombogenesis.* Lipids, 1993. **28**(9): p. 811-7.
59.   Li, B., C. Birdwell, and J. Whelan, *Antithetic relationship of dietary arachidonic acid and eicosapentaenoic acid on eicosanoid production in vivo.* J Lipid Res, 1994. **35**(10): p. 1869-77.
60.   Schiavone, A., et al., *Influence of dietary lipid source and strain on fatty acid composition of Muscovy duck meat.* J Anim Physiol Anim Nutr (Berl), 2004. **88**(3-4): p. 88-93.
61.   Krauss, R.M., et al., *AHA Dietary Guidelines: revision 2000: A statement for healthcare professionals from the Nutrition Committee of the American Heart Association.* Circulation, 2000. **102**(18): p. 2284-99.
62.   Kinsell, L.W., et al., *Dietary modification of serum cholesterol and phospholipid levels.* J Clin Endocrinol Metab, 1952. **12**(7): p. 909-13.
63.   Leren, P., *The effect of plasma cholesterol lowering diet in male survivors of myocardial infarction. A controlled clinical trial.* Acta Med Scand Suppl, 1966. **466**: p. 1-92.
64.   Leren, P., *The Oslo diet-heart study. Eleven-year report.* Circulation, 1970. **42**(5): p. 935-42.
65.   Pearce, M.L. and S. Dayton, *Incidence of cancer in men on a diet high in polyunsaturated fat.* Lancet, 1971. **1**(7697): p. 464-7.
66.   Turpeinen, O., et al., *Dietary prevention of coronary heart disease: the Finnish Mental Hospital Study.* Int J Epidemiol, 1979. **8**(2): p. 99-118.

67. Frantz, I.D., Jr., et al., *Test of effect of lipid lowering by diet on cardiovascular risk. The Minnesota Coronary Survey.* Arteriosclerosis, 1989. **9**(1): p. 129-35.
68. Rose, G.A., W.B. Thomson, and R.T. Williams, *Corn Oil in Treatment of Ischaemic Heart Disease.* Br Med J, 1965. **1**(5449): p. 1531-3.
69. Dolecek, T.A., *Epidemiological evidence of relationships between dietary polyunsaturated fatty acids and mortality in the multiple risk factor intervention trial.* Proc Soc Exp Biol Med, 1992. **200**(2): p. 177-82.
70. Dolecek, T.A. and G. Granditis, *Dietary polyunsaturated fatty acids and mortality in the Multiple Risk Factor Intervention Trial (MRFIT).* World Rev Nutr Diet, 1991. **66**: p. 205-16.
71. Kelley, D.S., et al., *Effects of dietary arachidonic acid on human immune response.* Lipids, 1997. **32**(4): p. 449-56.
72. Ferretti, A., et al., *Increased dietary arachidonic acid enhances the synthesis of vasoactive eicosanoids in humans.* Lipids, 1997. **32**(4): p. 435-9.
73. Dyerberg, J. and H.O. Bang, *Haemostatic function and platelet polyunsaturated fatty acids in Eskimos.* Lancet, 1979. **2**(8140): p. 433-5.
74. Dyerberg, J. and H.O. Bang, *Lipid metabolism, atherogenesis, and haemostasis in Eskimos: the role of the prostaglandin-3 family.* Haemostasis, 1979. **8**(3-5): p. 227-33.
75. Mezzano, D., et al., *Cardiovascular risk factors in vegetarians. Normalization of hyperhomocysteinemia with vitamin B(12) and reduction of platelet aggregation with n-3 fatty acids.* Thromb Res, 2000. **100**(3): p. 153-60.
76. Phinney, S.D., *Metabolism of exogenous and endogenous arachidonic acid in cancer.* Adv Exp Med Biol, 1996. **399**: p. 87-94.
77. Chen, X., et al., *Five-lipoxygenase pathway of arachidonic acid metabolism in carcino-genesis and cancer chemoprevention.* Curr Cancer Drug Targets, 2006. **6**(7): p. 613-22.
78. Ritch, C.R., et al., *Dietary fatty acids correlate with prostate cancer biopsy grade and volume in Jamaican men.* J Urol, 2007. **177**(1): p. 97-101; discussion 101.
79. Sugano, M. and F. Hirahara, *Polyunsaturated fatty acids in the food chain in Japan.* Am J Clin Nutr, 2000. **71**(1 Suppl): p. 189S-96S.
80. Singh, R.B., et al., *Recommendations for the prevention of coronary artery disease in Asians: a scientific statement of the International College of Nutrition.* J Cardiovasc Risk, 1996. **3**(6): p. 489-94.
81. Deutsche Gessellschaft fur Ernahrung. Referenzwerte fur die Nahrstoffzufuhr, Umschau Braus GmbH: Frankfurt am Main Germany, 2000, 227pp.
82. Simopoulos, A.P., *Evolutionary aspects of omega-3 fatty acids in the food supply.* Prostaglandins Leukot Essent Fatty Acids, 1999. **60**(5-6): p. 421-9.
83. ISSFAL. *Recommendations for intake of polyunsaturated fatty acids in healthy adults.* ISSFAL Board Statement # 3 2004 [cited 2006 June 19]; Available from: http://www.issfal.org.uk/lipid-matters/issfal-policy-statements/issfal-policy-statement-3-2.html.
84. Li, D., et al., *Contribution of meat fat to dietary arachidonic acid.* Lipids, 1998. **33**(4): p. 437-40.
85. Malau-Aduli, A.E., et al., *Breed comparison of the fatty acid composition of muscle phospholipids in Jersey and Limousin cattle.* J Anim Sci, 1998. **76**(3): p. 766-73.
86. Garg, A., et al., *Comparison of a high-carbohydrate diet with a high-monounsaturated-fat diet in patients with non-insulin-dependent diabetes mellitus.* N Engl J Med, 1988. **319**(13): p. 829-34.
87. Brash, A.R., *Arachidonic acid as a bioactive molecule.* J Clin Invest, 2001. **107**(11): p. 1339-45.
88. Seyberth, H.W., et al., *Increased arachidonate in lipids after administration to man: effects on prostaglandin biosynthesis.* Clin Pharmacol Ther, 1975. **18**(5 Pt 1): p. 521-9.
89. Broadhurst, C.L., S.C. Cunnane, and M.A. Crawford, *Rift Valley lake fish and shellfish provided brain-specific nutrition for early Homo.* Br J Nutr, 1998. **79**(1): p. 3-21.
90. Crawford, M.A., *Cerebral evolution.* Nutr Health, 2002. **16**(1): p. 29-34.
91. Crawford, M.A., et al., *Evidence for the unique function of docosahexaenoic acid during the evolution of the modern hominid brain.* Lipids, 1999. **34 Suppl**: p. S39-47.
92. Dannenberger, D., et al., *Diet alters the fatty acid composition of individual phospholipid classes in beef muscle.* J Agric Food Chem, 2007. **55**(2): p. 452-60.
93. Rule, D.C., et al., *Comparison of muscle fatty acid profiles and cholesterol concentrations of bison, beef cattle, elk, and chicken.* J Anim Sci, 2002. **80**(5): p. 1202-11.
94. Crawford, M.A., *Fatty-acid ratios in free-living and domestic animals. Possible implications for atheroma.* Lancet, 1968. **1**(7556): p. 1329-33.
95. Crawford, M.A., M.M. Gale, and M.H. Woodford, *Linoleic acid and linolenic acid elongation products in muscle tissue of Sncerus caffer and other ruminant species.* Biochem J, 1969. **115**(1): p. 25-7.
96. Crawford, M.A., M.M. Gale, and M.H. Woodford, *The polyenoic acids and their elongation products in the muscle tissue of Phacochoerus aethiopicus: a re-evaluation of "animal fat".* Biochem J, 1969. **114**(4): p. 68P.
97. Gale, M.M., M.A. Crawford, and M. Woodford, *The fatty acid composition of adipose and muscle tissue in domestic and free-living ruminants.* Biochem J, 1969. **113**(2): p. 6P.
98. Medeiros, L.B., JR etal, *Nutritional Content of Game Meat.* 1989, University of Wyoming, Laramie.
99. Komprda, T., et al., *Arachidonic acid and long-chain n-3 polyunsaturated fatty acid contents in meat of selected poultry and fish species in relation to dietary fat sources.* J Agric Food Chem, 2005. **53**(17): p. 6804-12.
100. Hebeisen, D.F., et al., *Increased concentrations of omega-3 fatty acids in milk and platelet rich plasma of grass-fed cows.* Int J Vitam Nutr Res, 1993. **63**(3): p. 229-33.
101. Hauswirth, C.B., M.R. Scheeder, and J.H. Beer, *High omega-3 fatty acid content in alpine cheese: the basis for an alpine paradox.* Circulation, 2004. **109**(1): p. 103-7.
102. Hites, R.A., et al., *Global assessment of organic contaminants in farmed salmon.* Science, 2004. **303**(5655): p. 226-9.

103. Nelson, G.J., et al., *The effect of dietary arachidonic acid on plasma lipoprotein distributions, apoproteins, blood lipid levels, and tissue fatty acid composition in humans.* Lipids, 1997. **32**(4): p. 427-33.

104. Osher, E., et al., *The 5 lipoxygenase system in the vasculature: emerging role in health and disease.* Mol Cell Endocrinol, 2006. **252**(1-2): p. 201-6.

105. Hakonarson, H., et al., *Effects of a 5-lipoxygenase-activating protein inhibitor on biomarkers associated with risk of myocardial infarction: a randomized trial.* Jama, 2005. **293**(18): p. 2245-56.

106. Soumaoro, L.T., et al., *Expression of 5-lipoxygenase in human colorectal cancer.* World J Gastroenterol, 2006. **12**(39): p. 6355-60.

107. Takase, B., et al., *Arachidonic acid metabolites in acute myocardial infarction.* Angiology, 1996. **47**(7): p. 649-61.

108. Hu, F.B., et al., *Dietary intake of alpha-linolenic acid and risk of fatal ischemic heart disease among women.* Am J Clin Nutr, 1999. **69**(5): p. 890-7.

109. Harris, W.S., *Alpha-linolenic acid: a gift from the land?* Circulation, 2005. **111**(22): p. 2872-4.

110. Leaf, A. and P.C. Weber, *A new era for science in nutrition.* Am J Clin Nutr, 1987. **45**(5 Suppl): p. 1048-53.

111. Ellis, K.A., et al., *Comparing the fatty acid composition of organic and conventional milk.* J Dairy Sci, 2006. **89**(6): p. 1938-50.

112. Crawford, M., *Fat animals - Fat Humans*, in *World Health - The Magazine of the World Health Organization.* 1991. p. 23-5.

113. Djousse, L., et al., *Relation between dietary linolenic acid and coronary artery disease in the National Heart, Lung, and Blood Institute Family Heart Study.* Am J Clin Nutr, 2001. **74**(5): p. 612-9.

114. Djousse, L., et al., *Dietary linolenic acid is inversely associated with calcified atherosclerotic plaque in the coronary arteries: the National Heart, Lung, and Blood Institute Family Heart Study.* Circulation, 2005. **111**(22): p. 2921-6.

115. Demark-Wahnefried, W., et al., *Pilot study of dietary fat restriction and flaxseed supplementation in men with prostate cancer before surgery: exploring the effects on hormonal levels, prostate-specific antigen, and histopathologic features.* Urology, 2001. **58**(1): p. 47-52.

116. Brouwer, I.A., M.B. Katan, and P.L. Zock, *Dietary alpha-linolenic acid is associated with reduced risk of fatal coronary heart disease, but increased prostate cancer risk: a meta-analysis.* J Nutr, 2004. **134**(4): p. 919-22.

117. Leitzmann, M.F., et al., *Dietary intake of n-3 and n-6 fatty acids and the risk of prostate cancer.* Am J Clin Nutr, 2004. **80**(1): p. 204-16.

118. Schuurman, A.G., et al., *Association of energy and fat intake with prostate carcinoma risk: results from The Netherlands Cohort Study.* Cancer, 1999. **86**(6): p. 1019-27.

119. Koralek, D.O., et al., *A prospective study of dietary alpha-linolenic acid and the risk of prostate cancer (United States).* Cancer Causes Control, 2006. **17**(6): p. 783-91.

120. Rose, D.P., *Effects of dietary fatty acids on breast and prostate cancers: evidence from in vitro experiments and animal studies.* Am J Clin Nutr, 1997. **66**(6 Suppl): p. 1513S-1522S.

121. Demark-Wahnefried, W. *Abstract 1510: Flaxseed slows prostate tumor growth.* in *American Society of Clinical Oncology.* 2007. Chicago, IL.

122. de Lorgeril, M. and P. Salen, *alpha-linolenic acid, coronary heart disease, and prostate cancer.* J Nutr, 2004. **134**(12): p. 3385; author reply 3386.

123. *National heart Foundation of Australia. A Review of the Relationship between Dietary Fat and Cardiovascular Disease.* Aust J Nutr Diet, 1999. **56**: p. S5-22.

124. de Deckere, E.A., et al., *Health aspects of fish and n-3 polyunsaturated fatty acids from plant and marine origin.* Eur J Clin Nutr, 1998. **52**(10): p. 749-53.

125. Sargent, J.R. and R.J. Henderson, *Lipid metabolism in marine animals.* Biochem Soc Trans, 1980. **8**(3): p. 296-7.

126. Simopoulos, A.P. and N. Salem, Jr., *Egg yolk as a source of long-chain polyunsaturated fatty acids in infant feeding.* Am J Clin Nutr, 1992. **55**(2): p. 411-4.

127. Siscovick, D.S., et al., *Dietary intake and cell membrane levels of long-chain n-3 polyunsaturated fatty acids and the risk of primary cardiac arrest.* Jama, 1995. **274**(17): p. 1363-7.

128. Iso, H., et al., *Intake of fish and n3 fatty acids and risk of coronary heart disease among Japanese: the Japan Public Health Center-Based (JPHC) Study Cohort I.* Circulation, 2006. **113**(2): p. 195-202.

129. Marchioli, R., et al., *Early protection against sudden death by n-3 polyunsaturated fatty acids after myocardial infarction: time-course analysis of the results of the Gruppo Italiano per lo Studio della Sopravvivenza nell'Infarto Miocardico (GISSI)-Prevenzione.* Circulation, 2002. **105**(16): p. 1897-903.

130. Raeder, M.B., et al., *Associations between cod liver oil use and symptoms of depression: The Hordaland Health Study.* J Affect Disord, 2006.

131. McNamara, R.K., et al., *Selective Deficits in the Omega-3 Fatty Acid Docosahexaenoic Acid in the Postmortem Orbitofrontal Cortex of Patients with Major Depressive Disorder.* Biol Psychiatry, 2006.

132. Nemets, B., Z. Stahl, and R.H. Belmaker, *Addition of omega-3 fatty acid to maintenance medication treatment for recurrent unipolar depressive disorder.* Am J Psychiatry, 2002. **159**(3): p. 477-9.

133. Schaefer, E.J., et al., *Plasma phosphatidylcholine docosahexaenoic acid content and risk of dementia and Alzheimer disease: the Framingham Heart Study.* Arch Neurol, 2006. **63**(11): p. 1545-50.

134. Freund-Levi, Y., et al., *Omega-3 fatty acid treatment in 174 patients with mild to moderate Alzheimer disease: OmegAD study: a randomized double-blind trial.* Arch Neurol, 2006. **63**(10): p. 1402-8.

135. Lukiw, W.J., et al., *A role for docosahexaenoic acid-derived neuroprotectin D1 in neural cell survival and Alzheimer disease.* J Clin Invest, 2005. **115**(10): p. 2774-83.

136. Wolk, A., et al., *Long-term fatty fish consumption and renal cell carcinoma incidence in women.* Jama, 2006. **296**(11): p. 1371-6.

137. Kimura, Y., *[Fish, n-3 polyunsaturated fatty acid and colorectal cancer prevention: a review of experimental and epidemiological studies]*. Nippon Koshu Eisei Zasshi, 2006. **53**(10): p. 735-48.
138. Johnson, E.J. and E.J. Schaefer, *Potential role of dietary n-3 fatty acids in the prevention of dementia and macular degeneration*. Am J Clin Nutr, 2006. **83**(6 Suppl): p. 1494S-1498S.
139. Chua, B., et al., *Dietary fatty acids and the 5-year incidence of age-related maculopathy*. Arch Ophthalmol, 2006. **124**(7): p. 981-6.
140. Conklin, S.M., et al., *Serum omega-3 fatty acids are associated with variation in mood, personality and behavior in hypercholesterolemic community volunteers*. Psychiatry Res, 2007.
141. Fan, Y.Y., et al., *Chemopreventive n-3 fatty acids activate RXRalpha in colonocytes*. Carcinogenesis, 2003. **24**(9): p. 1541-8.
142. Clarke, S.D., et al., *Fatty acid regulation of gene expression. Its role in fuel partitioning and insulin resistance*. Ann N Y Acad Sci, 1997. **827**: p. 178-87.
143. Clarke, S.D., et al., *Fatty acid regulation of gene expression: a genomic explanation for the benefits of the mediterranean diet*. Ann N Y Acad Sci, 2002. **967**: p. 283-98.
144. Caygill, C.P., A. Charlett, and M.J. Hill, *Fat, fish, fish oil and cancer*. Br J Cancer, 1996. **74**(1): p. 159-64.
145. Han, S.N., et al., *Effect of hydrogenated and saturated, relative to polyunsaturated, fat on immune and inflammatory responses of adults with moderate hypercholesterolemia*. J Lipid Res, 2002. **43**(3): p. 445-52.
146. Dyerberg, J., et al., *Eicosapentaenoic acid and prevention of thrombosis and atherosclerosis?* Lancet, 1978. **2**(8081): p. 117-9.
147. Couet, C., et al., *Effect of dietary fish oil on body fat mass and basal fat oxidation in healthy adults*. Int J Obes Relat Metab Disord, 1997. **21**(8): p. 637-43.
148. Hill, A.M., et al., *Combining fish-oil supplements with regular aerobic exercise improves body composition and cardiovascular disease risk factors*. Am J Clin Nutr, 2007. **85**(5): p. 1267-74.
149. Kris-Etherton, P.M., W.S. Harris, and L.J. Appel, *Omega-3 fatty acids and cardiovascular disease: new recommendations from the American Heart Association*. Arterioscler Thromb Vasc Biol, 2003. **23**(2): p. 151-2.
150. Stark, K.D., et al., *Fatty acid compositions of serum phospholipids of postmenopausal women: a comparison between Greenland Inuit and Canadians before and after supplementation with fish oil*. Nutrition, 2002. **18**(7-8): p. 627-30.
151. Dewailly, E., et al., *Cardiovascular disease risk factors and n-3 fatty acid status in the adult population of James Bay Cree*. Am J Clin Nutr, 2002. **76**(1): p. 85-92.
152. Bjerregaard, P. and J. Dyerberg, *Mortality from ischaemic heart disease and cerebrovascular disease in Greenland*. Int J Epidemiol, 1988. **17**(3): p. 514-9.
153. Iso, H., et al., *Serum fatty acids and fish intake in rural Japanese, urban Japanese, Japanese American and Caucasian American men*. Int J Epidemiol, 1989. **18**(2): p. 374-81.
154. Erkkila, A.T., et al., *n-3 Fatty acids and 5-y risks of death and cardiovascular disease events in patients with coronary artery disease*. Am J Clin Nutr, 2003. **78**(1): p. 65-71.
155. Emken, E.A., *Nutrition and biochemistry of trans and positional fatty acid isomers in hydrogenated oils*. Annu Rev Nutr, 1984. **4**: p. 339-76.
156. Mozaffarian, D., et al., *Trans fatty acids and cardiovascular disease*. N Engl J Med, 2006. **354**(15): p. 1601-13.
157. *Federal Research Notice. Food Labeling: Trans fatty acids in Nutrition Labeling: Consumer Research to Consider Nutrient Content and Health Claims and Possible Footnote and Disclosure Statements: Final Rule and Proposed Rule.* July 11, 2003 [cited 68 No. 153]; 41433-41506].
158. Ascherio, A., Stampfer, MJ. *Background and Scientific Review: Trans fatty acids and coronary heart disease*. [cited 2007; Available from: http://www.hsph.harvard.edu/reviews/transfats.html.
159. Harnack, L., et al., *Trends in the trans-fatty acid composition of the diet in a metropolitan area: the Minnesota Heart Survey*. J Am Diet Assoc, 2003. **103**(9): p. 1160-6.
160. Booyens, J., C.C. Louwrens, and I.E. Katzeff, *The role of unnatural dietary trans and cis unsaturated fatty acids in the epidemiology of coronary artery disease*. Med Hypotheses, 1988. **25**(3): p. 175-82.
161. Acar, N., et al., *Modification of the monoaminergic neurotransmitters in frontal cortex and hippocampus by dietary trans alpha-linolenic acid in piglets*. Neurosci Lett, 2002. **331**(3): p. 198-202.
162. Niu, S.L., D.C. Mitchell, and B.J. Litman, *Trans fatty acid derived phospholipids show increased membrane cholesterol and reduced receptor activation as compared to their cis analogs*. Biochemistry, 2005. **44**(11): p. 4458-65.
163. Riserus, U., *Trans fatty acids and insulin resistance*. Atheroscler Suppl, 2006. **7**(2): p. 37-9.
164. Hu, F.B., et al., *Dietary fat intake and the risk of coronary heart disease in women*. N Engl J Med, 1997. **337**(21): p. 1491-9.
165. Salmeron, J., et al., *Dietary fat intake and risk of type 2 diabetes in women*. Am J Clin Nutr, 2001. **73**(6): p. 1019-26.
166. Morris, M.C., et al., *Dietary fats and the risk of incident Alzheimer disease*. Arch Neurol, 2003. **60**(2): p. 194-200.
167. Morris, M.C., et al., *Dietary fat intake and 6-year cognitive change in an older biracial community population*. Neurology, 2004. **62**(9): p. 1573-9.
168. Slattery, M.L., et al., *Trans-fatty acids and colon cancer*. Nutr Cancer, 2001. **39**(2): p. 170-5.
169. Kavanagh, K., Rudel, LL. *Trans Fat Leads to Weight Gain Even on the Same Total Calories, Animal Study Shows.* 2006 [cited 2006 Nov 27]; Available from: https://www1.wfubmc.edu/news/NewsArticle.htm?Articleid=1869.
170. Chavarro, J.E., et al., *Dietary fatty acid intakes and the risk of ovulatory infertility*. Am J Clin Nutr, 2007. **85**(1): p. 231-7.
171. Leth, T., Bysted, A etal. *The effect of regulation on trans fatty acid content in Danish food* in *First International Symposium on Trans Fatty Acids and health*. 2005. Rungstedgaard, Denmark.

172.   Stender, S. and J. Dyerberg, *Influence of trans fatty acids on health.* Ann Nutr Metab, 2004. **48**(2): p. 61-6.
173.   *Food Labeling: Trans Fatty Acids in Nutrition Labeling, Nutrient Content Claims, and health Claims. Final Rule.* 2003, July 11, Food and Drug Administration, HHS. p. 1-74.
174.   Minino, A., Heron, M. *Deaths: preliminary data for 2004.* National Center for Health Statistics. [cited 2007 Feb 12]; Available from: http://www.cdc.gov/nchs/products/pubs/pubd/hestats/prelimdeaths04/preliminarydeaths04.htm.
175.   Eaton, S.B. and M. Konner, *Paleolithic nutrition. A consideration of its nature and current implications.* N Engl J Med, 1985. **312**(5): p. 283-9.
176.   Eaton, S.B., M. Konner, and M. Shostak, *Stone agers in the fast lane: chronic degenerative diseases in evolutionary perspective.* Am J Med, 1988. **84**(4): p. 739-49.
177.   Eaton, S.B., et al., *An evolutionary perspective enhances understanding of human nutritional requirements.* J Nutr, 1996. **126**(6): p. 1732-40.
178.   Eaton, C.B., *Hyperlipidemia.* Prim Care, 2005. **32**(4): p. 1027-55, viii.
179.   Boucher, P., et al., *Effect of dietary cholesterol on low density lipoprotein-receptor, 3-hydroxy-3-methylglutaryl-CoA reductase, and low density lipoprotein receptor-related protein mRNA expression in healthy humans.* Lipids, 1998. **33**(12): p. 1177-86.
180.   McNamara, D.J., *The impact of egg limitations on coronary heart disease risk: do the numbers add up?* J Am Coll Nutr, 2000. **19**(5 Suppl): p. 540S-548S.
181.   Hu, F.B. and W.C. Willett, *Optimal diets for prevention of coronary heart disease.* Jama, 2002. **288**(20): p. 2569-78.
182.   Fernandez, M.L., *Dietary cholesterol provided by eggs and plasma lipoproteins in healthy populations.* Curr Opin Clin Nutr Metab Care, 2006. **9**(1): p. 8-12.
183.   Kratz, M., *Dietary cholesterol, atherosclerosis and coronary heart disease.* Handb Exp Pharmacol, 2005(170): p. 195-213.
184.   Howell, W.H., et al., *Plasma lipid and lipoprotein responses to dietary fat and cholesterol: a meta-analysis.* Am J Clin Nutr, 1997. **65**(6): p. 1747-64.
185.   U.S. Department of Agricultural Research Service. 1997. *Data Tables: results from the USDA's 1994-1996 Continuing Survey of Food Intakes by Individuals and 1994-1996 Diet and Health Knowledge Survey [Online]* ARS Food Surveys Research Group.   [cited; Available from: http:barc.usda.gov/bhnrc/foodsurvey/home.htm. {visited 2006, August 10th}.
186.   McDonald, B.E., *The Canadian experience: why Canada decided against an upper limit for cholesterol.* J Am Coll Nutr, 2004. **23**(6 Suppl): p. 616S-620S.
187.   Hu, F.B., et al., *A prospective study of egg consumption and risk of cardiovascular disease in men and women.* Jama, 1999. **281**(15): p. 1387-94.
188.   Murray, R., Granner DK etal, *Harper's Illustrated Biochemistry, Thirty-seventh edition.* 2006: McGraw Hill Companies, INC.
189.   Erkkila, A.T. and A.H. Lichtenstein, *Fiber and cardiovascular disease risk: how strong is the evidence?* J Cardiovasc Nurs, 2006. **21**(1): p. 3-8.
190.   DeVries, J.W., *On defining dietary fibre.* Proc Nutr Soc, 2003. **62**(1): p. 37-43.
191.   Asp, N.G., *Classification and methodology of food carbohydrates as related to nutritional effects.* Am J Clin Nutr, 1995. **61**(4 Suppl): p. 930S-937S.
192.   Wahlqvist, M.L., E.G. Wilmshurst, and E.N. Richardson, *The effect of chain length on glucose absorption and the related metabolic response.* Am J Clin Nutr, 1978. **31**(11): p. 1998-2001.
193.   Bantle, J.P., et al., *Postprandial glucose and insulin responses to meals containing different carbohydrates in normal and diabetic subjects.* N Engl J Med, 1983. **309**(1): p. 7-12.
194.   Dahlqvist, A. and B. Borgstrom, *Digestion and absorption of disaccharides in man.* Biochem J, 1961. **81**: p. 411-8.
195.   Eaton, S.B., *The ancestral human diet: what was it and should it be a paradigm for contemporary nutrition?* Proc Nutr Soc, 2006. **65**(1): p. 1-6.
196.   Pereira, M.A., et al., *Dietary fiber and risk of coronary heart disease: a pooled analysis of cohort studies.* Arch Intern Med, 2004. **164**(4): p. 370-6.
197.   Anderson, J.W., et al., *Carbohydrate and fiber recommendations for individuals with diabetes: a quantitative assessment and meta-analysis of the evidence.* J Am Coll Nutr, 2004. **23**(1): p. 5-17.
198.   Landin, K., et al., *Guar gum improves insulin sensitivity, blood lipids, blood pressure, and fibrinolysis in healthy men.* Am J Clin Nutr, 1992. **56**(6): p. 1061-5.
199.   Fehily, A.M., et al., *A randomised controlled trial to investigate the effect of a high fibre diet on blood pressure and plasma fibrinogen.* J Epidemiol Community Health, 1986. **40**(4): p. 334-7.
200.   Shamliyan, T.A., et al., *Are your patients with risk of CVD getting the viscous soluble fiber they need?* J Fam Pract, 2006. **55**(9): p. 761-9.
201.   Khan, A.R., et al., *Effect of guar gum on blood lipids.* Am J Clin Nutr, 1981. **34**(11): p. 2446-9.
202.   Pietinen, P., et al., *Intake of dietary fiber and risk of coronary heart disease in a cohort of Finnish men. The Alpha-Tocopherol, Beta-Carotene Cancer Prevention Study.* Circulation, 1996. **94**(11): p. 2720-7.
203.   Lupton, J.R. and N.D. Turner, *Dietary fiber and coronary disease: does the evidence support an association?* Curr Atheroscler Rep, 2003. **5**(6): p. 500-5.
204.   McDowell, M.A., et al., *Energy and macronutrient intakes of persons ages 2 months and over in the United States: Third National Health and Nutrition Examination Survey, Phase 1, 1988-91.* Adv Data, 1994(255): p. 1-24.
205.   Ludwig, D.S., *The glycemic index: physiological mechanisms relating to obesity, diabetes, and cardiovascular disease.* Jama, 2002. **287**(18): p. 2414-23.

206. Bray, G.A., S.J. Nielsen, and B.M. Popkin, *Consumption of high-fructose corn syrup in beverages may play a role in the epidemic of obesity.* Am J Clin Nutr, 2004. **79**(4): p. 537-43.

207. Havel, P.J., *Dietary fructose: implications for dysregulation of energy homeostasis and lipid/carbohydrate metabolism.* Nutr Rev, 2005. **63**(5): p. 133-57.

208. Elliott, S.S., et al., *Fructose, weight gain, and the insulin resistance syndrome.* Am J Clin Nutr, 2002. **76**(5): p. 911-22.

209. Murakami, K., et al., *Dietary fiber intake, dietary glycemic index and load, and body mass index: a cross-sectional study of 3931 Japanese women aged 18-20 years.* Eur J Clin Nutr, 2007.

210. Belpoggi, F., et al., *Results of long-term carcinogenicity bioassay on Sprague-Dawley rats exposed to aspartame administered in feed.* Ann N Y Acad Sci, 2006. **1076**: p. 559-77.

211. U.S. Department of Agriculture, Economic Research Service. *Food Consumption (per capita) data system, sugars/sweeteners.* 2002 [cited 2006 August 15]; Available from: http://www.ers.usda.gov/Data/foodconsumption/datasystem.asp.

212. Block, G., *Foods Contributing to energy intake in the US: data from NHANES III and NHANES 1999-2000.* Journal of Agricultural Food Composition and Analyis, 2004. **17**: p. 439-447.

213. Krebs-Smith, S.M., et al., *Low energy reporters vs others: a comparison of reported food intakes.* Eur J Clin Nutr, 2000. **54**(4): p. 281-7.

214. Eaton, S.B., S.B. Eaton, 3rd, and M.J. Konner, *Paleolithic nutrition revisited: a twelve-year retrospective on its nature and implications.* Eur J Clin Nutr, 1997. **51**(4): p. 207-16.

215. Cordain, L., et al., *Macronutrient estimations in hunter-gatherer diets.* Am J Clin Nutr, 2000. **72**(6): p. 1589-92.

216. Cordain, L., et al., *Plant-animal subsistence ratios and macronutrient energy estimations in worldwide hunter-gatherer diets.* Am J Clin Nutr, 2000. **71**(3): p. 682-92.

217. Merchant, A.T., et al., *Carbohydrate intake and HDL in a multiethnic population.* Am J Clin Nutr, 2007. **85**(1): p. 225-30.

218. Malik, V.S., M.B. Schulze, and F.B. Hu, *Intake of sugar-sweetened beverages and weight gain: a systematic review.* Am J Clin Nutr, 2006. **84**(2): p. 274-88.

219. Suter, P.M., *Carbohydrates and dietary fiber.* Handb Exp Pharmacol, 2005(170): p. 231-61.

220. Jones, J.M., et al., *Becoming Proactive With the Whole-Grains Message.* Nutr Today, 2004. **39**(1): p. 10-17.

221. *Dietary Goals for the United States.* 1977, US Senate Select Committee on Nutrition and Human Needs. Washington, DC.

222. Grundy, S.M., et al., *Rationale of the diet-heart statement of the American Heart Association. Report of Nutrition Committee.* Circulation, 1982. **65**(4): p. 839A-854A.

223. Schulze, M.B., et al., *Glycemic index, glycemic load, and dietary fiber intake and incidence of type 2 diabetes in younger and middle-aged women.* Am J Clin Nutr, 2004. **80**(2): p. 348-56.

224. Qi, L., et al., *Whole-grain, bran, and cereal fiber intakes and markers of systemic inflammation in diabetic women.* Diabetes Care, 2006. **29**(2): p. 207-11.

225. Del Prato, S., et al., *Effect of sustained physiologic hyperinsulinaemia and hyperglycaemia on insulin secretion and insulin sensitivity in man.* Diabetologia, 1994. **37**(10): p. 1025-35.

226. Liu, S., et al., *A prospective study of dietary glycemic load, carbohydrate intake, and risk of coronary heart disease in US women.* Am J Clin Nutr, 2000. **71**(6): p. 1455-61.

227. Gross, L.S., et al., *Increased consumption of refined carbohydrates and the epidemic of type 2 diabetes in the United States: an ecologic assessment.* Am J Clin Nutr, 2004. **79**(5): p. 774-9.

228. Hu, Y., et al., *Relations of glycemic index and glycemic load with plasma oxidative stress markers.* Am J Clin Nutr, 2006. **84**(1): p. 70-6; quiz 266-7.

229. Liu, R.H., *Potential synergy of phytochemicals in cancer prevention: mechanism of action.* J Nutr, 2004. **134**(12 Suppl): p. 3479S-3485S.

230. Griel, A.E., E.H. Ruder, and P.M. Kris-Etherton, *The changing roles of dietary carbohydrates: from simple to complex.* Arterioscler Thromb Vasc Biol, 2006. **26**(9): p. 1958-65.

231. O'Dea, K., et al., *The effects of diet differing in fat, carbohydrate, and fiber on carbohydrate and lipid metabolism in type II diabetes.* J Am Diet Assoc, 1989. **89**(8): p. 1076-86.

232. Cooper, G.M., *The cell: a molecular approach, 2nd edition.* 2000, Sinauer Associates Inc.

233. Young, S.N., *Behavioral effects of dietary neurotransmitter precursors: basic and clinical aspects.* Neurosci Biobehav Rev, 1996. **20**(2): p. 313-23.

234. Connor, W.E., et al., *The plasma lipids, lipoproteins, and diet of the Tarahumara indians of Mexico.* Am J Clin Nutr, 1978. **31**(7): p. 1131-42.

235. *Report of the National Cholesterol Education Program Expert Panel on Detection, Evaluation, and Treatment of High Blood Cholesterol in Adults. The Expert Panel.* Arch Intern Med, 1988. **148**(1): p. 36-69.

236. Hu, F.B., et al., *Dietary protein and risk of ischemic heart disease in women.* Am J Clin Nutr, 1999. **70**(2): p. 221-7.

237. Yamashita, T., et al., *Arterial compliance, blood pressure, plasma leptin, and plasma lipids in women are improved with weight reduction equally with a meat-based diet and a plant-based diet.* Metabolism, 1998. **47**(11): p. 1308-14.

238. Ashton, E. and M. Ball, *Effects of soy as tofu vs meat on lipoprotein concentrations.* Eur J Clin Nutr, 2000. **54**(1): p. 14-9.

239. Merchant, A.T., et al., *Protein intake is inversely associated with abdominal obesity in a multi-ethnic population.* J Nutr, 2005. **135**(5): p. 1196-201.

240. Li, D., et al., *Lean meat and heart health.* Asia Pac J Clin Nutr, 2005. **14**(2): p. 113-9.

241. Halton, T.L., et al., *Low-carbohydrate-diet score and the risk of coronary heart disease in women.* N Engl J Med, 2006. **355**(19): p. 1991-2002.

242. Whelton, P.K., et al., *Primary prevention of hypertension: clinical and public health advisory from The National High Blood Pressure Education Program.* Jama, 2002. **288**(15): p. 1882-8.

243. James, W.P., A. Ralph, and C.P. Sanchez-Castillo, *The dominance of salt in manufactured food in the sodium intake of affluent societies.* Lancet, 1987. **1**(8530): p. 426-9.

244. Karppanen, H., P. Karppanen, and E. Mervaala, *Why and how to implement sodium, potassium, calcium, and magnesium changes in food items and diets?* J Hum Hypertens, 2005. **19 Suppl 3**: p. S10-9.

245. Eaton, S.B. and S.B. Eaton, 3rd, *Paleolithic vs. modern diets--selected pathophysiological implications.* Eur J Nutr, 2000. **39**(2): p. 67-70.

246. Karppanen, H. and E. Mervaala, *Sodium intake and hypertension.* Prog Cardiovasc Dis, 2006. **49**(2): p. 59-75.

247. Akita, S., et al., *Effects of the Dietary Approaches to Stop Hypertension (DASH) diet on the pressure-natriuresis relationship.* Hypertension, 2003. **42**(1): p. 8-13.

248. Adrogue, H.J. and N.E. Madias, *Sodium and potassium in the pathogenesis of hypertension.* N Engl J Med, 2007. **356**(19): p. 1966-78.

249. Tuomilehto, J., et al., *Urinary sodium excretion and cardiovascular mortality in Finland: a prospective study.* Lancet, 2001. **357**(9259): p. 848-51.

250. Cook, N.R., et al., *Long term effects of dietary sodium reduction on cardiovascular disease outcomes: observational follow-up of the trials of hypertension prevention (TOHP).* Bmj, 2007. **334**(7599): p. 885.

251. Cohen, H.W., et al., *Sodium intake and mortality in the NHANES II follow-up study.* Am J Med, 2006. **119**(3): p. 275 e7-14.

252. Vaskonen, T., *Dietary minerals and modification of cardiovascular risk factors.* J Nutr Biochem, 2003. **14**(9): p. 492-506.

253. Jee, S.H., et al., *The effect of magnesium supplementation on blood pressure: a meta-analysis of randomized clinical trials.* Am J Hypertens, 2002. **15**(8): p. 691-6.

254. Griffith, L.E., et al., *The influence of dietary and nondietary calcium supplementation on blood pressure: an updated metaanalysis of randomized controlled trials.* Am J Hypertens, 1999. **12**(1 Pt 1): p. 84-92.

255. Geleijnse, J.M., F.J. Kok, and D.E. Grobbee, *Blood pressure response to changes in sodium and potassium intake: a metaregression analysis of randomised trials.* J Hum Hypertens, 2003. **17**(7): p. 471-80.

256. Karppanen, H., *An antihypertensive salt: crucial role of Mildred Seelig in its development.* J Am Coll Nutr, 1994. **13**(5): p. 493-5.

257. Willcox, J.K., S.L. Ash, and G.L. Catignani, *Antioxidants and prevention of chronic disease.* Crit Rev Food Sci Nutr, 2004. **44**(4): p. 275-95.

258. Benzie, I.F., *Evolution of antioxidant defence mechanisms.* Eur J Nutr, 2000. **39**(2): p. 53-61.

259. Brighenti, F., et al., *Total antioxidant capacity of the diet is inversely and independently related to plasma concentration of high-sensitivity C-reactive protein in adult Italian subjects.* Br J Nutr, 2005. **93**(5): p. 619-25.

260. Nam, N.H., *Naturally occurring NF-kappaB inhibitors.* Mini Rev Med Chem, 2006. **6**(8): p. 945-51.

261. Freedman, J.E., et al., *Select flavonoids and whole juice from purple grapes inhibit platelet function and enhance nitric oxide release.* Circulation, 2001. **103**(23): p. 2792-8.

262. Covas, M.I., et al., *The effect of polyphenols in olive oil on heart disease risk factors: a randomized trial.* Ann Intern Med, 2006. **145**(5): p. 333-41.

263. Vinson, J.A., et al., *Phenol antioxidant quantity and quality in foods: fruits.* J Agric Food Chem, 2001. **49**(11): p. 5315-21.

264. Satyanarayana, S., et al., *Antioxidant activity of the aqueous extracts of spicy food additives--evaluation and comparison with ascorbic acid in in-vitro systems.* J Herb Pharmacother, 2004. **4**(2): p. 1-10.

265. Aherne, S.A. and N.M. O'Brien, *Dietary flavonols: chemistry, food content, and metabolism.* Nutrition, 2002. **18**(1): p. 75-81.

266. *USDA Database for Flavonoid Content of Selected Foods.* March 2003. [cited Aug 15, 2006]; Available from: http://www.nal.usda.gov/fnic/foodcomp

267. Pellegrini, N., et al., *Total antioxidant capacity of plant foods, beverages and oils consumed in Italy assessed by three different in vitro assays.* J Nutr, 2003. **133**(9): p. 2812-9.

268. Hertog, M.G., et al., *Flavonoid intake and long-term risk of coronary heart disease and cancer in the seven countries study.* Arch Intern Med, 1995. **155**(4): p. 381-6.

269. Williamson, G., et al., *Human metabolic pathways of dietary flavonoids and cinnamates.* Biochem Soc Trans, 2000. **28**(2): p. 16-22.

270. Kuhnau, J., *The flavonoids. A class of semi-essential food components: their role in human nutrition.* World Rev Nutr Diet, 1976. **24**: p. 117-91.

271. Rapola, J.M., et al., *Randomised trial of alpha-tocopherol and beta-carotene supplements on incidence of major coronary events in men with previous myocardial infarction.* Lancet, 1997. **349**(9067): p. 1715-20.

272. Podmore, I.D., et al., *Vitamin C exhibits pro-oxidant properties.* Nature, 1998. **392**(6676): p. 559.

273. Wright, M.E., et al., *Higher baseline serum concentrations of vitamin E are associated with lower total and cause-specific mortality in the Alpha-Tocopherol, Beta-Carotene Cancer Prevention Study.* Am J Clin Nutr, 2006. **84**(5): p. 1200-7.

274. Byrne, C., et al., *Predictors of dietary heterocyclic amine intake in three prospective cohorts.* Cancer Epidemiol Biomarkers Prev, 1998. **7**(6): p. 523-9.

275. Ghebremeskel, K. and M.A. Crawford, *Nutrition and health in relation to food production and processing.* Nutr Health, 1994. **9**(4): p. 237-53.

276. Fitzgerald, W., Lamborg, CH etal. *Modern and Historic Atmospheric Mercury Fluxes in Both Hemispheres: Global and Regional Mercury Cycling Implications.* in *Abstracts 6th International Conference on Mercury as a Global Pollutant* Oct 15-19, 2001. Minamata, Japan.

277.   Clarkson, T.W., J.J. Strain, and M.C. Archer, *Nutrition-toxicology: evolutionary aspects. Introduction. Conference held June 1999, Coleraine, Northern Ireland.* Eur J Nutr, 2000. **39**(2): p. 49-52.
278.   Oken, E., et al., *Maternal fish consumption, hair mercury, and infant cognition in a U.S. Cohort.* Environ Health Perspect, 2005. **113**(10): p. 1376-80.
279.   Gochfeld, M. and J. Burger, *Good fish/bad fish: a composite benefit-risk by dose curve.* Neurotoxicology, 2005. **26**(4): p. 511-20.
280.   Mozaffarian, D. and E.B. Rimm, *Fish intake, contaminants, and human health: evaluating the risks and the benefits.* Jama, 2006. **296**(15): p. 1885-99.
281.   Bourre, J.M., *Where to find omega-3 fatty acids and how feeding animals with diet enriched in omega-3 fatty acids to increase nutritional value of derived products for human: what is actually useful ?* J Nutr Health Aging, 2005. **9**(4): p. 232-42.
282.   Mozaffarian, D., et al., *Cardiac benefits of fish consumption may depend on the type of fish meal consumed: the Cardiovascular Health Study.* Circulation, 2003. **107**(10): p. 1372-7.
283.   US Department of Health and Human Services and Environmental Protection Agency. *Mercury Levels in Commercial Fish and Shellfish.* [cited December 12, 2005]; Available from: http://www.cfsan.fda.gov/~frf/sea-mehg.html.
284.   *Chicago Tribune Investigation: The Mercury Menace, FDA Updates Mercury Findings.* 2006 [cited Jan 7, 2006]; Available from: http://www.chicagotribune.com/media/graphic/2006-01/21650321.gif
285.   Burger, J. and M. Gochfeld, *Mercury in canned tuna: white versus light and temporal variation.* Environ Res, 2004. **96**(3): p. 239-49.
286.   Mahaffey, K., Clickner, RP. *Blood Organic Mercury and Dietray Mercury Intake: NHANES, 1999 and 2000.* 2003 [cited 2007 Feb 23]; Available from: http://dx.doi.org/.
287.   *Environmental protection Agency. What you need to know about mercury in fish and shellfish.* . 2001 Feb 2006 [cited Feb 12, 2006]; Available from: http://www.epa.gov/waterscience/fishadvice/advice.html.
288.   *Blood mercury levels in young children and childbearing-aged women--United States, 1999-2002.* MMWR Morb Mortal Wkly Rep, 2004. **53**(43): p. 1018-20.
289.   Birch, E.E., et al., *Visual acuity and the essentiality of docosahexaenoic acid and arachidonic acid in the diet of term infants.* Pediatr Res, 1998. **44**(2): p. 201-9.
290.   Birch, E.E., et al., *Visual acuity and cognitive outcomes at 4 years of age in a double-blind, randomized trial of long-chain polyunsaturated fatty acid-supplemented infant formula.* Early Hum Dev, 2007.
291.   McNamara, R.K. and S.E. Carlson, *Role of omega-3 fatty acids in brain development and function: potential implications for the pathogenesis and prevention of psychopathology.* Prostaglandins Leukot Essent Fatty Acids, 2006. **75**(4-5): p. 329-49.
292.   *U.S. Environmental Protection Agency Fact Sheet. Polychlorinated Biphenyls (PCBs) Update: Impact on Fish Advisories 1999.* [cited 2006 Aug 9]; Available from: http://www.epa.gov/OST/fish.
293.   Lee, D.H., et al., *A strong dose-response relation between serum concentrations of persistent organic pollutants and diabetes: results from the National Health and Examination Survey 1999-2002.* Diabetes Care, 2006. **29**(7): p. 1638-44.
294.   Lee, D.H., et al., *Association between serum concentrations of persistent organic pollutants and insulin resistance among nondiabetic adults: results from the National Health and Nutrition Examination Survey 1999-2002.* Diabetes Care, 2007. **30**(3): p. 622-8.
295.   Fierens, S., et al., *Dioxin/polychlorinated biphenyl body burden, diabetes and endometriosis: findings in a population-based study in Belgium.* Biomarkers, 2003. **8**(6): p. 529-34.
296.   U.S. Department of Health and Human Services, Agency for Toxic Substances and Disease. . [cited 2006 Aug 10]; Available from: http://www.atsdr.cdc.gov
297.   Melanson, S.F., et al., *Measurement of organochlorines in commercial over-the-counter fish oil preparations: implications for dietary and therapeutic recommendations for omega-3 fatty acids and a review of the literature.* Arch Pathol Lab Med, 2005. **129**(1): p. 74-7.
298.   *PCBs in Food: The Risks and Benefits of Salmon and Other Foods.* [cited 2006 Jan 2]; Available from: http://www.salmonoftheamericas.com/topic_pcbs_food.html.
299.   *EWG report: PCBs in farmed salmon.* . [cited Aug 10 2006]; Available from: www.ewg.org/reports/farmedPCBs/printversion.php.
300.   Hamilton, M.C., et al., *Lipid composition and contaminants in farmed and wild salmon.* Environ Sci Technol, 2005. **39**(22): p. 8622-9.
301.   *Department of Health and Human Services, Agency for Toxic Substances and Disease Registry.* [cited Aug 10, 2006]; Available from: http://www.atsdr.cdc.gov.
302.   Larsson, S.C., L. Bergkvist, and A. Wolk, *Processed meat consumption, dietary nitrosamines and stomach cancer risk in a cohort of Swedish women.* Int J Cancer, 2006. **119**(4): p. 915-9.
303.   Tricker, A.R. and R. Preussmann, *Carcinogenic N-nitrosamines in the diet: occurrence, formation, mechanisms and carcinogenic potential.* Mutat Res, 1991. **259**(3-4): p. 277-89.
304.   Wong, K.Y., et al., *Dietary exposure to heterocyclic amines in a Chinese population.* Nutr Cancer, 2005. **52**(2): p. 147-55.
305.   Layton, D.W., et al., *Cancer risk of heterocyclic amines in cooked foods: an analysis and implications for research.* Carcinogenesis, 1995. **16**(1): p. 39-52.
306.   Sinha, R., et al., *Heterocyclic amine content in beef cooked by different methods to varying degrees of doneness and gravy made from meat drippings.* Food Chem Toxicol, 1998. **36**(4): p. 279-87.
307.   Henkel, J., *Sugar Substitutes, Americans Opt for Sweetness and Lite'* FDA Consumer, 1999(Nov-Dec): p. 12-16.
308.   Gallus, S., et al., *Artificial sweeteners and cancer risk in a network of case-control studies.* Ann Oncol, 2007. **18**(1): p. 40-44.

309.   Weihrauch, M.R. and V. Diehl, *Artificial sweeteners--do they bear a carcinogenic risk?* Ann Oncol, 2004. **15**(10): p. 1460-5.

310.   Fowler, S., Williams, K etal. *Diet Soft Drink Consumption is Associated with Increased Incidence of Overweight and Obesity in the San Antonio Heart Study.* in American Diabetic Association 65th Annual Assembly. 2005.
       311. Dhingra, R., et al, *Soft Drink Consumption and Risk of Developing Cardiometabolic Risk Factors and the Metabolic Syndrome in Middle-Aged Adults in the Community.* Circulation, 2007.

312.   Davidson, T.L. and S.E. Swithers, *A Pavlovian approach to the problem of obesity.* Int J Obes Relat Metab Disord, 2004. **28**(7): p. 933-5.

313.   Pierce, WD. *Overeating by Young Obese-prone and Lean Rats Caused by Tastes Associated with Low Energy Foods.* Obesity 2007:15:1969-79.

PART THREE

DIET AND THE 7 KEY METABOLIC PROCESSES

DIET AND THE SEVEN KEY METABOLIC PROCESSES

In Part 3, we introduce and examine seven fundamental metabolic processes with wide-ranging health consequences:

- Inflammation
- Blood clotting
- Cholesterol metabolism
- Fat accumulation
- Insulin metabolism
- Oxidative stress
- Cellular replication

Balanced regulation of *each* of these key processes is crucial for optimal health. The standard American diet, by promoting *imbalance in all seven* of these metabolic processes, predisposes Americans to the "Big 7" epidemic U.S. diseases.

DIET AND INFLAMMATION

Key concepts you should take away from this chapter
• Persistent inflammation predisposes to development of the Big 7 U.S. epidemic diseases • The standard American diet promotes inflammation **Specifically:** • Excessive consumption of ω-6 fatty acids and relative deficiency of ω-3 fatty acids promotes inflammation • Consumption of trans fatty acids promotes inflammation • Relative deficiency of monounsaturated fatty acids promotes inflammation • Excessive consumption of non-fiber carbohydrates and relative deficiency of fiber promotes inflammation • Consumption of polyphenolic antioxidants reduces inflammation • Consumption of certain toxins, including PCBs and mercury, promotes inflammation • Moderate intake of alcohol, especially antioxidant-rich red wines and ales, reduces inflammation • Excess abdominal fat accumulation promotes inflammation

INFLAMMATION IN HEALTH AND DISEASE

The role of persistent low-grade inflammation in the development of a wide range of chronic diseases, from heart disease to Alzheimer's dementia to depression, has become well-established over the last two decades [1-3]. In fact, tissue damage resulting from unchecked inflammation is perhaps the *primary* underlying process involved in *all* of the Big 7 U.S. epidemic diseases, as well as the primary driver of the aging process [4-6]. Inflammation, or increased activity of the immune system, is a complex process involving a variety of mechanisms that converge by triggering the release of potent pro-inflammatory mediators [3]. These inflammatory mediators account for the redness, warmth, swelling, and pain at the site of a new injury, and stimulate immune cells to destroy invading bacteria and viruses [7].

While infection is the classic instigator, a wide variety of stimuli can instigate an inflammatory response. Whatever the initiating event, the immune system responds in the same manner, by releasing a limited number of potent inflammatory mediators [6]. Although these mediators are essential for fighting off infections, *excessive* production leads to unnecessary tissue damage. Persistent over-activity of the immune system, as evidenced by high levels of inflammatory mediators, plays a key role in development of the Big 7 epidemic U.S. diseases [4-6].

Author's Note: *Inflammation is a primary determinant of the "Big 7" U.S. epidemic diseases.*

Three categories of inflammatory mediators play important roles in the development of the Big 7 U.S. epidemic diseases: arachidonic acid metabolites, pro-inflammatory cytokines, and acute phase proteins.

Pro-inflammatory Mediator Classes

CLASS	MEDIATORS	ABBREVIATIONS
Arachidonic acid metabolites (ArA)	Leukotriene B4, Thromboxane A2, Prostaglandin E2	LTB4, TXA2, PGE2
Cytokines	Interleukin-1, Interleukin-6, Tumor Necrosis Factor	IL-1, IL-6, TNF
Acute phase proteins	C-reactive protein, fibrinogen	CRP, fibrinogen

INFLAMMATORY BALANCE

Pro-inflammatory and *anti*-inflammatory mediators are in a constant struggle to determine the "inflammatory balance." Generally, when an instigating inflammatory stimulus is removed, anti-inflammatory mediators regain control and inflammation resolves. However, when the balance shifts towards excessive inflammation, tissue damage results. If an imbalance persists, chronic inflammatory mediated tissue damage and fibrosis occur, ultimately leading to disease [5, 6]. Depending on the organs or tissues involved, this imbalance may manifest as diverse diseases [4, 6].

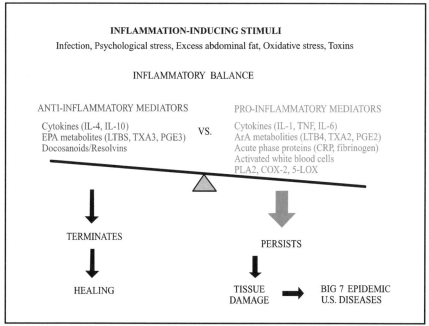

INFLAMMATION-INDUCING STIMULI
Infection, Psychological stress, Excess abdominal fat, Oxidative stress, Toxins

INFLAMMATORY BALANCE

ANTI-INFLAMMATORY MEDIATORS

Cytokines (IL-4, IL-10)
EPA metabolites (LTBS, TXA3, PGE3)   VS.
Docosanoids/Resolvins

PRO-INFLAMMATORY MEDIATORS

Cytokines (IL-1, TNF, IL-6)
ArA metabolities (LTB4, TXA2, PGE2)
Acute phase proteins (CRP, fibrinogen)
Activated white blood cells
PLA2, COX-2, 5-LOX

TERMINATES

PERSISTS

HEALING

TISSUE
DAMAGE

BIG 7 EPIDEMIC
U.S. DISEASES

Figure 1: Inflammatory Balance and the three step paradigm describing the common mechanism of chronic progressive diseases. RED signifies pro-inflammatory properties, BLUE signifies anti-inflammatory properties. Adapted from Forrester [6].

Inflammatory Mediators Involved in Development of the Big 7 Epidemic U.S. Diseases

Heart Disease	LTB4, TXA2, IL-1,IL-6, TNF, CRP, fibrinogen
Diabetes mellitus	IL-6, CRP
Alzheimer's dementia	PGE2,TXA2, IL-1,IL-6, TNF, CRP
Arthritis*	PGE2, LTB4, Il-1, IL-6, TNF, CRP
Depression	PGE2, IL-1, IL-6, TNF, CRP
Breast, Colon, Prostate Cancer	PGE2, LTB4, CRP **(colon)**
Obesity	**

[1-3, 8-39]* Includes both rheumatoid and degenerative arthritis. **Excess adipose tissue releases inflammatory mediators that predispose to disease.

PRO-INFLAMMATORY ω-6 ARACHIDONIC ACID METABOLITES

Omega-6 arachidonic acid (ArA), which is present in both plasma and cell membranes, can be converted to pro-inflammatory hormone-like mediators known as eicosonoids via the action of two enzymes known as 5-lipoxygenase (5-LOX) and cyclooxygenase (COX) [41].

ω-6 ARACHIDONIC ACID CASCADE

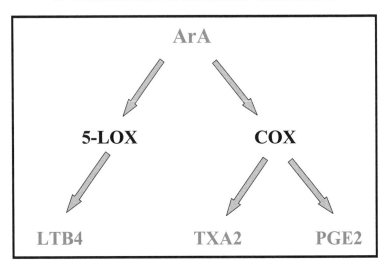

Figure 2: Arachidonic acid cascade. The enzymes 5-lipoxygenase (5-LOX) and cyclooxygenases (COX-1 and COX-2) convert ω-6 arachidonic acid into pro-inflammatory mediators. The red color of LTB4, TXA2, and PGE2 signifies pro-inflammatory properties.

The arachidonic acid metabolites LTB4, TXA2 and PGE2 favor inflammation, tissue destruction, blood clotting, and cell growth and division[8-19]. Excessive production of these compounds contributes to the development of several of the Big 7 epidemic diseases.

ω-6 Arachidonic Acid Metabolites and Disease

ArA Metabolite	Function	Associated diseases
Leukotriene B4 (LTB4)	Immune cell activation, tissue damage, fibrosis, cartilage degradation, coronary plaque rupture, pain, swelling	Heart disease and heart attack, rheumatoid and degenerative arthritis, Alzheimer's dementia, various cancers
Thromboxane A2 (TXA2)	Blood clotting (platelet aggregation), vasoconstriction, immune cell activation	Heart attack, stroke, Alzheimer's dementia
Prostaglandin E2 (PGE2)	Pain, cartilage degradation, bone resorption, cell growth and division, angiogenesis	Breast, colon, prostate cancers, Rheumatoid and degenerative arthritis, osteoporosis, depression, Alzheimer's dementia

[8-19, 40, 41]

PRO-INFLAMMATORY CYTOKINES

A transcription factor is a protein that acts as a "switch" to "turn on" the expression of certain genes [42, 43]. One nuclear factor in particular, known as *Nuclear Factor-Kappa B* (NF-kB), plays an especially important role in coordinating the inflammatory response to stressors [42-44]. NF-kB has been described as a "smoke sensor" because it is activated by a wide variety of stressful stimuli including infection, inflammatory mediators, oxidative stress, toxins, and psychological stress [42, 43]. Whatever the initiating stimulus, activation results in expression of a vast array of inflammatory genes, including the key pro-inflammatory cytokines interleukin-1 (IL-1), tumor necrosis factor (TNF), and interleukin-6 (IL-6) [42, 44]. Pro-inflammatory cytokines are signaling molecules that initiate, amplify, and perpetuate the inflammatory response [45]. Via this mechanism, unrestrained NF-kB activation and pro-inflammatory cytokine activation cause tissue destruction and disease [46-51]. Exaggerated pro-inflammatory cytokine responses play a key role in development and progression of the Big 7 U.S. epidemic diseases [47-49].

Pro-inflammatory Cytokines and Disease

Cytokine	Function	Associated diseases
Interleukin-1 (IL-1)	Immune cell activation, tissue damage, fibrosis, cartilage degradation, coronary plaque rupture, pain, swelling, promotes inflammatory mediator production (PLA2, 5-LOX, COX-2, LTB4, TXA2, PGE2, CRP), anhedonia, lethargy	Heart disease and heart attack, stroke, rheumatoid and degenerative arthritis, Alzheimer's dementia, depression
Tumor Necrosis Factor (TNF)	Immune cell activation, tissue damage, fibrosis, cartilage degradation, coronary plaque rupture, pain, swelling, promotes inflammatory mediator production (PLA2, 5-LOX, COX-2, LTB4, TXA2, PGE2, CRP), angiogenesis	Heart disease and heart attack, rheumatoid arthritis, Alzheimer's dementia, depression, certain cancers
Interleukin-6 (IL-6)	Stimulates production of CRP and fibrinogen, promotes insulin resistance	Heart disease, heart attack, rheumatoid arthritis, diabetes, Alzheimer's dementia and cognitive decline, depression

[2, 3, 17, 20-26, 28]

PRO-INFLAMMATORY C-REACTIVE PROTEIN (CRP)

C-reactive protein (CRP), a molecule involved in innate immunity and inflammation, is secreted by the liver in response to circulating IL-6 and, to a lesser extent, IL-1 and TNF [52, 53]. Plasma CRP levels, which are normally low, can increase up to 100-fold within 24-72 hours in response to cytokine (IL-6, IL-1, TNFa) -mediated reaction to infection or inflammation. Thus, CRP is a highly sensitive, but nonspecific, marker of even low grade inflammation [54]. As such, CRP levels are commonly used to monitor the activity of various inflammatory diseases. For instance, rising CRP levels in a patient with rheumatoid arthritis may correlate with a disease exacerbation or poor response to treatment. In addition, CRP directly damages blood vessels and other tissues [55, 56].

Elevated CRP levels predict higher overall mortality, as well as an increased risk of developing the Big 7 U.S. epidemic diseases [1, 32-36]. CRP may be a stronger predictor of heart attack than even LDL "bad" cholesterol levels [1]. Strikingly, modest CRP elevations may predict the risk of developing Alzheimer's disease 25 years later [31]!

C-reactive Protein and Disease

	Function	Associated diseases
C-reactive protein (CRP)	Attracts and activates immune cells, stimulates phagocytosis of pathogens and release of cytokines, activates platelets and blood vessels, promotes coronary plaque rupture	Heart disease, heart attack, stroke, Alzheimer's dementia, prediabetes, diabetes, rheumatoid and degenerative arthritis, depression

[1, 31-36, 38, 39, 52, 55, 57, 58]

DIET AND INFLAMMATION

Dietary molecules regulate the inflammatory response to noxious stimuli. Certain dietary constituents prime the immune system to overreact and generate disproportionate quantities of inflammatory mediators in response to minor stressors. Excessive accumulation of these mediators favors tissue destruction and disease. Other nutrients suppress misguided inflammatory responses and allow the immune system to mount a precise and self-limited response to threats. Without all the extra distractions, a balanced immune system can focus on legitimate threats and appropriately eliminate toxins and infections while minimizing unnecessary tissue damage.

Several features of the typical American diet promote constant misdirected inflammation, unnecessary tissue damage, and ultimately contribute to disease and premature death.

INFLAMMATORY PROPERTIES OF THE 15 DIETARY MOLECULAR CATEGORIES

POLYUNSATURATED FATS AND INFLAMMATION

The characteristic American dietary pattern of polyunsaturated fatty acid intake: massive ω-6 LA, moderate ArA, and deficient ω-3 ALA, EPA, and DHA, results in blood and tissue "ArA overload." (See pages 110-113). Excessive blood and tissue ArA accumulation favors generation of pro-inflammatory ArA metabolites.

A significant portion of dietary ω-6 LA is converted to its long-chain pro-inflammatory counterpart ω-6 arachidonic acid (ArA) by the human liver and other tissues [60]. Via this mechanism, massive U.S. intake of ω-6 linoleic acid (LA) contributes to characteristic American blood and tissue "ArA overload" [61].

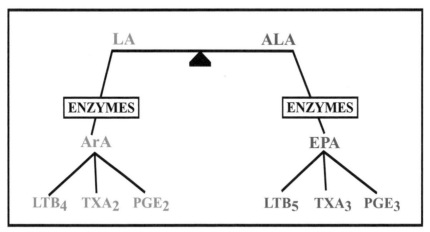

Figure 3: Dietary ω-6 LA and ω-3 ALA compete for the *same* enzymes which ultimately convert them to hormone-like mediators known as eicosaniods. In general, eicosaniods derived from ω-6 LA are pro-inflammatory, while those derived from ω-3 ALA are comparatively anti-inflammatory.

Because ω-3 alpha linolenic acid (ALA) blocks conversion of ω-6 LA to pro-inflammatory ArA, deficient U.S. dietary ω-3 ALA intake magnifies "ArA overload" [61]. Like ω-3 ALA, ω-3 EPA and DHA reduce conversion of ω-6 LA to pro-inflammatory ArA [62, 63]. In addition, ω-3 EPA competes *directly* with ω-6 ArA throughout the body [63-65]. Membrane and plasma ω-3 EPA can be derived directly from dietary EPA or converted from its precursor ω-3 ALA. Like ω-6 arachidonic acid, ω-3 EPA is converted to mediators by 5-LOX and COX [63, 66].

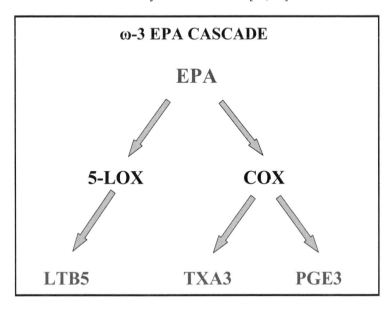

ω-3 EPA CASCADE

EPA

5-LOX   **COX**

LTB5   **TXA3**   **PGE3**

Figure 4: Eicosapentaenoic acid cascade. The enzymes 5-lipoxygenase (5-LOX) and cyclooxygenases (COX-1 and COX-2) convert eicosapentaenoic acid into eicosanoids with little or no inflammatory activity. The blue color of LTB5, TXA3, and PGE3 signifies that ω-3 EPA-derived mediators are anti-inflammatory in comparison to ω-6 ArA-derived mediators.

However, although ω-3 EPA-derived mediators are similar in shape to ω-6 ArA-derived mediators, they are anti-inflammatory and anticoagulant in comparison [63, 67-74].

By competing with ω-6 ArA, ω-3 EPA limits generation of pro-inflammatory mediators [66]. Thus, dietary deficiency of EPA and DHA further magnifies ω-6 "ArA overload"[63]. The net effect of consuming ω-3 EPA, and to a lesser extent ω-3 ALA, is reduced inflammation [63, 67].

Interestingly, the 22 carbon ω-3 fatty acid DHA, which can be consumed directly, or synthesized from dietary EPA or ALA, has been shown to generate a new class of compounds termed "docosanoids" with potent anti-inflammatory and neuroprotective attributes [75-78]. These actions may account for some of the preventative and mitigating properties of DHA in Alzheimer's dementia, depression, and other diseases [77, 79-84]. In addition, by inhibiting NF-kB and via other mechanisms, ω-3 EPA and DHA reduce production of the pro-inflammatory cytokines IL-1, IL-6, and TNF [67, 85-100].

Thus, the characteristic American dietary pattern of excessive ω-6 LA (and ArA) and deficient intake of ω-3 ALA, EPA, and DHA generates "ArA overload" and ultimately disproportionate ArA-derived eicosanoids (LTB4, TXA2, PGE2), pro-inflammatory cytokines (IL-1, TNF, IL-6) and acute phase proteins. Limiting intake of ω-6 LA and ArA and boosting intake of ω-3 ALA, EPA, and DHA reduces inflammation and can prevent or mitigate disease.

MONOUNSATURATED FATS (MUFAs) AND INFLAMMATION

Oleic acid and other monounsaturated fatty acids reduce generation of the potent pro-inflammatory ArA metabolite known as leukotriene B4 [101-107]. Therefore, fruits, nuts, and oils rich in oleic acid but deficient in ω-6 linoleic acid have anti-inflammatory properties. Excellent examples include avocados, olives and olive oil, macadamias, almonds, and cashews [108]. Likewise, replacing ω-6 LA-rich safflower, sunflower, corn, cottonseed, and soybean oils with oleic acid-rich olive oil suppresses inflammation.

TRANS FATS AND INFLAMMATION

Trans fatty acids increase production of pro-inflammatory cytokines and acute phase proteins via unknown mechanisms [109-111]. Reduction or elimination of trans fats from the diet can have *profound* anti-inflammatory effects.

CARBOHYDRATES AND INFLAMMATION

On average, Americans consume 16 times as many non-fiber carbohydrates as fiber, more than 3 times the ratio consumed throughout most of the history of mankind (see Part 2, page 65). Excessive non-fiber carbohydrate and inadequate fiber intake increases generation of pro-inflammatory cytokines and acute-phase proteins including IL-6, TNF,

CRP, and fibrinogen [112-116]. Increasing fiber intake and reducing sugar and starch intake can reduce systemic inflammation.

PHYTOCHEMICALS AND INFLAMMATION

Polyphenolic antioxidants from certain fruits, vegetables, spices, and teas interfere with the conversion of ω-6 arachidonic acid into pro-inflammatory metabolites by blocking 5-lipoxygenase (5-LOX) and cyclooxygenase (COX) enzymes. Polyphenolic antioxidants also reduce production of pro-inflammatory cytokines, phospholipase A2 (PLA2), 5-LOX, COX-2, and other important inflammatory proteins by blocking NF-kB activation [117, 118]. Antioxidants with especially potent anti-inflammatory actions include curcumin (turmeric, curry powder), hydroxytyrosol (olives), capsaicin (hot pepper), anthocyanins (berries), quercetin (onions, apples, tea), salicylates (fruits, vegetables, spices), resveratrol (red wine), and EGCG (green tea) [80, 119-134]. These and other anti-inflammatory actions likely account for the strong inverse association between dietary antioxidant capacity and C-reactive protein levels [118]. Habitual consumption of a variety of foods and beverages rich in polyphenolic antioxidants can have profound anti-inflammatory properties.

DIETARY TOXINS AND INFLAMMATION

Consumption of PCBs, mercury, and other toxins promotes inflammatory mediator production [135-137].

ALCOHOL AND INFLAMMATION

Moderate alcohol consumption, especially red wines and ales, inhibits NF-kB activation and reduces generation of the pro-inflammatory cytokines and acute phase proteins IL-1, TNF, IL-6, and CRP [138-142].

ABDOMINAL FAT ACCUMULATION AND INFLAMMATION

Individuals have highly variable amounts of abdominal fat stores ranging from a few milliliters to six liters [143]. Like immune cells, fat cells secrete the pro-inflammatory cytokines IL-1, TNF, and IL-6 during times of stress [115, 144, 145]. Importantly, fat cells that surround abdominal organs secrete far greater amounts of cytokines than other fat cells [144]. Via this mechanism, excess fat, especially abdominal fat, contributes to systemic inflammation and disease [4].

Inflammatory Properties of Dietary Molecular Categories

	NF-kB Activation	Pro-inflammatory ω-6 ArA metabolites (LTB4, TXA2,PGE2)	Pro-inflammatory cytokines (IL-1, IL-6, TNF)	Pro-inflammatory acute phase proteins (CRP, fibrinogen)
Monounsaturated fats	−	↓	↓	−
ω-6 Linoleic acid	↑	↑↑	↑	−
ω-6 Arachidonic acid	↑	↑↑↑	↑	−
ω-3 Alpha linolenic acid	↓	↓↓	↓	↓
ω-3 EPA + DHA	↓↓↓	↓↓↓	↓↓↓	↓
Trans fats	−	−	↑↑↑	↑
Nonfiber Carbohydrates	↑	−	↑	↑
Fiber	↓	−	↓	↓↓↓
Polyphenolic antioxidants	↓	↓↓↓	↓	↓
Toxins: PCBs, mercury	↑	−	↑	↑
Alcohol (Moderate)	↓	↓	↓	↓

Chart Key: ↑, ↑, and ↑ signify mild, moderate, and profound pro-inflammatory properties. ↓, ↓, and ↓ signify mild, moderate, and profound anti-inflammatory properties. The chart represents *long-term* dietary intake. Saturated fats, dietary cholesterol, protein, sodium, and artificial sweeteners have minimal or unknown effects on inflammation. Chart References: throughout text and [73, 146, 147].

SUMMARY

Excessive consumption of pro-inflammatory dietary molecules, especially ω-6 LA and ArA, trans fats, and non-fiber carbohydrates by most Americans contributes to inflammatory-mediated disease. Relative deficiencies of anti-inflammatory dietary molecules, especially ω-3 ALA, EPA and DHA, MUFAs, fibers, and polyphenolic antioxidants, further contributes to uncontrolled inflammation and disease. Boosting intake of ω-3 ALA, EPA and DHA, MUFAs, fiber, and polyphenolic antioxidants while limiting ω-6 LA and ArA, trans fats, toxins, and NFCs can reduce inflammation and the risk of developing the Big 7 diseases.

References

1. Ridker, P.M., *High-sensitivity C-reactive protein, inflammation, and cardiovascular risk: from concept to clinical practice to clinical benefit.* Am Heart J, 2004. **148**(1 Suppl): p. S19-26.
2. Dziedzic, T., *Systemic inflammatory markers and risk of dementia.* Am J Alzheimers Dis Other Demen, 2006. **21**(4): p. 258-62.
3. Schiepers, O.J., M.C. Wichers, and M. Maes, *Cytokines and major depression.* Prog Neuropsychopharmacol Biol Psychiatry, 2005. **29**(2): p. 201-17.
4. Bengmark, S., *Acute and "chronic" phase reaction-a mother of disease.* Clin Nutr, 2004. **23**(6): p. 1256-66.
5. Finch, C.E. and E.M. Crimmins, *Inflammatory exposure and historical changes in human life-spans.* Science, 2004. **305**(5691): p. 1736-9.
6. Forrester, J.S., *Common ancestors: chronic progressive diseases have the same pathogenesis.* Clin Cardiol, 2004. **27**(4): p. 186-90.
7. Kumar, V., Abbas, AK etal, *Robbins and Cotran: Pathologic Basis of Disease, Seventh edition.* 2005, Philadelphia: Elsevier Inc.
8. Radmark, O., *5-lipoxygenase-derived leukotrienes: mediators also of atherosclerotic inflammation.* Arterioscler Thromb Vasc Biol, 2003. **23**(7): p. 1140-2.
9. Dwyer, J.H., et al., *Arachidonate 5-lipoxygenase promoter genotype, dietary arachidonic acid, and atherosclerosis.* N Engl J Med, 2004. **350**(1): p. 29-37.
10. Henderson, B., E.R. Pettipher, and G.A. Higgs, *Mediators of rheumatoid arthritis.* Br Med Bull, 1987. **43**(2): p. 415-28.
11. Dogne, J.M., J. Hanson, and D. Pratico, *Thromboxane, prostacyclin and isoprostanes: therapeutic targets in atherogenesis.* Trends Pharmacol Sci, 2005. **26**(12): p. 639-44.
12. Scali, C., et al., *Neutrophils CD11b and fibroblasts PGE(2) are elevated in Alzheimer's disease.* Neurobiol Aging, 2002. **23**(4): p. 523-30.
13. Minghetti, L., *Cyclooxygenase-2 (COX-2) in inflammatory and degenerative brain diseases.* J Neuropathol Exp Neurol, 2004. **63**(9): p. 901-10.
14. Kojima, F., S. Kato, and S. Kawai, *Prostaglandin E synthase in the pathophysiology of arthritis.* Fundam Clin Pharmacol, 2005. **19**(3): p. 255-61.
15. Mezzetti, A., *Pharmacological modulation of plaque instability.* Lupus, 2005. **14**(9): p. 769-72.
16. Chen, X., et al., *Five-lipoxygenase pathway of arachidonic acid metabolism in carcino-genesis and cancer chemoprevention.* Curr Cancer Drug Targets, 2006. **6**(7): p. 613-22.
17. Maes, M., *Evidence for an immune response in major depression: a review and hypothesis.* Prog Neuropsychopharmacol Biol Psychiatry, 1995. **19**(1): p. 11-38.
18. Furstenberger, G., et al., *What are cyclooxygenases and lipoxygenases doing in the driver's seat of carcinogenesis?* Int J Cancer, 2006. **119**(10): p. 2247-54.
19. Marks, F., K. Muller-Decker, and G. Furstenberger, *A causal relationship between unscheduled eicosanoid signaling and tumor development: cancer chemoprevention by inhibitors of arachidonic acid metabolism.* Toxicology, 2000. **153**(1-3): p. 11-26.
20. Woods, A., et al., *Genetics of inflammation and risk of coronary artery disease: the central role of interleukin-6.* Eur Heart J, 2000. **21**(19): p. 1574-83.
21. Biasucci, L.M., et al., *Increasing levels of interleukin (IL)-1Ra and IL-6 during the first 2 days of hospitalization in unstable angina are associated with increased risk of in-hospital coronary events.* Circulation, 1999. **99**(16): p. 2079-84.
22. Ridker, P.M., et al., *Elevation of tumor necrosis factor-alpha and increased risk of recurrent coronary events after myocardial infarction.* Circulation, 2000. **101**(18): p. 2149-53.
23. Kolb, H. and T. Mandrup-Poulsen, *An immune origin of type 2 diabetes?* Diabetologia, 2005. **48**(6): p. 1038-50.
24. Pickup, J.C., *Inflammation and activated innate immunity in the pathogenesis of type 2 diabetes.* Diabetes Care, 2004. **27**(3): p. 813-23.
25. Cacquevel, M., et al., *Cytokines in neuroinflammation and Alzheimer's disease.* Curr Drug Targets, 2004. **5**(6): p. 529-34.
26. Maes, M., *Major depression and activation of the inflammatory response system.* Adv Exp Med Biol, 1999. **461**: p. 25-46.
27. Field, M., et al., *Interleukin-6 localisation in the synovial membrane in rheumatoid arthritis.* Rheumatol Int, 1991. **11**(2): p. 45-50.
28. Eastgate, J.A., et al., *Correlation of plasma interleukin 1 levels with disease activity in rheumatoid arthritis.* Lancet, 1988. 2(8613): p. 706-9.
29. Grundy, S.M., *Inflammation, metabolic syndrome, and diet responsiveness.* Circulation, 2003. **108**(2): p. 126-8.
30. Hu, F.B., et al., *Inflammatory markers and risk of developing type 2 diabetes in women.* Diabetes, 2004. **53**(3): p. 693-700.
31. Schmidt, R., et al., *Early inflammation and dementia: a 25-year follow-up of the Honolulu-Asia Aging Study.* Ann Neurol, 2002. **52**(2): p. 168-74.
32. Kuo, H.K., et al., *Relation of C-reactive protein to stroke, cognitive disorders, and depression in the general population: systematic review and meta-analysis.* Lancet Neurol, 2005. **4**(6): p. 371-80.

33. Masi, A.T., J.C. Aldag, and J. Sipes, *Do elevated levels of serum C-reactive protein predict rheumatoid arthritis in men: correlations with pre-RA status and baseline positive rheumatoid factors.* J Rheumatol, 2001. **28**(10): p. 2359-61.
34. Nielen, M.M., et al., *Increased levels of C-reactive protein in serum from blood donors before the onset of rheumatoid arthritis.* Arthritis Rheum, 2004. **50**(8): p. 2423-7.
35. Sowers, M., et al., *C-reactive protein as a biomarker of emergent osteoarthritis.* Osteoarthritis Cartilage, 2002. **10**(8): p. 595-601.
36. Erlinger, T.P., et al., *C-reactive protein and the risk of incident colorectal cancer.* Jama, 2004. **291**(5): p. 585-90.
37. Kop, W.J., et al., *Inflammation and coagulation factors in persons > 65 years of age with symptoms of depression but without evidence of myocardial ischemia.* Am J Cardiol, 2002. **89**(4): p. 419-24.
38. Ford, D.E. and T.P. Erlinger, *Depression and C-reactive protein in US adults: data from the Third National Health and Nutrition Examination Survey.* Arch Intern Med, 2004. **164**(9): p. 1010-4.
39. Penninx, B.W., et al., *Inflammatory markers and depressed mood in older persons: results from the Health, Aging and Body Composition study.* Biol Psychiatry, 2003. **54**(5): p. 566-72.
40. Sugaya, K., et al., *New anti-inflammatory treatment strategy in Alzheimer's disease.* Jpn J Pharmacol, 2000. **82**(2): p. 85-94.
41. Funk, C.D., *Prostaglandins and leukotrienes: advances in eicosanoid biology.* Science, 2001. **294**(5548): p. 1871-5.
42. Lee, J.I. and G.J. Burckart, *Nuclear factor kappa B: important transcription factor and therapeutic target.* J Clin Pharmacol, 1998. **38**(11): p. 981-93.
43. Ahn, K.S. and B.B. Aggarwal, *Transcription Factor NF-{kappa}B: A Sensor for Smoke and Stress Signals.* Ann N Y Acad Sci, 2005. **1056**: p. 218-33.
44. Nam, N.H., *Naturally occurring NF-kappaB inhibitors.* Mini Rev Med Chem, 2006. **6**(8): p. 945-51.
45. Park, W.Y., et al., *Cytokine balance in the lungs of patients with acute respiratory distress syndrome.* Am J Respir Crit Care Med, 2001. **164**(10 Pt 1): p. 1896-903.
46. Arend, W.P. and C. Gabay, *Cytokines in the rheumatic diseases.* Rheum Dis Clin North Am, 2004. **30**(1): p. 41-67, v-vi.
47. Brand, K., et al., *Activated transcription factor nuclear factor-kappa B is present in the atherosclerotic lesion.* J Clin Invest, 1996. **97**(7): p. 1715-22.
48. Kaltschmidt, B., et al., *Transcription factor NF-kappaB is activated in primary neurons by amyloid beta peptides and in neurons surrounding early plaques from patients with Alzheimer disease.* Proc Natl Acad Sci U S A, 1997. **94**(6): p. 2642-7.
49. Roshak, A.K., et al., *Manipulation of distinct NFkappaB proteins alters interleukin-1beta-induced human rheumatoid synovial fibroblast prostaglandin E2 formation.* J Biol Chem, 1996. **271**(49): p. 31496-501.
50. Sakurada, S., T. Kato, and T. Okamoto, *Induction of cytokines and ICAM-1 by proinflammatory cytokines in primary rheumatoid synovial fibroblasts and inhibition by N-acetyl-L-cysteine and aspirin.* Int Immunol, 1996. **8**(10): p. 1483-93.
51. Borish, L.C. and J.W. Steinke, *2. Cytokines and chemokines.* J Allergy Clin Immunol, 2003. **111**(2 Suppl): p. S460-75.
52. Du Clos, T.W. and C. Mold, *C-reactive protein: an activator of innate immunity and a modulator of adaptive immunity.* Immunol Res, 2004. **30**(3): p. 261-77.
53. Volanakis, J.E., *Human C-reactive protein: expression, structure, and function.* Mol Immunol, 2001. **38**(2-3): p. 189-97.
54. Chait, A., et al., *Thematic review series: The immune system and atherogenesis. Lipoprotein-associated inflammatory proteins: markers or mediators of cardiovascular disease?* J Lipid Res, 2005. **46**(3): p. 389-403.
55. Wilson, A.M., M.C. Ryan, and A.J. Boyle, *The novel role of C-reactive protein in cardiovascular disease: risk marker or pathogen.* Int J Cardiol, 2006. **106**(3): p. 291-7.
56. Willerson, J.T. and P.M. Ridker, *Inflammation as a cardiovascular risk factor.* Circulation, 2004. **109**(21 Suppl 1): p. II2-10.
57. Szalai, A.J., *The antimicrobial activity of C-reactive protein.* Microbes Infect, 2002. **4**(2): p. 201-5.
58. Gershov, D., et al., *C-Reactive protein binds to apoptotic cells, protects the cells from assembly of the terminal complement components, and sustains an antiinflammatory innate immune response: implications for systemic autoimmunity.* J Exp Med, 2000. **192**(9): p. 1353-64.
59. Merchant, A.T., et al., *Intake of n-6 and n-3 fatty acids and fish and risk of community-acquired pneumonia in US men.* Am J Clin Nutr, 2005. **82**(3): p. 668-74.
60. Hussein, N., et al., *Long-chain conversion of [13C]linoleic acid and alpha-linolenic acid in response to marked changes in their dietary intake in men.* J Lipid Res, 2005. **46**(2): p. 269-80.
61. Budowski, P. and M.A. Crawford, *a-Linolenic acid as a regulator of the metabolism of arachidonic acid: dietary implications of the ratio, n-6:n-3 fatty acids.* Proc Nutr Soc, 1985. **44**(2): p. 221-9.
62. Emken, E.A., *Nutrition and biochemistry of trans and positional fatty acid isomers in hydrogenated oils.* Annu Rev Nutr, 1984. **4**: p. 339-76.
63. Lands, W.E., *Dietary fat and health: the evidence and the politics of prevention: careful use of dietary fats can improve life and prevent disease.* Ann N Y Acad Sci, 2005. **1055**: p. 179-92.
64. Li, B., C. Birdwell, and J. Whelan, *Antithetic relationship of dietary arachidonic acid and eicosapentaenoic acid on eicosanoid production in vivo.* J Lipid Res, 1994. **35**(10): p. 1869-77.
65. Iritani, N. and S. Fujikawa, *Competitive incorporation of dietary omega-3 and omega-6 polyunsaturated fatty acids into the tissue phospholipids in rats.* J Nutr Sci Vitaminol (Tokyo), 1982. **28**(6): p. 621-9.
66. Kinsella, J.E., K.S. Broughton, and J.W. Whelan, *Dietary unsaturated fatty acids: interactions and possible needs in relation to eicosanoid synthesis.* J Nutr Biochem, 1990. **1**(3): p. 123-41.
67. Gil, A., *Polyunsaturated fatty acids and inflammatory diseases.* Biomed Pharmacother, 2002. **56**(8): p. 388-96.

68.   Goldman, D.W., W.C. Pickett, and E.J. Goetzl, *Human neutrophil chemotactic and degranulating activities of leukotriene B5 (LTB5) derived from eicosapentaenoic acid.* Biochem Biophys Res Commun, 1983. **117**(1): p. 282-8.

69.   Hawkes, J.S., M.J. James, and L.G. Cleland, *Separation and quantification of PGE3 following derivatization with panacyl bromide by high pressure liquid chromatography with fluorometric detection.* Prostaglandins, 1991. **42**(4): p. 355-68.

70.   Hawkes, J.S., M.J. James, and L.G. Cleland, *Biological activity of prostaglandin E3 with regard to oedema formation in mice.* Agents Actions, 1992. **35**(1-2): p. 85-7.

71.   Simopoulos, A.P., *Omega-3 fatty acids in inflammation and autoimmune diseases.* J Am Coll Nutr, 2002. **21**(6): p. 495-505.

72.   James, M.J., et al., *Interaction between fish and vegetable oils in relation to rat leucocyte leukotriene production.* J Nutr, 1991. **121**(5): p. 631-7.

73.   Camandola, S., et al., *Nuclear factor kB is activated by arachidonic acid but not by eicosapentaenoic acid.* Biochem Biophys Res Commun, 1996. **229**(2): p. 643-7.

74.   Serhan, C.N., *Novel omega -- 3-derived local mediators in anti-inflammation and resolution.* Pharmacol Ther, 2005. **105**(1): p. 7-21.

75.   Hong, S., et al., *Novel docosatrienes and 17S-resolvins generated from docosahexaenoic acid in murine brain, human blood, and glial cells. Autacoids in anti-inflammation.* J Biol Chem, 2003. **278**(17): p. 14677-87.

76.   Serhan, C.N., *Novel eicosanoid and docosanoid mediators: resolvins, docosatrienes, and neuroprotectins.* Curr Opin Clin Nutr Metab Care, 2005. **8**(2): p. 115-21.

77.   Marcheselli, V.L., et al., *Novel docosanoids inhibit brain ischemia-reperfusion-mediated leukocyte infiltration and pro-inflammatory gene expression.* J Biol Chem, 2003. **278**(44): p. 43807-17.

78.   Mukherjee, P.K., et al., *Neuroprotectin D1: a docosahexaenoic acid-derived docosatriene protects human retinal pigment epithelial cells from oxidative stress.* Proc Natl Acad Sci U S A, 2004. **101**(22): p. 8491-6.

79.   Freund-Levi, Y., et al., *Omega-3 fatty acid treatment in 174 patients with mild to moderate Alzheimer disease: OmegAD study: a randomized double-blind trial.* Arch Neurol, 2006. **63**(10): p. 1402-8.

80.   Cheong, E., et al., *Synthetic and naturally occurring COX-2 inhibitors suppress proliferation in a human oesophageal adenocarcinoma cell line (OE33) by inducing apoptosis and cell cycle arrest.* Carcinogenesis, 2004. **25**(10): p. 1945-52.

81.   McNamara, R.K., et al., *Selective Deficits in the Omega-3 Fatty Acid Docosahexaenoic Acid in the Postmortem Orbitofrontal Cortex of Patients with Major Depressive Disorder.* Biol Psychiatry, 2006.

82.   Raeder, M.B., et al., *Associations between cod liver oil use and symptoms of depression: The Hordaland Health Study.* J Affect Disord, 2006.

83.   Schaefer, E.J., et al., *Plasma phosphatidylcholine docosahexaenoic acid content and risk of dementia and Alzheimer disease: the Framingham Heart Study.* Arch Neurol, 2006. **63**(11): p. 1545-50.

84.   Kiecolt-Glaser, J.K., et al., *Depressive symptoms, omega-6:omega-3 fatty acids, and inflammation in older adults.* Psychosom Med, 2007. **69**(3): p. 217-24.

85.   Rola-Pleszczynski, M. and I. Lemaire, *Leukotrienes augment interleukin 1 production by human monocytes.* J Immunol, 1985. **135**(6): p. 3958-61.

86.   Denys, A., A. Hichami, and N.A. Khan, *n-3 PUFAs modulate T-cell activation via protein kinase C-alpha and -epsilon and the NF-kappaB signaling pathway.* J Lipid Res, 2005. **46**(4): p. 752-8.

87.   Meydani, S.N., et al., *Immunologic effects of national cholesterol education panel step-2 diets with and without fish-derived N-3 fatty acid enrichment.* J Clin Invest, 1993. **92**(1): p. 105-13.

88.   Endres, S., et al., *The effect of dietary supplementation with n-3 polyunsaturated fatty acids on the synthesis of interleukin-1 and tumor necrosis factor by mononuclear cells.* N Engl J Med, 1989. **320**(5): p. 265-71.

89.   Kremer, J.M., et al., *Dietary fish oil and olive oil supplementation in patients with rheumatoid arthritis. Clinical and immunologic effects.* Arthritis Rheum, 1990. **33**(6): p. 810-20.

90.   Meydani, S.N., et al., *Oral (n-3) fatty acid supplementation suppresses cytokine production and lymphocyte proliferation: comparison between young and older women.* J Nutr, 1991. **121**(4): p. 547-55.

91.   Molvig, J., et al., *Dietary supplementation with omega-3-polyunsaturated fatty acids decreases mononuclear cell proliferation and interleukin-1 beta content but not monokine secretion in healthy and insulin-dependent diabetic individuals.* Scand J Immunol, 1991. **34**(4): p. 399-410.

92.   Cooper, A.L., et al., *Effect of dietary fish oil supplementation on fever and cytokine production in human volunteers.* Clin Nutr, 1993. **12**(6): p. 321-8.

93.   Robinson, D.R., et al., *Dietary marine lipids suppress continuous expression of interleukin-1 beta gene transcription.* Lipids, 1996. **31 Suppl**: p. S23-31.

94.   Gallai, V., et al., *Cytokine secretion and eicosanoid production in the peripheral blood mononuclear cells of MS patients undergoing dietary supplementation with n-3 polyunsaturated fatty acids.* J Neuroimmunol, 1995. **56**(2): p. 143-53.

95.   Caughey, G.E., et al., *The effect on human tumor necrosis factor alpha and interleukin 1 beta production of diets enriched in n-3 fatty acids from vegetable oil or fish oil.* Am J Clin Nutr, 1996. **63**(1): p. 116-22.

96.   Wu, D., et al., *Effect of concomitant consumption of fish oil and vitamin E on production of inflammatory cytokines in healthy elderly humans.* Ann N Y Acad Sci, 2004. **1031**: p. 422-4.

97.   Trebble, T., et al., *Inhibition of tumour necrosis factor-alpha and interleukin 6 production by mononuclear cells following dietary fish-oil supplementation in healthy men and response to antioxidant co-supplementation.* Br J Nutr, 2003. **90**(2): p. 405-12.

98.   Zampelas, A., et al., *Fish consumption among healthy adults is associated with decreased levels of inflammatory markers related to cardiovascular disease: the ATTICA study.* J Am Coll Cardiol, 2005. **46**(1): p. 120-4.

99. Ciubotaru, I., Y.S. Lee, and R.C. Wander, *Dietary fish oil decreases C-reactive protein, interleukin-6, and triacylglycerol to HDL-cholesterol ratio in postmenopausal women on HRT.* J Nutr Biochem, 2003. **14**(9): p. 513-21.
100. Lopez-Garcia, E., et al., *Consumption of (n-3) fatty acids is related to plasma biomarkers of inflammation and endothelial activation in women.* J Nutr, 2004. **134**(7): p. 1806-11.
101. James, M.J., R.A. Gibson, and L.G. Cleland, *Dietary polyunsaturated fatty acids and inflammatory mediator production.* Am J Clin Nutr, 2000. **71**(1 Suppl): p. 343S-8S.
102. Jakschik, B.A., A.R. Morrison, and H. Sprecher, *Products derived from 5,8,11-eicosatrienoic acid by the 5-lipoxygenase-leukotriene pathway.* J Biol Chem, 1983. **258**(21): p. 12797-800.
103. Stenson, W.F., S.M. Prescott, and H. Sprecher, *Leukotriene B formation by neutrophils from essential fatty acid-deficient rats.* J Biol Chem, 1984. **259**(19): p. 11784-9.
104. Cleland, L.G., et al., *Inhibition of human neutrophil leukotriene B4 synthesis in essential fatty acid deficiency: role of leukotriene A hydrolase.* Lipids, 1994. **29**(3): p. 151-5.
105. Cleland, L.G., et al., *Dietary (n-9) eicosatrienoic acid from a cultured fungus inhibits leukotriene B4 synthesis in rats and the effect is modified by dietary linoleic acid.* J Nutr, 1996. **126**(6): p. 1534-40.
106. James, M.J., et al., *Effect of dietary supplementation with n-9 eicosatrienoic acid on leukotriene B4 synthesis in rats: a novel approach to inhibition of eicosanoid synthesis.* J Exp Med, 1993. **178**(6): p. 2261-5.
107. Radmark, O., et al., *Leukotriene A4 hydrolase in human leukocytes. Purification and properties.* J Biol Chem, 1984. **259**(20): p. 12339-45.
108. U.S. Department of Agriculture, A.R.S. *USDA Nutrient Database for Standard Reference. Release 18, Nutrient Data Laboratory Home Page.* [cited Jan 1, 2006 Available from: http://www.nal.usda.gov/fnic/foodcomp.
109. Han, S.N., et al., *Effect of hydrogenated and saturated, relative to polyunsaturated, fat on immune and inflammatory responses of adults with moderate hypercholesterolemia.* J Lipid Res, 2002. **43**(3): p. 445-52.
110. Lopez-Garcia, E., et al., *Consumption of trans fatty acids is related to plasma biomarkers of inflammation and endothelial dysfunction.* J Nutr, 2005. **135**(3): p. 562-6.
111. Mozaffarian, D., et al., *Dietary intake of trans fatty acids and systemic inflammation in women.* Am J Clin Nutr, 2004. **79**(4): p. 606-12.
112. Kirwan, J.P., et al., *Human aging is associated with altered TNF-alpha production during hyperglycemia and hyperinsulinemia.* Am J Physiol Endocrinol Metab, 2001. **281**(6): p. E1137-43.
113. King, D.E., B.M. Egan, and M.E. Geesey, *Relation of dietary fat and fiber to elevation of C-reactive protein.* Am J Cardiol, 2003. **92**(11): p. 1335-9.
114. Liu, S., et al., *Relation between a diet with a high glycemic load and plasma concentrations of high-sensitivity C-reactive protein in middle-aged women.* Am J Clin Nutr, 2002. **75**(3): p. 492-8.
115. McCarty, M.F., *Low-insulin-response diets may decrease plasma C-reactive protein by influencing adipocyte function.* Med Hypotheses, 2005. **64**(2): p. 385-7.
116. Ajani, U.A., E.S. Ford, and A.H. Mokdad, *Dietary fiber and C-reactive protein: findings from national health and nutrition examination survey data.* J Nutr, 2004. **134**(5): p. 1181-5.
117. Hoshiko, S., O. Radmark, and B. Samuelsson, *Characterization of the human 5-lipoxygenase gene promoter.* Proc Natl Acad Sci U S A, 1990. **87**(23): p. 9073-7.
118. Brighenti, F., et al., *Total antioxidant capacity of the diet is inversely and independently related to plasma concentration of high-sensitivity C-reactive protein in adult Italian subjects.* Br J Nutr, 2005. **93**(5): p. 619-25.
119. Ringman, J.M., et al., *A potential role of the curry spice curcumin in Alzheimer's disease.* Curr Alzheimer Res, 2005. **2**(2): p. 131-6.
120. Funk, J.L., et al., *Efficacy and mechanism of action of turmeric supplements in the treatment of experimental arthritis.* Arthritis Rheum, 2006. **54**(11): p. 3452-64.
121. Bengmark, S., *Curcumin, an atoxic antioxidant and natural NFkappaB, cyclooxygenase-2, lipooxygenase, and inducible nitric oxide synthase inhibitor: a shield against acute and chronic diseases.* JPEN J Parenter Enteral Nutr, 2006. **30**(1): p. 45-51.
122. Kim, C.S., et al., *Capsaicin exhibits anti-inflammatory property by inhibiting IkB-a degradation in LPS-stimulated peritoneal macrophages.* Cell Signal, 2003. **15**(3): p. 299-306.
123. Hou, D.X., et al., *Anthocyanidins inhibit cyclooxygenase-2 expression in LPS-evoked macrophages: structure-activity relationship and molecular mechanisms involved.* Biochem Pharmacol, 2005. **70**(3): p. 417-25.
124. Xu, X.M., et al., *Suppression of inducible cyclooxygenase 2 gene transcription by aspirin and sodium salicylate.* Proc Natl Acad Sci U S A, 1999. **96**(9): p. 5292-7.
125. Wu, K.K., et al., *Aspirin inhibits interleukin 1-induced prostaglandin H synthase expression in cultured endothelial cells.* Proc Natl Acad Sci U S A, 1991. **88**(6): p. 2384-7.
126. Mutoh, M., et al., *Suppression by flavonoids of cyclooxygenase-2 promoter-dependent transcriptional activity in colon cancer cells: structure-activity relationship.* Jpn J Cancer Res, 2000. **91**(7): p. 686-91.
127. Baumann, J., F. von Bruchhausen, and G. Wurm, *Flavonoids and related compounds as inhibition of arachidonic acid peroxidation.* Prostaglandins, 1980. **20**(4): p. 627-39.
128. Subbaramaiah, K., et al., *Resveratrol inhibits cyclooxygenase-2 transcription and activity in phorbol ester-treated human mammary epithelial cells.* J Biol Chem, 1998. **273**(34): p. 21875-82.
129. de la Lastra, C.A. and I. Villegas, *Resveratrol as an anti-inflammatory and anti-aging agent: mechanisms and clinical implications.* Mol Nutr Food Res, 2005. **49**(5): p. 405-30.
130. Hussain, T., et al., *Green tea constituent epigallocatechin-3-gallate selectively inhibits COX-2 without affecting COX-1 expression in human prostate carcinoma cells.* Int J Cancer, 2005. **113**(4): p. 660-9.
131. Ahmed, S., et al., *Green tea polyphenol epigallocatechin-3-gallate inhibits the IL-1 beta-induced activity and expression of cyclooxygenase-2 and nitric oxide synthase-2 in human chondrocytes.* Free Radic Biol Med, 2002. **33**(8): p. 1097-105.

132. Kundu, J.K., et al., *Inhibition of phorbol ester-induced COX-2 expression by epigallocatechin gallate in mouse skin and cultured human mammary epithelial cells.* J Nutr, 2003. **133**(11 Suppl 1): p. 3805S-3810S.

133. Petroni, A., et al., *Inhibition of leukocyte leukotriene B4 production by an olive oil-derived phenol identified by mass-spectrometry.* Thromb Res, 1997. **87**(3): p. 315-22.

134. de la Puerta, R., V. Ruiz Gutierrez, and J.R. Hoult, *Inhibition of leukocyte 5-lipoxygenase by phenolics from virgin olive oil.* Biochem Pharmacol, 1999. **57**(4): p. 445-9.

135. Hennig, B., et al., *Proinflammatory properties of coplanar PCBs: in vitro and in vivo evidence.* Toxicol Appl Pharmacol, 2002. **181**(3): p. 174-83.

136. Hennig, B., et al., *PCB-induced oxidative stress in endothelial cells: modulation by nutrients.* Int J Hyg Environ Health, 2002. **205**(1-2): p. 95-102.

137. Monnet-Tschudi, F., et al., *Involvement of environmental mercury and lead in the etiology of neurodegenerative diseases.* Rev Environ Health, 2006. **21**(2): p. 105-17.

138. Mandrekar, P., D. Catalano, and G. Szabo, *Inhibition of lipopolysaccharide-mediated NFkappaB activation by ethanol in human monocytes.* Int Immunol, 1999. **11**(11): p. 1781-90.

139. Blanco-Colio, L.M., et al., *Red wine intake prevents nuclear factor-kappaB activation in peripheral blood mononuclear cells of healthy volunteers during postprandial lipemia.* Circulation, 2000. **102**(9): p. 1020-6.

140. Szabo, G., P. Mandrekar, and D. Catalano, *Inhibition of superantigen-induced T cell proliferation and monocyte IL-1 beta, TNF-alpha, and IL-6 production by acute ethanol treatment.* J Leukoc Biol, 1995. **58**(3): p. 342-50.

141. Nelson, S., et al., *The effects of acute and chronic alcoholism on tumor necrosis factor and the inflammatory response.* J Infect Dis, 1989. **160**(3): p. 422-9.

142. Volpato, S., et al., *Relationship of alcohol intake with inflammatory markers and plasminogen activator inhibitor-1 in well-functioning older adults: the Health, Aging, and Body Composition study.* Circulation, 2004. **109**(5): p. 607-12.

143. Thomas, E.L., et al., *Magnetic resonance imaging of total body fat.* J Appl Physiol, 1998. **85**(5): p. 1778-85.

144. Fried, S.K., D.A. Bunkin, and A.S. Greenberg, *Omental and subcutaneous adipose tissues of obese subjects release interleukin-6: depot difference and regulation by glucocorticoid.* J Clin Endocrinol Metab, 1998. **83**(3): p. 847-50.

145. Maachi, M., et al., *Systemic low-grade inflammation is related to both circulating and adipose tissue TNFalpha, leptin and IL-6 levels in obese women.* Int J Obes Relat Metab Disord, 2004. **28**(8): p. 993-7.

146. Hennig, B., et al., *Linoleic acid activates nuclear transcription factor-kappa B (NF-kappa B) and induces NF-kappa B-dependent transcription in cultured endothelial cells.* Am J Clin Nutr, 1996. **63**(3): p. 322-8.

147. Yerneni, K.K., et al., *Hyperglycemia-induced activation of nuclear transcription factor kappaB in vascular smooth muscle cells.* Diabetes, 1999. **48**(4): p. 855-64.

DIET AND BLOOD CLOTTING

Key Concepts you should take away from this chapter:
• The formation of blood clots in arteries and veins, *known as thrombosis*, plays a key role in the development of heart attacks, strokes, and other thrombotic diseases • The standard American diet promotes thrombosis **Specifically:** • Excessive consumption of ω-6 and relative deficiency of ω-3 fatty acids promotes thrombosis • Consumption of trans fatty acids promotes thrombosis • Excessive consumption of saturated fats and relative deficiency of monounsaturated fats promotes thrombosis • Excessive consumption of non-fiber carbohydrates and relative deficiency of fiber promotes thrombosis • Consumption of polyphenolic antioxidants reduces thrombosis • Moderate alcohol consumption reduces thrombosis • Excess abdominal fat accumulation promotes thrombosis

BACKGROUND AND TERMINOLOGY

Blood *clotting*, also known as **coagulation**, refers to the transformation of blood from a liquid to a solid state. **Platelets**, small disk-shaped structures capable of clumping together, or *aggregating*, are the major players involved in blood clotting. *Pro*-coagulant mediators stimulate platelets to aggregate; *anti*-coagulant mediators prevent platelet aggregation. Excessive activity of pro-coagulant mediators or insufficient activity of anti-coagulant mediators can lead to **thrombosis**, or formation of a blood clot in an artery or vein. Arterial thrombosis plays a crucial role in both heart attacks and ischemic strokes, two of the three major U.S. causes of death [1-3].

COAGULATION BALANCE

"Coagulation balance" refers to the delicate equilibrium between pro-coagulant and anti-coagulant forces necessary for maintaining optimal blood flow to tissues. Tipping the balance toward excessive anti-coagulant mediators leads to bleeding while tipping the balance toward excessive pro-coagulant mediators leads to thrombosis.

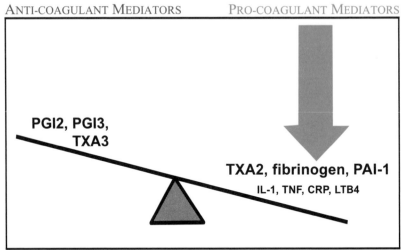

Figure 1: Coagulation Balance.

In general, U.S. coagulation balance has tipped markedly towards coagulation and thrombosis, which helps explain the epidemic nature of heart attacks, strokes, and other thrombotic diseases [4-7].

INFLAMMATION AND THROMBOSIS

Thrombosis and inflammation are intimately related, and several inflammatory mediators promote thrombosis and vice versa [4, 8, 9]. Important dual pro-inflammatory and pro-thrombotic mediators influenced by the diet include fibrinogen, C-reactive protein (CRP), pro-inflammatory cytokines (IL-1, IL-6, TNF), plasminogen activator inhibitor (PAI-1), and thromboxane A2 (TXA2).

FIBRINOGEN, C-REACTIVE PROTEIN, AND INFLAMMATORY CYTOKINES

Fibrinogen, like C-reactive protein, is an acute phase protein released by the liver in response to inflammatory stimuli. During an inflammatory response, circulating IL-6 and other pro-inflammatory cytokines stimulate the liver to secrete fibrinogen, which increases 2 to 20-fold. When inflammation subsides, fibrinogen levels return to normal. However, in chronic inflammatory states plasma fibrinogen stays elevated indefinitely.

Fibrinogen binds platelets and promotes platelet aggregation, and when activated, traps these aggregated platelets and red blood cells to form a clot [7]. In addition, fibrinogen is the primary determinant of plasma viscosity, a feature closely correlated with risk of thrombotic diseases [10]. Via these mechanisms, even modest elevations of fibrinogen increase the risk of heart attack and stroke [11-15]. In addition, fibrinogen and other inflammatory mediators including CRP, IL-1 and TNF activate the cells lining the inner walls of blood vessels, known as endothelial cells. Because endothelial cell activation favors local blood clot formation, these inflammatory mediators *indirectly* promote thrombosis [16, 17].

PLASMINOGEN ACTIVATOR INHIBITOR-1

Most clots are quickly dissolved in a process called fibrinolysis, which restores normal blood flow. However, abdominal fat cells secrete large amounts of a protein known as plasminogen activator inhibitor-1 (PAI-1), which inhibits the *destruction* of blood clots. Fat cell secretion of PAI-1 partly accounts for the increased risk of heart attack, stroke, and other thrombotic diseases in overweight and obese individuals [18-20].

THROMBOXANE A2

Upon platelet stimulation, enzymes known as cyclooxygenases (COX) convert membrane ω-6 arachidonic acid (ArA) to thromboxane A2 (TXA2), a mediator with potent platelet aggregatory effects [21-23]. Via this mechanism, accumulation of ω-6 ArA predisposes to thrombosis.

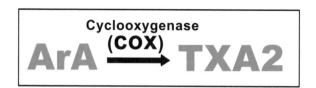

Figure 2: ω-6 Arachidonate is converted to thromboxaneA2 by the enzyme cyclooxygenase.

DIETARY NUTRIENTS AND COAGULATION BALANCE

Because inflammation and thrombosis are intimately related processes, and many mediators have dual pro-inflammatory and pro-thrombotic properties, several of the same dietary imbalances that promote persistent inflammation also promote thrombosis. The remainder of this section explores which characteristics of the standard U.S. diet promote thrombotic disease, and suggests dietary strategies for restoring balance.

OMEGA-6 AND OMEGA-3 IMBALANCE AND THROMBOSIS

The standard American dietary pattern of excessive ω-6 linoleic acid (LA) and ArA consumption, coupled with a deficient intake of ω-3 ALA, EPA and DHA, results in ArA accumulation in platelets, plasma, adipose tissue, and other tissues. This "ArA Overload" promotes platelet aggregation and favors thrombosis during periods of inflammation or oxidative stress [24, 25].

Dietary intake of ω-3 ALA, EPA and DHA, especially when combined with *long-term* reduction of ω-6 LA and ArA intake, results in partial replacement of ω-6 ArA with ω-3 EPA in plasma as well as platelet membranes [26-29]. EPA-enriched platelets release TXA3 in place of ArA-derived TXA2 [30]. Unlike ω-6 ArA-derived TXA2, TXA3 has minimal platelet aggregatory effects [21, 30-32]. Thus, in comparison to ArA-enriched platelets, EPA-enriched platelets have reduced net thrombotic tendency [21, 22, 29-34].

Plasma levels of ω-3 EPA and DHA and ω-6 ArA vary dramatically across populations with different dietary patterns [21, 26, 31, 34-42]. As extreme examples, contrast the high ω-6, low ω-3 diets of Americans which result in an ArA:EPA ratio of approximately 22 to 1, the relatively high ω-3, low ω-6 diets of rural Japanese or modern Greenland Eskimos which result in a ArA:EPA ratio of about 1 to 1, and the very high ω-3, low ω-6 diets of *traditional* Greenland Eskimos studied by Dyerberg in 1975 with an ArA:EPA ratio of 1 to 9 [26, 35].

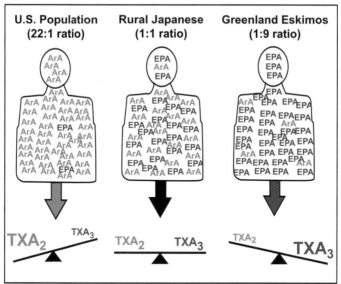

Figure 3: Illustration of the remarkable differences in plasma ArA and EPA among populations consuming vastly different diets. The red colors of ArA and TXA2 reflect pro-coagulant properties; the blue colors of EPA and TXA3 reflect their comparatively anti-coagulant properties.

Thus, "ArA Overload" seen in the U.S. population above results in disproportionate TXA2 production and *promotes* platelet aggregation while EPA accumulation in the other populations *prevents* platelet aggregation. In fact, the traditional Eskimo population studied by Dyerberg had nearly *double* the bleeding time as their western counterparts. In some cases, aspirin administration actually shortened the bleeding time [21]! (see Addendum and Figure 5, page 116). This reduced platelet aggregation protects traditional Greenland Eskimos from thrombotic diseases [43].

Like plasma ω-3 EPA and DHA and ω-6 ArA levels, large cross-cultural differences in coronary heart disease (CHD) rates exist, with CHD mortality ranging from 20 to 200 deaths per 100,000 people each year [35, 40-42]. A strong inverse association between dietary, blood, and tissue levels of EPA and DHA and coronary heart disease mortality has been demonstrated across multiple populations and individuals [26, 35-37, 40-50]. Depending on dietary characteristics, ArA accounts for between 10% and 96% of plasma twenty carbon polyunsaturated fatty acids (total ArA plus EPA). Intriguingly, plasma ArA:EPA ratios are inversely associated with CHD mortality rates in a near linear fashion [21, 26, 35-42, 49, 50]!

Plasma ω-6 ArA and ω-3 EPA as a Percentage of Total ArA + EPA, ArA:EPA Ratio, and Cardiovascular Disease Mortality

Population	ω-6 ArA	ω-3 EPA	ArA/ EPA Ratio	CHD- Related Deaths
Caucasian American	96%	4%	22:1	Very High
Japanese American	93%	7%	13:1	High
Quebecers (Urban Canadian)	93%	7%	13:1	High
Swedish	92%	8%	11:1	Moderate
Spanish	87%	13%	7:1	Moderate
Urban Japan	69%	31%	2:1	Low
Inuit Nunavik	67%	33%	2:1	Low
Rural Japan (elders)	56%	44%	1:1	Very Low
Greenland Inuit (2001)	52%	48%	1:1	Very Low
Greenland Eskimos (1975)	10%	90%	1:9	Very, Very Low

[26, 35-42]

Of note, the highest recorded plasma ArA:EPA ratio of 40 to 1, belonging to a Danish population with known CHD, was nearly 400 times as high as the Greenland Eskimo population examined by Dyerberg in 1975 [39]! Higher plasma ArA:EPA ratios in younger generations of Eskimos and Japanese reflect the westernization of dietary habits, with less fish and more linoleic acid intake than their elder counterparts [35, 36, 44].

Dietary intakes of the short-chain polyunsaturated fatty acids ALA and LA can alter the plasma ArA:EPA ratio [27, 28, 51]. In the Lyon Diet Heart Study, the plasma ArA:EPA ratio of the experimental group following a ω-3 ALA-rich, low LA Mediterranean diet, dropped from 9.1:1 to 6.8:1 while no change was observed in the control group consuming the standard high LA, low ALA western diet. Interestingly, this drop in the ArA:EPA ratio was accompanied by a 55-65% reduction in CHD events and overall mortality despite minimal changes in serum cholesterol levels [51-54]!

Like plasma, *platelet* membrane ArA and EPA concentrations vary widely amongst different populations, with ArA:EPA ratios ranging from a high of 45:1 in western populations to a low of 1:1 in some Eskimo populations [31, 33]. *Long-term* dietary replacement of ω-6 LA and ArA with ω-3 ALA, EPA and DHA has the potential to markedly reduce the ArA:EPA ratio, TXA2 production, and the risk of thrombotic disease [21, 26, 28, 30, 31, 33, 45, 55-57]. This shift away from a prothrombotic state is believed to partially account for the much lower risk of cardiovascular death seen in traditional Eskimos compared with western counterparts [43].

When combined with established anti-inflammatory and anti-arrythmic properties, the anti-thrombotic attributes of ω-3 EPA and DHA help explain the strong inverse relationships between dietary fatty fish or fish oil consumption, plasma and tissue EPA and DHA, and CHD mortality across and amongst multiple populations [40-42, 44, 45, 47-50, 58-62].

TRANS FATS

Trans fats increase thrombotic tendency by multiple mechanisms [63, 64]. These pro-thrombotic effects, when coupled with adverse effects on inflammation, cholesterol metabolism, and insulin metabolism, may account for the robust association between trans fat intake and CHD mortality [65].

SATURATED FATS

Saturated fatty acids, and stearic acid (18:0) in particular, may promote platelet aggregation and coronary thrombosis [66]. This relationship helps explain the positive correlation between excessive saturated fat intake and coronary heart disease, which remains after adjusting for effects on blood cholesterol [48, 66].

MONOUNSATURATED FATS (MUFAs)

Long-term consumption of MUFAs reduces the risk of thrombosis via inhibiting platelet aggregation and a variety of other mechanisms [67-69]. Thus, replacement of trans and saturated fats with MUFAs may reduce thrombotic diseases.

CARBOHYDRATES

On average, Americans consume more than sixteen grams of non-fiber carbohydrates (NFC) for every gram of fiber. These low fiber, high NFC diets increase blood glucose and insulin responses, elevate plasma fibrinogen, and promote thrombosis [70-72]. Conversely, high intake of fiber, especially soluble fiber, has been associated with reductions in both fibrinogen and PAI-1 levels, and reduced risk of venous thrombosis, heart attack, and stroke. [73-79].

POLYPHENOLIC ANTIOXIDANTS

Polyphenolic antioxidants, salicylates, and other phytochemicals present in plant-derived foods, especially fruits, vegetables, spices, teas, and dark chocolate, inhibit platelet aggregation by blocking conversion of arachidonic acid into TXA2 via COX-1 inhibition [80-91]. Habitual consumption of foods and beverages rich in these phytochemicals tips the coagulation balance away from thrombosis and may contribute to the well-known cardioprotective effects of plant-derived foods.

ALCOHOL

Light to moderate alcohol consumption inhibits platelet aggregation and reduces fibrinogen levels, two mechanisms which may account for its cardioprotective properties [92-94]. However, benefits of alcohol must be weighed against increased risk of alcoholism, breast cancer, violent behavior, and motor vehicle accidents [65].

ABDOMINAL FAT, INFLAMMATION, AND THROMBOSIS

Abdominal fat tissue contributes to a pro-thrombotic state by secreting large amounts of PAI-1 and pro-inflammatory cytokines, which in turn leads to elevated blood levels of fibrinogen [93, 95]. These mechanisms may account for the strong association between excess abdominal fat and heart attacks, strokes, and deep venous thrombosis.

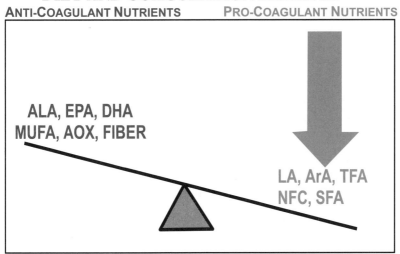

DIET AND COAGULATION BALANCE

ANTI-COAGULANT NUTRIENTS | **PRO-COAGULANT NUTRIENTS**

**ALA, EPA, DHA
MUFA, AOX, FIBER**

**LA, ArA, TFA
NFC, SFA**

Figure 4: Nutrients and Coagulation Balance. Excessive U.S. consumption of pro-coagulant nutrients coupled with deficient intake of anti-coagulant nutrients favors development of thrombotic disease.

SUMMARY

In conclusion, scientific advances have clearly demonstrated a strong correlation exists between diet, coagulation balance, and thrombosis. These differences can be vast, as illustrated by the enormous differences between populations consuming dissimilar diets. By reducing pro-thrombotic features of the American diet, Americans can restore a more natural coagulation balance. Beneficial dietary changes include:

- Long-term reduction of the ω-3 LA to ω-3 ALA ratio to no more than 4 to 1
- Increasing ω-3 EPA and DHA, while limiting ω-6 ArA intake
- Reducing or eliminating consumption of trans fatty acids
- Reducing saturated fatty acid intake, while boosting MUFA consumption
- Increasing consumption of fiber, while reducing the NFC to fiber ratio
- Increasing consumption of fruits, vegetables, spices, teas, dark chocolate, and other foods rich in polyphenolic antioxidants, salicylates, and other beneficial compounds

Author's Note: Paradoxical Decrease In Bleeding Times Of Greenland Eskimos After Aspirin Administration: *For the sake of simplicity, the above chapter listed TXA2 as the sole ω-6 ArA-derived mediator of platelet aggregation. In reality, the situation is more complex. Activated platelets chiefly convert PLA2-released ArA to TXA2. However, endothelial cells mainly convert ArA to prostacyclin (PGI2), an eicosanoid with anti-aggregatory and vasodilatory effects which counter some of the effects of TXA2. In contrast, ω-3 EPA enriched platelets and endothelial cells convert EPA into TXA3 and PGI3 respectively [21, 32]. Because TXA3 has little or no pro-coagulant properties, and PGI3 and PGI2 have equivalent anti-coagulant properties, partial substitution of EPA for ArA results in reduced net thrombotic tendency [21, 32].*

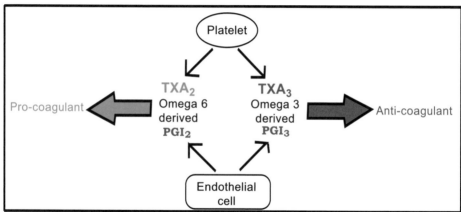

Figure 5: Partial substitution of omega-6 ArA with omega-3 EPA reduces the formation of TXA2, interferes with platelet aggregation, and increases bleeding time. The red color signifies platelet aggregation; the blue color signifies reduced platelet aggregation.

ASPIRIN AND BLEEDING TIME

By reducing the potent pro-thrombotic mediator TXA2 and moderately anti-thrombotic mediator PGI2, aspirin administration to an individual with classic "ArA Overload" results in a net reduction of platelet aggregation and increases bleeding time. In contrast, by reducing formation of minimally active TXA3 and moderately anti-thrombotic PGI3, aspirin may actually reduce bleeding time in an individual consuming a very high ω-3, low ω-6 diet [21].

References:

1. Farb, A., et al., *Sudden coronary death. Frequency of active coronary lesions, inactive coronary lesions, and myocardial infarction.* Circulation, 1995. **92**(7): p. 1701-9.
2. Davies, M.J. and A. Thomas, *Thrombosis and acute coronary-artery lesions in sudden cardiac ischemic death.* N Engl J Med, 1984. **310**(18): p. 1137-40.
3. Lewandowski, C. and W. Barsan, *Treatment of acute ischemic stroke.* Ann Emerg Med, 2001. **37**(2): p. 202-16.
4. Devaraj, S., R.S. Rosenson, and I. Jialal, *Metabolic syndrome: an appraisal of the pro-inflammatory and procoagulant status.* Endocrinol Metab Clin North Am, 2004. **33**(2): p. 431-53, table of contents.
5. Appel, S.J., J.S. Harrell, and M.L. Davenport, *Central obesity, the metabolic syndrome, and plasminogen activator inhibitor-1 in young adults.* J Am Acad Nurse Pract, 2005. **17**(12): p. 535-41.
6. Nieuwdorp, M., et al., *Hypercoagulability in the metabolic syndrome.* Curr Opin Pharmacol, 2005. **5**(2): p. 155-9.
7. Vorster, H.H., J.H. Cummings, and F.J. Veldman, *Diet and haemostasis: time for nutrition science to get more involved.* Br J Nutr, 1997. **77**(5): p. 671-84.
8. Kannel, W.B., *Overview of hemostatic factors involved in atherosclerotic cardiovascular disease.* Lipids, 2005. **40**(12): p. 1215-20.
9. Danese, S., E. Dejana, and C. Fiocchi, *Immune regulation by microvascular endothelial cells: directing innate and adaptive immunity, coagulation, and inflammation.* J Immunol, 2007. **178**(10): p. 6017-22.
10. Woodward, M., et al., *Does sticky blood predict a sticky end? Associations of blood viscosity, haematocrit and fibrinogen with mortality in the West of Scotland.* Br J Haematol, 2003. **122**(4): p. 645-50.
11. Scarabin, P.Y., et al., *Associations of fibrinogen, factor VII and PAI-1 with baseline findings among 10,500 male participants in a prospective study of myocardial infarction--the PRIME Study. Prospective Epidemiological Study of Myocardial Infarction.* Thromb Haemost, 1998. **80**(5): p. 749-56.
12. Ma, J., et al., *A prospective study of fibrinogen and risk of myocardial infarction in the Physicians' Health Study.* J Am Coll Cardiol, 1999. **33**(5): p. 1347-52.
13. Wilhelmsen, L., et al., *Fibrinogen as a risk factor for stroke and myocardial infarction.* N Engl J Med, 1984. **311**(8): p. 501-5.
14. Thompson, S.G., et al., *Hemostatic factors and the risk of myocardial infarction or sudden death in patients with angina pectoris. European Concerted Action on Thrombosis and Disabilities Angina Pectoris Study Group.* N Engl J Med, 1995. **332**(10): p. 635-41.
15. Resch, K.L., et al., *Fibrinogen and viscosity as risk factors for subsequent cardiovascular events in stroke survivors.* Ann Intern Med, 1992. **117**(5): p. 371-5.
16. Madge, L.A. and J.S. Pober, *TNF signaling in vascular endothelial cells.* Exp Mol Pathol, 2001. **70**(3): p. 317-25.
17. Verhamme, P. and M.F. Hoylaerts, *The pivotal role of the endothelium in haemostasis and thrombosis.* Acta Clin Belg, 2006. **61**(5): p. 213-9.
18. Alessi, M.C., et al., *Production of plasminogen activator inhibitor 1 by human adipose tissue: possible link between visceral fat accumulation and vascular disease.* Diabetes, 1997. **46**(5): p. 860-7.
19. Shimomura, I., et al., *Enhanced expression of PAI-1 in visceral fat: possible contributor to vascular disease in obesity.* Nat Med, 1996. **2**(7): p. 800-3.
20. Juhan-Vague, I., M.C. Alessi, and P. Vague, *Increased plasma plasminogen activator inhibitor 1 levels. A possible link between insulin resistance and atherothrombosis.* Diabetologia, 1991. **34**(7): p. 457-62.
21. Dyerberg, J. and H.O. Bang, *Lipid metabolism, atherogenesis, and haemostasis in Eskimos: the role of the prostaglandin-3 family.* Haemostasis, 1979. **8**(3-5): p. 227-33.
22. Mezzano, D., et al., *Cardiovascular risk factors in vegetarians. Normalization of hyperhomocysteinemia with vitamin B(12) and reduction of platelet aggregation with n-3 fatty acids.* Thromb Res, 2000. **100**(3): p. 153-60.
23. Elwood, P.C., et al., *Ischemic heart disease and platelet aggregation. The Caerphilly Collaborative Heart Disease Study.* Circulation, 1991. **83**(1): p. 38-44.
24. Lagarde, M., C. Calzada, and E. Vericel, *Pathophysiologic role of redox status in blood platelet activation. Influence of docosahexaenoic acid.* Lipids, 2003. **38**(4): p. 465-8.
25. Diaz, B.L. and J.P. Arm, *Phospholipase A(2).* Prostaglandins Leukot Essent Fatty Acids, 2003. **69**(2-3): p. 87-97.
26. Stark, K.D., et al., *Fatty acid compositions of serum phospholipids of postmenopausal women: a comparison between Greenland Inuit and Canadians before and after supplementation with fish oil.* Nutrition, 2002. **18**(7-8): p. 627-30.
27. Renaud, S. and M. de Lorgeril, *Dietary lipids and their relation to ischaemic heart disease: from epidemiology to prevention.* J Intern Med Suppl, 1989. **731**: p. 39-46.
28. Renaud, S., *Linoleic acid, platelet aggregation and myocardial infarction.* Atherosclerosis, 1990. **80**(3): p. 255-6.
29. Li, D., et al., *Effect of dietary alpha-linolenic acid on thrombotic risk factors in vegetarian men.* Am J Clin Nutr, 1999. **69**(5): p. 872-82.
30. Dyerberg, J., et al., *Eicosapentaenoic acid and prevention of thrombosis and atherosclerosis?* Lancet, 1978. **2**(8081): p. 117-9.
31. Dyerberg, J., *Linolenate-derived polyunsaturated fatty acids and prevention of atherosclerosis.* Nutr Rev, 1986. **44**(4): p. 125-34.
32. Dyerberg, J. and H.O. Bang, *Dietary fat and thrombosis.* Lancet, 1978. **1**(8056): p. 152.

33. Mann, N., et al., *The effect of short-term diets rich in fish, red meat, or white meat on thromboxane and prostacyclin synthesis in humans.* Lipids, 1997. **32**(6): p. 635-44.

34. Bang, H.O., J. Dyerberg, and H.M. Sinclair, *The composition of the Eskimo food in north western Greenland.* Am J Clin Nutr, 1980. **33**(12): p. 2657-61.

35. Iso, H., et al., *Serum fatty acids and fish intake in rural Japanese, urban Japanese, Japanese American and Caucasian American men.* Int J Epidemiol, 1989. **18**(2): p. 374-81.

36. Dewailly, E., et al., *n-3 Fatty acids and cardiovascular disease risk factors among the Inuit of Nunavik.* Am J Clin Nutr, 2001. **74**(4): p. 464-73.

37. Dewailly, E.E., et al., *Relations between n-3 fatty acid status and cardiovascular disease risk factors among Quebecers.* Am J Clin Nutr, 2001. **74**(5): p. 603-11.

38. Chajes, V., et al., *Comparison of fatty acid profile in plasma phospholipids in women from Granada (southern Spain) and Malmo (southern Sweden).* Int J Vitam Nutr Res, 2001. **71**(4): p. 237-42.

39. Dyerberg, J., H.O. Bang, and N. Hjorne, *Fatty acid composition of the plasma lipids in Greenland Eskimos.* Am J Clin Nutr, 1975. **28**(9): p. 958-66.

40. Lands, W.E., *Dietary fat and health: the evidence and the politics of prevention: careful use of dietary fats can improve life and prevent disease.* Ann N Y Acad Sci, 2005. **1055**: p. 179-92.

41. Lands, W.E., *Diets could prevent many diseases.* Lipids, 2003. **38**(4): p. 317-21.

42. Lands, W.E., *Primary prevention in cardiovascular disease: moving out of the shadows of the truth about death.* Nutr Metab Cardiovasc Dis, 2003. **13**(3): p. 154-64.

43. Bjerregaard, P. and J. Dyerberg, *Mortality from ischaemic heart disease and cerebrovascular disease in Greenland.* Int J Epidemiol, 1988. **17**(3): p. 514-9.

44. Iso, H., et al., *Intake of fish and n3 fatty acids and risk of coronary heart disease among Japanese: the Japan Public Health Center-Based (JPHC) Study Cohort I.* Circulation, 2006. **113**(2): p. 195-202.

45. Siscovick, D.S., et al., *Dietary intake and cell membrane levels of long-chain n-3 polyunsaturated fatty acids and the risk of primary cardiac arrest.* Jama, 1995. **274**(17): p. 1363-7.

46. Dewailly, E., et al., *Cardiovascular disease risk factors and n-3 fatty acid status in the adult population of James Bay Cree.* Am J Clin Nutr, 2002. **76**(1): p. 85-92.

47. Sugano, M. and F. Hirahara, *Polyunsaturated fatty acids in the food chain in Japan.* Am J Clin Nutr, 2000. **71**(1 Suppl): p. 189S-96S.

48. Simon, J.A., et al., *Serum fatty acids and the risk of coronary heart disease.* Am J Epidemiol, 1995. **142**(5): p. 469-76.

49. Dolecek, T.A., *Epidemiological evidence of relationships between dietary polyunsaturated fatty acids and mortality in the multiple risk factor intervention trial.* Proc Soc Exp Biol Med, 1992. **200**(2): p. 177-82.

50. Dolecek, T.A. and G. Granditis, *Dietary polyunsaturated fatty acids and mortality in the Multiple Risk Factor Intervention Trial (MRFIT).* World Rev Nutr Diet, 1991. **66**: p. 205-16.

51. de Lorgeril, M. and P. Salen, *Modified cretan mediterranean diet in the prevention of coronary heart disease and cancer: an update.* World Rev Nutr Diet, 2007. **97**: p. 1-32.

52. de Lorgeril, M. and P. Salen, *The Mediterranean diet in secondary prevention of coronary heart disease.* Clin Invest Med, 2006. **29**(3): p. 154-8.

53. de Lorgeril, M., et al., *Mediterranean dietary pattern in a randomized trial: prolonged survival and possible reduced cancer rate.* Arch Intern Med, 1998. **158**(11): p. 1181-7.

54. de Lorgeril, M., et al., *Mediterranean diet, traditional risk factors, and the rate of cardiovascular complications after myocardial infarction: final report of the Lyon Diet Heart Study.* Circulation, 1999. **99**(6): p. 779-85.

55. Hussein, N., et al., *Long-chain conversion of [13C]linoleic acid and alpha-linolenic acid in response to marked changes in their dietary intake in men.* J Lipid Res, 2005. **46**(2): p. 269-80.

56. Ferretti, A., et al., *Ingestion of marine oil reduces excretion of 11-dehydrothromboxane B2, an index of intravascular production of thromboxane A2.* Prostaglandins Leukot Essent Fatty Acids, 1993. **48**(4): p. 305-8.

57. Bemelmans, W.J., et al., *Effect of an increased intake of alpha-linolenic acid and group nutritional education on cardiovascular risk factors: the Mediterranean Alpha-linolenic Enriched Groningen Dietary Intervention (MARGARIN) study.* Am J Clin Nutr, 2002. **75**(2): p. 221-7.

58. Dwyer, J.H., et al., *Arachidonate 5-lipoxygenase promoter genotype, dietary arachidonic acid, and atherosclerosis.* N Engl J Med, 2004. **350**(1): p. 29-37.

59. Han, S.N., et al., *Effect of hydrogenated and saturated, relative to polyunsaturated, fat on immune and inflammatory responses of adults with moderate hypercholesterolemia.* J Lipid Res, 2002. **43**(3): p. 445-52.

60. Jabbar, R. and T. Saldeen, *A new predictor of risk for sudden cardiac death.* Ups J Med Sci, 2006. **111**(2): p. 169-77.

61. Reiffel, J.A. and A. McDonald, *Antiarrhythmic effects of omega-3 fatty acids.* Am J Cardiol, 2006. **98**(4A): p. 50i-60i.

62. Marchioli, R., et al., *Early protection against sudden death by n-3 polyunsaturated fatty acids after myocardial infarction: time-course analysis of the results of the Gruppo Italiano per lo Studio della Sopravvivenza nell'Infarto Miocardico (GISSI)-Prevenzione.* Circulation, 2002. **105**(16): p. 1897-903.

63. Almendingen, K., et al., *Effects of partially hydrogenated fish oil, partially hydrogenated soybean oil, and butter on hemostatic variables in men.* Arterioscler Thromb Vasc Biol, 1996. **16**(3): p. 375-80.

64. Muller, H., et al., *Partially hydrogenated soybean oil reduces postprandial t-PA activity compared with palm oil.* Atherosclerosis, 2001. **155**(2): p. 467-76.

65. Stampfer, M.J., et al., *Primary prevention of coronary heart disease in women through diet and lifestyle.* N Engl J Med, 2000. **343**(1): p. 16-22.

66. Renaud, S.C., *What is the epidemiologic evidence for the thrombogenic potential of dietary long-chain fatty acids?* Am J Clin Nutr, 1992. **56**(4 Suppl): p. 823S-824S.

67. Thomsen, C., et al., *Plasma levels of von Willebrand factor in non-insulin-dependent diabetes mellitus are influenced by dietary monounsaturated fatty acids.* Thromb Res, 1995. **77**(4): p. 347-56.
68. Smith, R.D., et al., *Long-term monounsaturated fatty acid diets reduce platelet aggregation in healthy young subjects.* Br J Nutr, 2003. **90**(3): p. 597-606.
69. Covas, M.I., *Olive oil and the cardiovascular system.* Pharmacol Res, 2007.
70. Kasim-Karakas, S.E., et al., *Responses of inflammatory markers to a low-fat, high-carbohydrate diet: effects of energy intake.* Am J Clin Nutr, 2006. **83**(4): p. 774-9.
71. Slaughter, T.F., *Hemostasis and glycemic control in the cardiac surgical patient.* Semin Cardiothorac Vasc Anesth, 2006. **10**(2): p. 176-9.
72. Lefebvre, P.J. and A.J. Scheen, *The postprandial state and risk of cardiovascular disease.* Diabet Med, 1998. **15 Suppl 4**: p. S63-8.
73. Fehily, A.M., et al., *A randomised controlled trial to investigate the effect of a high fibre diet on blood pressure and plasma fibrinogen.* J Epidemiol Community Health, 1986. **40**(4): p. 334-7.
74. Koepp, P. and S. Hegewisch, *Effects of guar on plasma viscosity and related parameters in diabetic children.* Eur J Pediatr, 1981. **137**(1): p. 31-3.
75. Landin, K., et al., *Guar gum improves insulin sensitivity, blood lipids, blood pressure, and fibrinolysis in healthy men.* Am J Clin Nutr, 1992. **56**(6): p. 1061-5.
76. Frohn, M.J., *Left-leg varicose veins and deep-vein thrombosis.* Lancet, 1976. **2**(7993): p. 1019-20.
77. Latto, C., R.W. Wilkinson, and O.J. Gilmore, *Diverticular disease and varicose veins.* Lancet, 1973. **1**(7812): p. 1089-90.
78. Lupton, J.R. and N.D. Turner, *Dietary fiber and coronary disease: does the evidence support an association?* Curr Atheroscler Rep, 2003. **5**(6): p. 500-5.
79. Pietinen, P., et al., *Intake of dietary fiber and risk of coronary heart disease in a cohort of Finnish men. The Alpha-Tocopherol, Beta-Carotene Cancer Prevention Study.* Circulation, 1996. **94**(11): p. 2720-7.
80. Leger, C.L., et al., *A thromboxane effect of a hydroxytyrosol-rich olive oil wastewater extract in patients with uncomplicated type I diabetes.* Eur J Clin Nutr, 2005. **59**(5): p. 727-30.
81. Freedman, J.E., et al., *Select flavonoids and whole juice from purple grapes inhibit platelet function and enhance nitric oxide release.* Circulation, 2001. **103**(23): p. 2792-8.
82. Keevil, J.G., et al., *Grape juice, but not orange juice or grapefruit juice, inhibits human platelet aggregation.* J Nutr, 2000. **130**(1): p. 53-6.
83. Pearson, D.A., et al., *Flavanols and platelet reactivity.* Clin Dev Immunol, 2005. **12**(1): p. 1-9.
84. Rein, D., et al., *Cocoa inhibits platelet activation and function.* Am J Clin Nutr, 2000. **72**(1): p. 30-5.
85. Murphy, K.J., et al., *Dietary flavanols and procyanidin oligomers from cocoa (Theobroma cacao) inhibit platelet function.* Am J Clin Nutr, 2003. **77**(6): p. 1466-73.
86. Naemura, A., et al., *Anti-thrombotic effect of strawberries.* Blood Coagul Fibrinolysis, 2005. **16**(7): p. 501-9.
87. Ali, M. and M. Thomson, *Consumption of a garlic clove a day could be beneficial in preventing thrombosis.* Prostaglandins Leukot Essent Fatty Acids, 1995. **53**(3): p. 211-2.
88. Higgs, G.A., et al., *Pharmacokinetics of aspirin and salicylate in relation to inhibition of arachidonate cyclooxygenase and antiinflammatory activity.* Proc Natl Acad Sci U S A, 1987. **84**(5): p. 1417-20.
89. Flower, R.J., *Drugs which inhibit prostaglandin biosynthesis.* Pharmacol Rev, 1974. **26**(1): p. 33-67.
90. Blackwell, G.J., R.J. Flower, and J.R. Vane, *Some characteristics of the prostaglandin synthesizing system in rabbit kidney microsomes.* Biochim Biophys Acta, 1975. **398**(1): p. 178-90.
91. Haynes, D.R., et al., *Is aspirin a prodrug for antioxidant and cytokine-modulating oxymetabolites?* Agents Actions, 1993. **39**(1-2): p. 49-58.
92. Renaud, S. and M. de Lorgeril, *Wine, alcohol, platelets, and the French paradox for coronary heart disease.* Lancet, 1992. **339**(8808): p. 1523-6.
93. Krobot, K., et al., *Determinants of plasma fibrinogen: relation to body weight, waist-to-hip ratio, smoking, alcohol, age, and sex. Results from the second MONICA Augsburg survey 1989-1990.* Arterioscler Thromb, 1992. **12**(7): p. 780-8.
94. Di Castelnuovo, A., L. Iacoviello, and G. de Gaetano, *Alcohol and coronary heart disease.* N Engl J Med, 2003. **348**(17): p. 1719-22; author reply 1719-22.
95. Iso, H., et al., *Antigens of tissue plasminogen activator and plasminogen activator inhibitor 1: correlates in nonsmoking Japanese and Caucasian men and women.* Thromb Haemost, 1993. **70**(3): p. 475-80.
96. Osher, E., et al., *The 5 lipoxygenase system in the vasculature: emerging role in health and disease.* Mol Cell Endocrinol, 2006. **252**(1-2): p. 201-6.

DIET AND BLOOD CHOLESTEROL METABOLISM

Key concepts you should take away from this chapter:
• Blood cholesterol dysregulation predisposes to development of heart disease, stroke, and other cardiovascular diseases   • The standard American diet promotes cholesterol dysregulation   **Specifically**:   • *Dietary* cholesterol has little meaningful impact on *blood* cholesterol status   • Consumption of even small quantities of trans fatty acids promotes blood cholesterol dysregulation   • Excessive consumption of saturated fatty acids promotes blood cholesterol dysregulation   • Excessive consumption of non-fiber carbohydrates and relative deficiency of fiber promotes blood cholesterol dysregulation   • Relative deficiency of monounsaturated fatty acids promotes blood cholesterol dysregulation   • Short-chain omega-3 and omega-6 polyunsaturated fatty acids both improve cholesterol status but unbalanced consumption may predispose to disease via other mechanisms   • Excess abdominal fat accumulation promotes cholesterol dysregulation.   • Excessive inflammation promotes cholesterol dysregulation

BLOOD CHOLESTEROL IN HEALTH AND DISEASE

Over the last half-century, the role of elevated blood cholesterol in heart disease has become well established [1]. Efforts of health promotion agencies have successfully aligned cholesterol abnormalities with heart disease in the minds of the American people. However, only half of all heart attacks and strokes occur in individuals with high cholesterol levels, suggesting that other factors are at least as important [2, 3]. For instance, in the Lyon Diet Heart Study, patients eating a Mediterranean diet rich in omega-3 fatty acids suffered 55-65% fewer cardiac deaths as those consuming a diet similar to that recommended by American health promotion agencies at the time, despite minimal differences in blood cholesterol levels between the two groups [4-6]! Scientific advances over the last two decades have clearly demonstrated that coronary heart disease advances via multiple metabolic processes including excessive inflammation and blood clotting, oxidative stress, fat accumulation, and insulin resistance, in addition to cholesterol dysregulation [7-9]. In fact, certain inflammatory mediators may be stronger predictors of cardiac events than even blood cholesterol levels [2]. Despite these advances, the majority of Americans focus solely on cholesterol modification to reduce their risk of heart disease. This overemphasis on cholesterol and lack of public appreciation for other modifiable risk factors may be partly to blame for the steady rates of coronary heart disease, which have not declined over the last two decades [10]. However, it is important to keep in mind that cholesterol dysregulation *does* play a key role in the development of cardiovascular disease, and that preventing blood cholesterol abnormalities is a crucial health intervention.

Furthermore, many Americans erroneously believe that all cholesterol is "bad." In the human body, cholesterol is a necessary precursor for synthesis of steroid hormones, vitamin D, and bile acids, as well as an essential structural component of cell membranes [11]. Because cholesterol itself is insoluble in blood, combinations of proteins, fats, and cholesterol, collectively known as lipoproteins, are necessary to deliver cholesterol to various tissues of the body. From a heart disease perspective, there are several different "good" and "bad" subtypes of lipoproteins, each of which contributes to *total* cholesterol levels. The relative *ratios* of these lipoprotein subtypes are stronger predictors of coronary events than are *total* cholesterol levels [2]. At least six different lipoprotein subtypes are known to either favor or antagonize the progression of coronary heart disease. Understanding the effects of dietary molecules on these six lipoprotein subtypes is one key to preventing coronary events.

LDL CHOLESTEROL

Low density lipoprotein, commonly referred to as LDL or "bad cholesterol," is a lipoprotein that delivers cholesterol from the liver to tissues where it is converted to cortisol, testosterone, estrogen and other hormones, or it becomes a structural component of lipid membranes. Unfortunately, elevated blood levels of LDL can lead to deposition into blood vessel walls, a process that predisposes to heart disease and is an independent risk factor of future cardiac events [1].

Recent research has demonstrated that not all LDL subtypes are equivalent in this respect. Certain subtypes of LDL, especially "small and dense" LDL, oxidized LDL, and lipoprotein A (LpA) predispose to cardiovascular disease by damaging blood vessel walls, promoting blood clotting, and increasing inflammation. Elevated levels of these subtypes are more dangerous than other subtypes of LDL [2, 12-14]. In contrast to small and dense LDL, large and buoyant LDL particles protect from coronary disease [12, 15].

LDL SUBTYPES

Small and dense LDL
Large and buoyant LDL
Oxidized LDL
Lipoprotein(a) (LpA)

HDL CHOLESTEROL

High density lipoprotein, commonly referred to as HDL or "good cholesterol," protects against cardiovascular disease by removing excess cholesterol from damaged blood vessel walls, through inhibition of blood clotting, and by acting as an antioxidant [16, 17]. While low HDL predisposes to coronary heart disease, high HDL is strongly protective, and very high HDL is associated with longevity syndrome [2, 18]. HDL levels are reduced by systemic inflammation, by excess abdominal fat accumulation, and by insulin resistance [19-23]. In this respect, HDL represents an intersection linking several important metabolic pathways.

VERY LOW DENSITY LIPOPROTEIN

Very low density lipoprotein, or VLDL, serves as a highly concentrated vehicle for transporting a type of fat known as triglycerides through the bloodstream [1]. Elevated levels of triglycerides and VLDL predispose to coronary heart disease and independently increase the risk of cardiac events [24, 25].

Simplified Consequences of High Blood Levels of Lipoprotein Subtypes

Total LDL	"Bad"
Small, dense LDL	"Very bad"
Oxidized LDL	"Bad"
Lipoprotein A (LpA)	"Bad"
Large, buoyant LDL	"Good"
HDL	"Very good"
VLDL	"Bad"

VLDL contains triglycerides

Thus, the ideal blood lipoprotein pattern for preventing coronary heart disease, stroke and other cardiovascular diseases consists of:

- Low blood *total* LDL levels
- Predominance of large, buoyant LDL particles
- Low levels of small and dense, oxidized, and LpA varieties of LDL particles
- Low levels of VLDL particles (triglycerides)
- High or very high levels of HDL

Although this overall concept may be more difficult to grasp than the simple premise that "all cholesterol is bad," it allows for a more accurate estimation of the consequences of specific dietary nutrients on cardiovascular disease risk.

> *"Things should be as simple as possible but no simpler."* -Albert Einstein

DIET AND BLOOD CHOLESTEROL

Less than 20% of all blood cholesterol abnormalities are attributable to genetics. Rather, the majority of cholesterol dysregulation represents metabolic disturbances due to poor lifestyle choices [1]. Among these lifestyle factors, diet plays the preeminent role.

DIETARY CHOLESTEROL VERSUS *BLOOD* CHOLESTEROL

In order to understand the impact of diet on cholesterol regulation, it is crucial to appreciate the distinction between *dietary* cholesterol and *blood* cholesterol.

Dietary cholesterol has little impact on overall *blood* cholesterol status [26-30]. In fact, 70% of Americans halt production of cholesterol when *dietary* cholesterol is increased [27]. Via this mechanism, even large amounts of *dietary* cholesterol have minimal impact on *blood* cholesterol levels for the majority of the population [29]. The other 30%, who are known as *dietary* cholesterol "hyper-responders," respond with blood elevations of both LDL, or "bad" cholesterol, and HDL, or "good" cholesterol, with little or no change in the LDL to HDL ratio [26]. *Dietary* cholesterol may even reduce the atherogenicity of LDL particles by increasing their size and buoyancy [29, 31]. These facts likely explain why studies have failed to demonstrate a relationship between *dietary* cholesterol and heart disease and suggest that focusing on more high-yield dietary changes may be a more valuable means of reducing cardiovascular risk [32, 33]. Unfortunately, most Americans place at least as much emphasis on limiting *dietary* cholesterol as they do on making more significant dietary changes [34]. Dietary molecules with much more pronounced effects on *blood* cholesterol levels include trans fatty acids, saturated fatty acids, and nonfiber carbohydrates [32].

TRANS FATS

Trans fatty acids have the most adverse impact of all dietary molecules on cholesterol status. Trans fats raise LDL, triglycerides, and LpA and favor formation of atherogenic small and dense LDL particles while simultaneously reducing HDL [35-40]. These deleterious effects, along with adverse effects on inflammation, blood clotting, and insulin regulation, help explain the strong correlation between even small quantities of trans fatty acid intake and cardiac events [41, 42].

SATURATED FATS (SFAs)

Saturated fatty acids, in general, markedly increase LDL or "bad" cholesterol and moderately increase HDL, or "good" cholesterol. By increasing the LDL:HDL ratio, SFAs adversely affect overall cholesterol status. The intermediate chain SFAs, myristic and palmitic acid, have the most pronounced negative effects in this manner [43]. However, the 12 and 18 carbon, lauric and stearic acids may also increase cardiovascular events by adversely impacting insulin regulation, blood clotting, and other metabolic processes [44]. These cholesterol dysregulating effects, when combined with adverse effects on insulin regulation and blood clotting, help explain the association between saturated fatty acid consumption and cardiovascular disease [13, 45, 46].

NON-FIBER CARBOHYDRATES (NFCs)

Sugars and starches, collectively known as non-fiber carbohydrates (NFCs), modestly reduce LDL cholesterol levels but increase the proportion of the small and dense LDL subtype, which has been linked to increased risk of cardiac events [12, 47]. In addition, NFCs reduce HDL cholesterol and increase triglycerides [48-50]. In fact, NFCs disrupt the LDL/HDL ratio to a similar degree as saturated fats [13]. These negative effects, along with the adverse impact of excessive NFC intake on insulin regulation, fat accumulation, inflammation, blood clotting, and oxidative stress, help explain the association between excessive NFC consumption and cardiovascular events [51-56].

FIBERS

*In*soluble fiber has minimal impact on blood cholesterol regulation. In contrast, consumption of soluble fiber significantly reduces LDL levels [57]. However, both insoluble and soluble fibers have other beneficial metabolic effects and their consumption reduces the risk of developing heart disease and diabetes [58, 59].

MONOUNSATURATED FATS (MUFAs)

In general, replacing NFCs and saturated fats with MUFAs improves the ratio of LDL or "bad" cholesterol to HDL or "good" cholesterol. In addition, MUFAs reduce blood levels of VLDL (triglycerides) and reduce the formation of the oxidized LDL subtype [60, 61]. Overall, replacing nonfiber carbohydrates and saturated fats with MUFAs can have profoundly positive effects on blood cholesterol regulation and other metabolic parameters [13, 61].

POLYUNSATURATED FATS (PUFAs)

Omega-6 (ω-6) and omega-3 (ω-3) polyunsaturated fatty acids (PUFAs) have a complicated relationship with cardiovascular disease that extends far beyond their impact on blood cholesterol levels. PUFAs have important regulatory effects on inflammation, blood clotting, fat accumulation, insulin regulation, and oxidative stress. Omega-6 LA and ω-3 ALA both reduce LDL cholesterol to a similar degree while improving the LDL/HDL ratio [62]. In this respect, both appear to be beneficial. However, excess dietary LA may promote oxidative modification of LDL, damage to the blood vessel wall, and local blood clotting [63, 64]. In addition, excessive LA consumption out of proportion to ALA (>4:1 ratio) is associated with excessive inflammation, blood clotting tendency, and fat accumulation, three processes that play important roles in the development of cardiovascular disease [4-6, 65].

PROTEINS

Both animal and vegetable proteins appear to reduce LDL cholesterol. When substituted for nonfiber carbohydrates, proteins improve the LDL:HDL ratio [66-70]. Beneficial effects on both cholesterol and insulin metabolism may account for the modest cardioprotective properties of protein observed in the Nurses Health Study [71].

PHYTOCHEMICALS (plant chemicals)

A wide variety of polyphenolic antioxidants have demonstrated the ability to protect LDL cholesterol from oxidation [72, 73]. In addition, polyphenolic antioxidants in extra virgin olive oil appear to increase HDL cholesterol [73]. Other phytochemicals, especially phytosterols, reduce LDL cholesterol [74]. Via these and other mechanisms, polyphenolic antioxidants and other phytochemicals may reduce the risk of developing cardiovascular disease.

DIETARY NUTRIENTS AND LIPOPROTEIN SUBTYPES

Nutrients	LDL/HDL ratio	Small/ dense LDL	Large/ buoyant LDL	Oxidized LDL	LpA	VLDL (TG)	Overall effect
SFA	↑	-	-	-	-	-	Bad
MUFA	↓	-	↑	↓	-	↓	Good
Total PUFA	↓	-	-	-	-	↓	Good*
ω-6 LA	↓	-	-	↑	-	↓	Good*
ω-3ALA	↓	-	-	↓	-	↓	Good*
Trans	↑	↑	-	-	↑	↑	Very Bad
Cholesterol	Neutral**	-	↑	-	-	-	Neutral
NFC	↑	↑	↓	-	-	↑	Bad
Fiber	↓	-	-	-	-	-	Good
Protein	↓	-	-	-	-	-	Good
Polyphenolic antioxidants	↓	-	-	↓	-	-	Good
Phytosterols	↓	-	-	-	-	-	Good

Small, medium, and large arrows represent modest, moderate, profound effects, respectively. *= All PUFAs reduce LDL cholesterol levels. However, an excessive ω-6 LA to ω-3 ratio may predispose to heart disease via other mechanisms. **= Has a modest adverse effect on LDL/HDL ratio at low intakes.

CONCLUSION

Blood cholesterol regulation is an important feature of cardiovascular health. Diet plays a central role in regulating both the total amount and quality of different lipoproteins collectively known as blood cholesterol. In general, the standard U.S. diet strongly promotes cholesterol dysregulation. Reduction of trans fats, saturated fats, and non-fiber carbohydrates, in conjunction with increased intake of monounsaturated fats, fibers, proteins, phytosterols, and polyphenolic antioxidants can have a positive impact on cholesterol status. When combined with dietary strategies designed to reduce inflammation, blood clotting, fat accumulation, insulin dysregulation, and oxidative stress, these dietary features have the potential to prevent most cardiovascular diseases.

References:

1. Eaton, C.B., *Hyperlipidemia*. Prim Care, 2005. **32**(4): p. 1027-55, viii.
2. Ma, J., et al., *A prospective study of fibrinogen and risk of myocardial infarction in the Physicians' Health Study*. J Am Coll Cardiol, 1999. **33**(5): p. 1347-52.
3. Heller, R.F., et al., *How well can we predict coronary heart disease? Findings in the United Kingdom Heart Disease Prevention Project*. Br Med J (Clin Res Ed), 1984. **288**(6428): p. 1409-11.
4. de Lorgeril, M. and P. Salen, *Modified cretan mediterranean diet in the prevention of coronary heart disease and cancer: an update*. World Rev Nutr Diet, 2007. **97**: p. 1-32.
5. de Lorgeril, M., et al., *Mediterranean dietary pattern in a randomized trial: prolonged survival and possible reduced cancer rate*. Arch Intern Med, 1998. **158**(11): p. 1181-7.
6. de Lorgeril, M., et al., *Mediterranean diet, traditional risk factors, and the rate of cardiovascular complications after myocardial infarction: final report of the Lyon Diet Heart Study*. Circulation, 1999. **99**(6): p. 779-85.
7. Colwell, J.A. and R.W. Nesto, *The platelet in diabetes: focus on prevention of ischemic events*. Diabetes Care, 2003. **26**(7): p. 2181-8.
8. Mozaffarian, D., et al., *Cardiac benefits of fish consumption may depend on the type of fish meal consumed: the Cardiovascular Health Study*. Circulation, 2003. **107**(10): p. 1372-7.
9. Despres, J.P., et al., *Hyperinsulinemia as an independent risk factor for ischemic heart disease*. N Engl J Med, 1996. **334**(15): p. 952-7.
10. Ajani, U.A., E.S. Ford, and A.H. Mokdad, *Dietary fiber and C-reactive protein: findings from national health and nutrition examination survey data*. J Nutr, 2004. **134**(5): p. 1181-5.
11. Devaraj, S., R.S. Rosenson, and I. Jialal, *Metabolic syndrome: an appraisal of the pro-inflammatory and procoagulant status*. Endocrinol Metab Clin North Am, 2004. **33**(2): p. 431-53, table of contents.
12. Krauss, R.M., et al., *AHA Dietary Guidelines: revision 2000: A statement for healthcare professionals from the Nutrition Committee of the American Heart Association*. Circulation, 2000. **102**(18): p. 2284-99.
13. Mensink, R.P., et al., *Effects of dietary fatty acids and carbohydrates on the ratio of serum total to HDL cholesterol and on serum lipids and apolipoproteins: a meta-analysis of 60 controlled trials*. Am J Clin Nutr, 2003. **77**(5): p. 1146-55.
14. Suk Danik, J., et al., *Lipoprotein(a), measured with an assay independent of apolipoprotein(a) isoform size, and risk of future cardiovascular events among initially healthy women*. Jama, 2006. **296**(11): p. 1363-70.
15. Hurt-Camejo, E., et al., *Cellular consequences of the association of apoB lipoproteins with proteoglycans. Potential contribution to atherogenesis*. Arterioscler Thromb Vasc Biol, 1997. **17**(6): p. 1011-7.
16. Shah, P.K., et al., *Exploiting the vascular protective effects of high-density lipoprotein and its apolipoproteins: an idea whose time for testing is coming, part I*. Circulation, 2001. **104**(19): p. 2376-83.
17. Kontush, A., S. Chantepie, and M.J. Chapman, *Small, dense HDL particles exert potent protection of atherogenic LDL against oxidative stress*. Arterioscler Thromb Vasc Biol, 2003. **23**(10): p. 1881-8.
18. Castelli, W.P., *Cardiovascular disease and multifactorial risk: challenge of the 1980s*. Am Heart J, 1983. **106**(5 Pt 2): p. 1191-200.
19. Navab, M., et al., *The double jeopardy of HDL*. Ann Med, 2005. **37**(3): p. 173-8.
20. Arend, W.P. and C. Gabay, *Cytokines in the rheumatic diseases*. Rheum Dis Clin North Am, 2004. **30**(1): p. 41-67, v-vi.
21. Pruzanski, W., et al., *Comparative analysis of lipid composition of normal and acute-phase high density lipoproteins*. J Lipid Res, 2000. **41**(7): p. 1035-47.
22. Park, S.H., et al., *The relative effects of obesity and insulin resistance on cardiovascular risk factors in nondiabetic and normotensive men*. Korean J Intern Med, 2004. **19**(2): p. 75-80.
23. Batista, M.C., et al., *Apolipoprotein A-I, B-100, and B-48 metabolism in subjects with chronic kidney disease, obesity, and the metabolic syndrome*. Metabolism, 2004. **53**(10): p. 1255-61.
24. Hokanson, J.E. and M.A. Austin, *Plasma triglyceride level is a risk factor for cardiovascular disease independent of high-density lipoprotein cholesterol level: a meta-analysis of population-based prospective studies*. J Cardiovasc Risk, 1996. **3**(2): p. 213-9.
25. Abdel-Maksoud, M.F. and J.E. Hokanson, *The complex role of triglycerides in cardiovascular disease*. Semin Vasc Med, 2002. **2**(3): p. 325-33.
26. McNamara, D.J., *The impact of egg limitations on coronary heart disease risk: do the numbers add up?* J Am Coll Nutr, 2000. **19**(5 Suppl): p. 540S-548S.
27. Boucher, P., et al., *Effect of dietary cholesterol on low density lipoprotein-receptor, 3-hydroxy-3-methylglutaryl-CoA reductase, and low density lipoprotein receptor-related protein mRNA expression in healthy humans*. Lipids, 1998. **33**(12): p. 1177-86.
28. Hu, F.B. and W.C. Willett, *Optimal diets for prevention of coronary heart disease*. Jama, 2002. **288**(20): p. 2569-78.
29. Fernandez, M.L., *Dietary cholesterol provided by eggs and plasma lipoproteins in healthy populations*. Curr Opin Clin Nutr Metab Care, 2006. **9**(1): p. 8-12.

30.   Kratz, M., *Dietary cholesterol, atherosclerosis and coronary heart disease*. Handb Exp Pharmacol, 2005(170): p. 195-213.
31.   Greene, C.M., et al., *Plasma LDL and HDL characteristics and carotenoid content are positively influenced by egg consumption in an elderly population1*. Nutr Metab (Lond), 2006. **3**: p. 6.
32.   2005, D.o.A. *Dietary Guidelines Advisory Committee. Nutrition and your health: dietary guidelines for Americans*. Dietary Guidelines Advisory Committee report   [cited 2006 July 15]; Available from: http://health.gov/dietaryguidelines/dga2005/report/.
33.   Howell, W.H., et al., *Plasma lipid and lipoprotein responses to dietary fat and cholesterol: a meta-analysis*. Am J Clin Nutr, 1997. **65**(6): p. 1747-64.
34.   U.S. Department of Agricultural Research Service. 1997. *Data Tables: results from the USDA's 1994-1996 Continuing Survey of Food Intakes by Individuals and 1994-1996 Diet and Health Knowledge Survey [Online] ARS Food Surveys Research Group*.   [cited; Available from: http:barc.usda.gov/bhnrc/foodsurvey/home.htm. {visited 2006, August 10th}.
35.   Mensink, R.P. and M.B. Katan, *Effect of dietary trans fatty acids on high-density and low-density lipoprotein cholesterol levels in healthy subjects*. N Engl J Med, 1990. **323**(7): p. 439-45.
36.   de Roos, N.M., M.L. Bots, and M.B. Katan, *Replacement of dietary saturated fatty acids by trans fatty acids lowers serum HDL cholesterol and impairs endothelial function in healthy men and women*. Arterioscler Thromb Vasc Biol, 2001. **21**(7): p. 1233-7.
37.   Ferretti, A., et al., *Ingestion of marine oil reduces excretion of 11-dehydrothromboxane B2, an index of intravascular production of thromboxane A2*. Prostaglandins Leukot Essent Fatty Acids, 1993. **48**(4): p. 305-8.
38.   Lichtenstein, A.H., et al., *Effects of different forms of dietary hydrogenated fats on serum lipoprotein cholesterol levels*. N Engl J Med, 1999. **340**(25): p. 1933-40.
39.   Zock, P.L. and M.B. Katan, *Trans fatty acids, lipoproteins, and coronary risk*. Can J Physiol Pharmacol, 1997. **75**(3): p. 211-6.
40.   Mauger, J.F., et al., *Effect of different forms of dietary hydrogenated fats on LDL particle size*. Am J Clin Nutr, 2003. **78**(3): p. 370-5.
41.   Hu, F.B., et al., *Dietary fat intake and the risk of coronary heart disease in women*. N Engl J Med, 1997. **337**(21): p. 1491-9.
42.   Pietinen, P., et al., *Intake of fatty acids and risk of coronary heart disease in a cohort of Finnish men. The Alpha-Tocopherol, Beta-Carotene Cancer Prevention Study*. Am J Epidemiol, 1997. **145**(10): p. 876-87.
43.   Brighenti, F., et al., *Total antioxidant capacity of the diet is inversely and independently related to plasma concentration of high-sensitivity C-reactive protein in adult Italian subjects*. Br J Nutr, 2005. **93**(5): p. 619-25.
44.   Renaud, S.C., *What is the epidemiologic evidence for the thrombogenic potential of dietary long-chain fatty acids?* Am J Clin Nutr, 1992. **56**(4 Suppl): p. 823S-824S.
45.   Das, U.N., *A defect in the activity of Delta6 and Delta5 desaturases may be a factor predisposing to the development of insulin resistance syndrome*. Prostaglandins Leukot Essent Fatty Acids, 2005. **72**(5): p. 343-50.
46.   Keys, A., *Seven Countries: a multivariate analysis of death and coronary heart disease.*, Cambridge, Mass: Harvard University Press, 1980.
47.   Reaven, G.M., *Do high carbohydrate diets prevent the development or attenuate the manifestations (or both) of syndrome X? A viewpoint strongly against*. Curr Opin Lipidol, 1997. **8**(1): p. 23-7.
48.   Grundy, S.M., et al., *Comparison of three cholesterol-lowering diets in normolipidemic men*. Jama, 1986. **256**(17): p. 2351-5.
49.   Mancini, M., et al., *Studies of the mechanisms of carbohydrate-induced lipaemia in normal man*. Atherosclerosis, 1973. **17**(3): p. 445-54.
50.   Merchant, A.T., et al., *Carbohydrate intake and HDL in a multiethnic population*. Am J Clin Nutr, 2007. **85**(1): p. 225-30.
51.   Gross, L.S., et al., *Increased consumption of refined carbohydrates and the epidemic of type 2 diabetes in the United States: an ecologic assessment*. Am J Clin Nutr, 2004. **79**(5): p. 774-9.
52.   Schulze, M.B., et al., *Glycemic index, glycemic load, and dietary fiber intake and incidence of type 2 diabetes in younger and middle-aged women*. Am J Clin Nutr, 2004. **80**(2): p. 348-56.
53.   Del Prato, S., et al., *Effect of sustained physiologic hyperinsulinaemia and hyperglycaemia on insulin secretion and insulin sensitivity in man*. Diabetologia, 1994. **37**(10): p. 1025-35.
54.   Liu, S., et al., *A prospective study of dietary glycemic load, carbohydrate intake, and risk of coronary heart disease in US women*. Am J Clin Nutr, 2000. **71**(6): p. 1455-61.
55.   Liu, S., et al., *Relation between a diet with a high glycemic load and plasma concentrations of high-sensitivity C-reactive protein in middle-aged women*. Am J Clin Nutr, 2002. **75**(3): p. 492-8.
56.   Yerneni, K.K., et al., *Hyperglycemia-induced activation of nuclear transcription factor kappaB in vascular smooth muscle cells*. Diabetes, 1999. **48**(4): p. 855-64.
57.   Shamliyan, T.A., et al., *Are your patients with risk of CVD getting the viscous soluble fiber they need?* J Fam Pract, 2006. **55**(9): p. 761-9.
58.   Erkkila, A.T. and A.H. Lichtenstein, *Fiber and cardiovascular disease risk: how strong is the evidence?* J Cardiovasc Nurs, 2006. **21**(1): p. 3-8.
59.   Bazzano, L.A., et al., *Dietary fiber intake and reduced risk of coronary heart disease in US men and women: the National Health and Nutrition Examination Survey I Epidemiologic Follow-up Study*. Arch Intern Med, 2003. **163**(16): p. 1897-904.
60.   Berry, E.M., et al., *Effects of diets rich in monounsaturated fatty acids on plasma lipoproteins--the Jerusalem Nutrition Study. II. Monounsaturated fatty acids vs carbohydrates*. Am J Clin Nutr, 1992. **56**(2): p. 394-403.
61.   Covas, M.I., *Olive oil and the cardiovascular system*. Pharmacol Res, 2007.
62.   Harris, W.S., *n-3 fatty acids and serum lipoproteins: human studies*. Am J Clin Nutr, 1997. **65**(5 Suppl): p. 1645S-1654S.

DIET AND FAT ACCUMULATION

Key Concepts you should take away from this chapter:

• Excessive accumulation of fat, especially abdominal fat, predisposes to the development of the Big 7 epidemic U.S. diseases
• The standard American diet promotes excessive fat accumulation
• The calories in - calories out, or "energy balance" hypothesis of fat accumulation is obsolete and inadequate
• Three separate factors determine the *net* effect of any dietary nutrient on weight gain and fat accumulation:
    - caloric value
    - effect on satiety/hunger
    - metabolic properties
• American dietary practices promote fat accumulation at the molecular level
Specifically:
• Excessive consumption of non-fiber carbohydrates and relative deficiency of fiber promotes fat accumulation
• Excessive consumption of ω-6 and relative deficiency of ω-3 fatty acids promotes fat accumulation
• Relative deficiency of protein intake favors fat accumulation
• Consumption of artificial sweeteners favors fat accumulation

HISTORICAL PERSPECTIVE

For millions of years, the healthy diets and active lifestyles of our ancestors prevented excessive fat tissue accumulation. However, beginning with the Industrial Revolution 150-200 years ago, advances in transportation, manufacturing, and electronics have enabled Americans to become progressively less active. Simultaneously, modern food processing, selective plant breeding, crop manipulation, and animal rearing practices have radically altered the qualitative and quantitative balance of dietary molecules consumed by Americans [1]. These dietary changes occurred too recently to allow for adequate genetic adaptation [2, 3]. The fact that individuals who migrate to the U.S. develop much higher rates of overweight and obesity than their native counterparts confirms that environmental, rather than genetic changes are the primary driving force behind the U.S. obesity epidemic [4, 5]. Consequently, a staggering 66% of Americans are overweight and 33% are obese, with even higher rates predicted for the future [6].

FAT ACCUMULATION IN HEALTH AND DISEASE

In health, *modest* fat stores enable humans to meet caloric needs during periods of reduced nutrient intake or intense exercise, situations our ancestors presumably encountered more often than modern Americans [7]. Individuals have highly variable amounts of abdominal fat stores ranging from a few milliliters to an astonishing six liters [8]. Although fat has historically been regarded as metabolically inactive, scientists now know that fat cells secrete potent mediators which promote inflammation, blood clotting, insulin resistance, elevate blood pressure, and disturb blood cholesterol metabolism [9-15]. Fat tissue surrounding abdominal organs, known as visceral fat, is especially metabolically active. By secreting three times as many inflammatory and other mediators as other fat cells, excessive visceral fat tissue predisposes to heart disease, diabetes mellitus, Alzheimer's dementia, arthritis, depression, certain cancers, and many other illnesses [9, 10, 16]. These adverse metabolic properties of fat tissue may account for Hippocrates astute 400 B.C. observation that "Individuals who have a full body habitus die earlier than slim persons" [17].

THE MOLECULAR BASIS OF FAT EXPANSION: HYPERTROPHY AND HYPERPLASIA

The expansion of fat tissue progresses via two integrated molecular processes: hypertrophy and hyperplasia. Hypertrophy refers to the growth of *existing* fat cells. Hyperplasia refers to the formation of *new* fat cells from fat "stem cells."

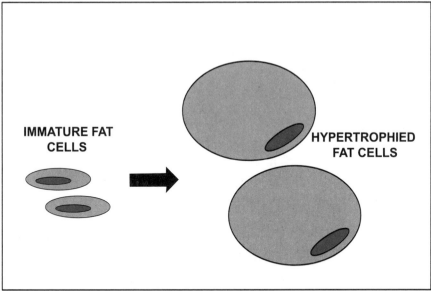

Figure 1: Hypertrophy.

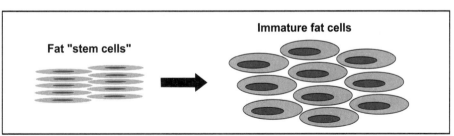

Figure 2: Hyperplasia.

Traditionally, the study of fat expansion has focused solely on hypertrophy of existing fat cells (adipocytes). However, because fully hypertrophied fat cells *cannot* divide, a limited quantity of fat tissue can accumulate via hypertrophy alone. ***Thus, any significant fat tissue expansion requires formation of new fat cells.***

Hyperplasia, or formation of new fat cells from fat "stem cells," has been referred to as "weightless" weight gain because new adipocytes *originally* possess 30 to 50 times less volume than fully hypertrophied counterparts [18]. Importantly, however, new fat cells are permanent, and play a key role in expansion of total fat mass [19, 20]. In fact, in obese individuals, the increased ***number*** of fat cells may account for a larger percentage of fat tissue expansion than does the increased *size* of existing fat cells [21]. Although hyperplasia is most active during infancy, adolescence, and during periods of rapid weight gain, it is now recognized that hyperplasia occurs *throughout life* [10, 18, 22, 23]! Because these new cells do not signal satiety as well as mature adipocytes, fat cell hyperplasia may impede future attempts to lose weight and maintain weight loss [24].

DIETARY CONTROL OF FAT ACCUMULATION

INADEQUACIES OF THE *CALORIES IN - CALORIES OUT* HYPOTHESIS OF WEIGHT GAIN

Most health promotion agencies expound the clear-cut "energy balance" hypothesis that weight gain is simply the result of the consumption of more calories than are burned [25]. While technically correct, the formula is often misinterpreted to suggest that the sole modifiable variables determining weight status are *calories* consumed and *energy* burned through activity. From this viewpoint, exercise and restricting calories are the only tools for limiting weight gain [25]. However, it is important to realize that in addition to simply providing calories, different nutrients also have highly variable effects on resting metabolic rate, satiety, satiation, and future caloric intake. In addition, certain nutrients promote fat tissue formation, while others promote formation of lean muscle mass. Via these mechanisms, subsets of fats, carbohydrates, and proteins have distinct, even opposite effects on the molecular processes which control energy metabolism and fat accumulation.

DIETARY FAT AND FAT ACCUMULATION: *QUALITY IS KEY*

The *calories in - calories out* hypothesis suggests that *all* fats, which each supply nine calories per gram, are created equal in terms of weight gain and development of adipose tissue. However, the fact that isocaloric (providing equal calories) diets with different fatty acid compositions result in vastly different amounts of fat expansion and body mass clearly refutes this overly simplified assumption [19, 26]. Different fatty acids have diverse effects on a wide variety of metabolic determinants including gene expression, membrane properties, metabolic signaling, hormone production, and resting metabolic rate [27]. Mounting evidence indicates that different subclasses of dietary fats also have distinct, even opposite effects on fat tissue development [18, 19, 26, 28, 29].

OMEGA-6/OMEGA-3 IMBALANCE: THE MISSING LINK IN THE U.S. OBESITY EPIDEMIC?

In particular, the balance between ω-6 and ω-3 polyunsaturated fatty acids plays a critical role in the molecular processes that govern *long-term* fat tissue accumulation via mechanisms independent of caloric value [18, 19, 28-31]. In general, ω-6 fatty acids promote and ω-3 fatty acids block expansion of fat tissue.

Arachidonic acid (ArA), the long-chain ω-6 fatty acid derivative, is a potent fat-promoting "booster" which stimulates fat cell hyperplasia and fat tissue expansion [18, 29, 30, 32-34]. Emerging evidence suggests that excessive ω-6 linoleic (LA) consumption and resulting ω-6 blood and tissue "ArA overload" play crucial roles in the U.S. epidemics of obesity and overweight [18, 19, 33].

By limiting conversion of ω-6 LA to fat-promoting ω-6 ArA, both the short chain ω-3 ALA, and longer chain ω-3 EPA and DHA restrict fat tissue expansion [18, 19]. In addition, long-chain ω-3 fatty acids EPA and DHA *directly* activate numerous "fat-burning" (lipolytic) genes which inhibit both fat cell hypertrophy and hyperplasia [18, 19, 28, 31, 35-39]. The lipolytic effects of ω-3 fatty acids have been demonstrated in both humans and animal models of fat accumulation [31, 38, 40, 41]. Overall, long-chain ω-3 EPA and DHA are more effective inhibitors of fat tissue expansion than ALA [41, 42]. Thus, the typical American dietary pattern of massive ω-6 LA, moderate ω-6 ArA, and deficient ω-3 ALA, EPA, and DHA intake, which results in blood and tissue "ArA overload," strongly promotes the molecular pathogenesis of fat expansion and predisposes to *long-term* weight gain and obesity.

THE ROLE OF INSULIN IN FAT ACCUMULATION

Insulin is a potent growth-promoting, or anabolic, hormone that favors the growth and accumulation of fat tissue through regulation of several metabolic pathways [43, 44]. At the cellular level, insulin promotes hypertrophy of existing fat cells by increasing fat deposits *and* hyperplasia by stimulating the conversion of fat "stem cells" into actual fat cells [44-46]. *Via these mechanisms, high plasma insulin levels strongly favor the expansion of total fat mass.* Dietary nutrients that boost plasma insulin levels generally favor weight gain and accumulation of fat tissue.

CARBOHYDRATES AND INSULIN METABOLISM

Like fats, different subsets of carbohydrates have distinct, even opposite effects on the molecular mechanisms responsible for fat accumulation. Excessive intake of sugars and refined starches triggers elevation of blood glucose and compensatory elevation of blood insulin levels [47-50]. Repeated elevation of blood insulin levels promotes conversion of non-fiber carbohydrates to saturated fats, fat cell hypertrophy and hyperplasia, and accumulation of fat tissue [43, 50-53]. In contrast, fibers stabilize blood sugar levels and reduce plasma insulin responses [54, 55]. By lowering serum insulin levels, fibers inhibit fat cell hypertrophy and hyperplasia, block fat tissue expansion, and favor weight loss [50, 56-58]. Thus, like fats, *both quality and amounts* of carbohydrates play crucial roles in energy metabolism and fat accumulation.

FATS AND INSULIN METABOLISM

Dietary fatty acids become incorporated into cell membranes. Due to their straight molecular structures, saturated and trans fats limit membrane fluidity by packing tightly together. This lack of fluidity *indirectly* raises insulin levels by reducing the sensitivity of insulin and glucose receptors [59]. In contrast, natural monounsaturated fats, which have a kinked configuration, cannot pack together as tightly, making membranes more fluid. The higher membrane fluidity of monounsaturated fats improves insulin sensitivity. Via indirectly elevating serum insulin levels, saturated and trans fats may insidiously promote and monounsaturated fats may inhibit weight gain. Interestingly, animal studies demonstrate that the isocaloric replacement of monounsaturated fats with trans fats leads to fat tissue expansion and redistribution of fat to the abdomen, independently of simply providing calories [26].

PROTEIN AND INSULIN METABOLISM

Like fiber, protein consumption stabilizes blood glucose and insulin responses [60-62]. In addition, the consumption of protein both directly and indirectly raises the metabolic rate by speeding metabolism and promoting the formation of lean body mass [61, 63, 64]. Therefore, long term replacement of *non-fiber* carbohydrates with proteins promotes weight loss [63, 65].

DIET, APPETITE CONTROL, AND FAT ACCUMULATION

Different classes of dietary molecules have different, even opposite effects on metabolism, appetite control, and *future* food consumption. For instance, high fiber meals not only limit the amount of food consumed at one sitting, but may also prolong the feeling of fullness, and reduce the amount of food consumed at the next meal. In addition, fibers can displace high-calorie foods while providing little or no calories. Fibers antagonize weight gain by controlling hunger, reducing the insulin response to foods, and by displacing calorie-dense foods [50, 55, 66, 67]. In contrast, non-fiber carbohydrate (NFC)-rich, fiber-poor foods and beverages provide little satiety, and excessive consumption favors overeating and weight gain [50, 68-71]. Like fiber, proteins reduce appetite and future caloric intake, and promote weight loss [61, 63, 65]. Thus, the typical low-fiber, high non-fiber carbohydrate, low protein U.S. dietary pattern contributes to appetite dysregulation, overeating, and weight gain.

ARTIFICIAL SWEETENERS AND APPETITE DYSREGULATION

Many Americans attempt to lose weight by consuming "diet" and "low-cal" foods and beverages containing artificial sweeteners. However, rather than promoting weight loss, intake of artificial sweeteners *may* actually promote *future* weight gain! For instance, in the San Antonio Heart Study, the risk of becoming overweight or obese increased 65% and 41% respectively, for each can of "diet" soda consumed per day. Ironically, "diet" drink intake was a stronger predictor of long-term weight gain than consumption of sugar-rich "regular" soda [72]. Later analysis demonstrated a dose-response association between artificial sweetener consumption and weight gain. Similarly, diet drink intake was associated with a variety of metabolic abnormalities, weight gain, and obesity in the

Framington Heart Study [73]. While the mechanism responsible for this long-term weight gain is poorly understood and controversial, animal studies suggest that artificial sweeteners may contribute to weight gain via appetite dysregulation, later overeating, and increased caloric consumption [74, 75]. Alternatively, people who consume calorie-free foods may also feel entitled to consume high-calorie junk foods concurrently with the "diet" food items [76]. Whatever the mechanism, it appears that artificial sweeteners are not the solution for the epidemics of weight gain and obesity in the U.S.

DIETARY NUTRIENTS AND *LONG-TERM* FAT ACCUMULATION

Nutrient	Energy density (Kcal/gram)	Hypertrophy	Hyperplasia	Appetite*	*Long-term Fat Balance*
Saturated fat	9	↑	↑	↓	↑
MUFA	9	-	-	↓	Neutral**
ω-6 LA	9	-	↑	↓	↑
ω-6 ArA	9	-	**↑**	↓	**↑**
ω-3 ALA	9	**↓**	**↓**	↓	**↓**
ω-3 EPA/DHA	9	**↓**	**↓**	↓	**↓**
Trans fat	9	↑	↑	↓	**↑**
NFCs	4	↑	↑	↑	**↑**
Fiber	<4	**↓**	**↓**	**↓**	**↓**
Protein	4	↓	↓	**↓**	↓
Sugar Substitute	0	-	-	**↑**	**↑**

References in text. * = Includes satiety, satiation and mental effects. ** = Better insulin sensitivity than SFA and TFA. - = neutral or unknown

CONCLUSION

Despite growing evidence that not all calories are created equal, health promotion agencies continue to champion the simplified strategy of "exercise more and eat less," while neglecting the role of choosing the *right* kinds of nutrients. In order to accurately predict any food item's *overall* impact on fat tissue development, one must consider not only caloric value, but also the impact of its molecular content on fat accumulation, energy metabolism, and satiety.

Several characteristics of the standard American diet, namely the very high ratios of non-fiber carbohydrate to fiber intake (16:1), ω-6 to ω-3 imbalance, excessive intake of trans fats, saturated fats, and artificial sweeteners, and relative deficiency of protein consumption, predispose to excessive fat accumulation and development of the Big 7 epidemic U.S. diseases.

References:

1. Ghebremeskel, K. and M.A. Crawford, *Nutrition and health in relation to food production and processing.* Nutr Health, 1994. **9**(4): p. 237-53.
2. Cordain, L., et al., *Origins and evolution of the Western diet: health implications for the 21st century.* Am J Clin Nutr, 2005. **81**(2): p. 341-54.
3. Cordain, L., *The Nutritional Characteristics of a Contemporary Diet.* JANA, 2002. **5**(3): p. 15-25.
4. Goel, M.S., et al., *Obesity among US immigrant subgroups by duration of residence.* Jama, 2004. **292**(23): p. 2860-7.
5. Lauderdale, D.S. and P.J. Rathouz, *Body mass index in a US national sample of Asian Americans: effects of nativity, years since immigration and socioeconomic status.* Int J Obes Relat Metab Disord, 2000. **24**(9): p. 1188-94.
6. Ogden, C.L., et al., *Prevalence of overweight and obesity in the United States, 1999-2004.* Jama, 2006. **295**(13): p. 1549-55.
7. Jeffcoat, R., *Obesity - A perspective based on the biochemical interrelationship of lipids and carbohydrates.* Med Hypotheses, 2007. **68**(5): p. 1159-71.
8. Thomas, E.L., et al., *Magnetic resonance imaging of total body fat.* J Appl Physiol, 1998. **85**(5): p. 1778-85.
9. Maachi, M., et al., *Systemic low-grade inflammation is related to both circulating and adipose tissue TNFalpha, leptin and IL-6 levels in obese women.* Int J Obes Relat Metab Disord, 2004. **28**(8): p. 993-7.
10. Hirsch, J., et al., *The fat cell.* Med Clin North Am, 1989. **73**(1): p. 83-96.
11. McCarty, M.F., *Low-insulin-response diets may decrease plasma C-reactive protein by influencing adipocyte function.* Med Hypotheses, 2005. **64**(2): p. 385-7.
12. Shimomura, I., et al., *Enhanced expression of PAI-1 in visceral fat: possible contributor to vascular disease in obesity.* Nat Med, 1996. **2**(7): p. 800-3.
13. Hotamisligil, G.S., et al., *Increased adipose tissue expression of tumor necrosis factor-alpha in human obesity and insulin resistance.* J Clin Invest, 1995. **95**(5): p. 2409-15.
14. Frederich, R.C., Jr., et al., *Tissue-specific nutritional regulation of angiotensinogen in adipose tissue.* Hypertension, 1992. **19**(4): p. 339-44.
15. Licata, G., et al., *Obesity: a main factor of metabolic syndrome?* Panminerva Med, 2006. **48**(2): p. 77-85.
16. Pender, J.R. and W.J. Pories, *Epidemiology of obesity in the United States.* Gastroenterol Clin North Am, 2005. **34**(1): p. 1-7.
17. Bengmark, S., *Acute and "chronic" phase reaction-a mother of disease.* Clin Nutr, 2004. **23**(6): p. 1256-66.
18. Ailhaud, G., et al., *Temporal changes in dietary fats: role of n-6 polyunsaturated fatty acids in excessive adipose tissue development and relationship to obesity.* Prog Lipid Res, 2006. **45**(3): p. 203-36.
19. Massiera, F., et al., *Arachidonic acid and prostacyclin signaling promote adipose tissue development: a human health concern?* J Lipid Res, 2003. **44**(2): p. 271-9.
20. Ailhaud, G., P. Grimaldi, and R. Negrel, *Cellular and molecular aspects of adipose tissue development.* Annu Rev Nutr, 1992. **12**: p. 207-33.
21. Knittle, J.L., et al., *The growth of adipose tissue in children and adolescents. Cross-sectional and longitudinal studies of adipose cell number and size.* J Clin Invest, 1979. **63**(2): p. 239-46.
22. Bougneres, P., et al., *In vivo resistance of lipolysis to epinephrine. A new feature of childhood onset obesity.* J Clin Invest, 1997. **99**(11): p. 2568-73.
23. Cleary, M.P., F.C. Phillips, and R.A. Morton, *Genotype and diet effects in lean and obese Zucker rats fed either safflower or coconut oil diets.* Proc Soc Exp Biol Med, 1999. **220**(3): p. 153-61.
24. Lofgren, P., et al., *Long-term prospective and controlled studies demonstrate adipose tissue hypercellularity and relative leptin deficiency in the postobese state.* J Clin Endocrinol Metab, 2005. **90**(11): p. 6207-13.
25. Lichtenstein, A.H., et al., *Diet and lifestyle recommendations revision 2006: a scientific statement from the American Heart Association Nutrition Committee.* Circulation, 2006. **114**(1): p. 82-96.
26. Kavanagh, K., Rudel, LL. *Trans Fat Leads to Weight Gain Even on the Same Total Calories, Animal Study Shows.* 2006 [cited 2006 Nov 27]; Available from: https://www1.wfubmc.edu/news/NewsArticle.htm?Articleid=1869.
27. Vessby, B., et al., *Desaturation and elongation of Fatty acids and insulin action.* Ann N Y Acad Sci, 2002. **967**: p. 183-95.
28. Madsen, L., R.K. Petersen, and K. Kristiansen, *Regulation of adipocyte differentiation and function by polyunsaturated fatty acids.* Biochim Biophys Acta, 2005. **1740**(2): p. 266-86.

29.	Ailhaud, G., *[Development of adipose tissue and dietary lipids: from basic science to medicine]*. Ann Endocrinol (Paris), 2005. **66**(2 Pt 3): p. 2S7-10.
30.	Javadi, M., et al., *The effect of six different C18 fatty acids on body fat and energy metabolism in mice*. Br J Nutr, 2004. **92**(3): p. 391-9.
31.	Couet, C., et al., *Effect of dietary fish oil on body fat mass and basal fat oxidation in healthy adults*. Int J Obes Relat Metab Disord, 1997. **21**(8): p. 637-43.
32.	Ailhaud, G., *Cell surface receptors, nuclear receptors and ligands that regulate adipose tissue development*. Clin Chim Acta, 1999. **286**(1-2): p. 181-90.
33.	Savva, S.C., et al., *Association of adipose tissue arachidonic acid content with BMI and overweight status in children from Cyprus and Crete*. Br J Nutr, 2004. **91**(4): p. 643-9.
34.	Gaillard, D., et al., *Requirement and role of arachidonic acid in the differentiation of pre-adipose cells*. Biochem J, 1989. **257**(2): p. 389-97.
35.	Guo, W., et al., *Eicosapentaenoic acid, but not oleic acid, stimulates beta-oxidation in adipocytes*. Lipids, 2005. **40**(8): p. 815-21.
36.	Parrish, C.C., D.A. Pathy, and A. Angel, *Dietary fish oils limit adipose tissue hypertrophy in rats*. Metabolism, 1990. **39**(3): p. 217-9.
37.	Raclot, T., et al., *Site-specific regulation of gene expression by n-3 polyunsaturated fatty acids in rat white adipose tissues*. J Lipid Res, 1997. **38**(10): p. 1963-72.
38.	Okuno, M., et al., *Perilla oil prevents the excessive growth of visceral adipose tissue in rats by down-regulating adipocyte differentiation*. J Nutr, 1997. **127**(9): p. 1752-7.
39.	Ruzickova, J., et al., *Omega-3 PUFA of marine origin limit diet-induced obesity in mice by reducing cellularity of adipose tissue*. Lipids, 2004. **39**(12): p. 1177-85.
40.	Hill, A.M., et al., *Combining fish-oil supplements with regular aerobic exercise improves body composition and cardiovascular disease risk factors*. Am J Clin Nutr, 2007. **85**(5): p. 1267-74.
41.	Nakatani, T., et al., *A low fish oil inhibits SREBP-1 proteolytic cascade, while a high-fish-oil feeding decreases SREBP-1 mRNA in mice liver: relationship to anti-obesity*. J Lipid Res, 2003. **44**(2): p. 369-79.
42.	Flachs, P., et al., *Polyunsaturated fatty acids of marine origin upregulate mitochondrial biogenesis and induce beta-oxidation in white fat*. Diabetologia, 2005. **48**(11): p. 2365-75.
43.	Kim, J.B., et al., *Nutritional and insulin regulation of fatty acid synthetase and leptin gene expression through ADD1/SREBP1*. J Clin Invest, 1998. **101**(1): p. 1-9.
44.	Lustig, R.H., *The 'skinny on childhood obesity: how our western environment starves kids' brains*. Pediatr Ann, 2006. **35**(12): p. 898-902, 905-7.
45.	Gagnon, A. and A. Sorisky, *The effect of glucose concentration on insulin-induced 3T3-L1 adipose cell differentiation*. Obes Res, 1998. **6**(2): p. 157-63.
46.	Smith, P.J., et al., *Insulin-like growth factor-I is an essential regulator of the differentiation of 3T3-L1 adipocytes*. J Biol Chem, 1988. **263**(19): p. 9402-8.
47.	Bantle, J.P., et al., *Postprandial glucose and insulin responses to meals containing different carbohydrates in normal and diabetic subjects*. N Engl J Med, 1983. **309**(1): p. 7-12.
48.	Dahlqvist, A. and B. Borgstrom, *Digestion and absorption of disaccharides in man*. Biochem J, 1961. **81**: p. 411-8.
49.	Wahlqvist, M.L., E.G. Wilmshurst, and E.N. Richardson, *The effect of chain length on glucose absorption and the related metabolic response*. Am J Clin Nutr, 1978. **31**(11): p. 1998-2001.
50.	Liu, S., et al., *Relation between changes in intakes of dietary fiber and grain products and changes in weight and development of obesity among middle-aged women*. Am J Clin Nutr, 2003. **78**(5): p. 920-7.
51.	Murakami, K., et al., *Dietary fiber intake, dietary glycemic index and load, and body mass index: a cross-sectional study of 3931 Japanese women aged 18-20 years*. Eur J Clin Nutr, 2007.
52.	Lau, C., et al., *Association between dietary glycemic index, glycemic load, and body mass index in the Inter99 study: is underreporting a problem?* Am J Clin Nutr, 2006. **84**(3): p. 641-5.
53.	Liu, S., et al., *A prospective study of dietary glycemic load, carbohydrate intake, and risk of coronary heart disease in US women*. Am J Clin Nutr, 2000. **71**(6): p. 1455-61.
54.	Jenkins, D.J., et al., *Unabsorbable carbohydrates and diabetes: Decreased post-prandial hyperglycaemia*. Lancet, 1976. **2**(7978): p. 172-4.
55.	Jenkins, D.J., et al., *Decrease in postprandial insulin and glucose concentrations by guar and pectin*. Ann Intern Med, 1977. **86**(1): p. 20-3.
56.	Howarth, N.C., E. Saltzman, and S.B. Roberts, *Dietary fiber and weight regulation*. Nutr Rev, 2001. **59**(5): p. 129-39.
57.	Ludwig, D.S., et al., *Dietary fiber, weight gain, and cardiovascular disease risk factors in young adults*. Jama, 1999. **282**(16): p. 1539-46.
58.	Roberts, S.B. and M.B. Heyman, *Dietary composition and obesity: do we need to look beyond dietary fat?* J Nutr, 2000. **130**(2S Suppl): p. 267S.
59.	Storlien, L.H., et al., *Dietary fats and insulin action*. Diabetologia, 1996. **39**(6): p. 621-31.
60.	Gannon, M.C. and F.Q. Nuttall, *Effect of a high-protein, low-carbohydrate diet on blood glucose control in people with type 2 diabetes*. Diabetes, 2004. **53**(9): p. 2375-82.
61.	Leidy, H.J., et al., *Higher Protein Intake Preserves Lean Mass and Satiety with Weight Loss in Pre-obese and Obese Women*. Obesity (Silver Spring), 2007. **15**(2): p. 421-9.
62.	Boden, G., et al., *Effect of a low-carbohydrate diet on appetite, blood glucose levels, and insulin resistance in obese patients with type 2 diabetes*. Ann Intern Med, 2005. **142**(6): p. 403-11.
63.	Blaak, E.E., *Prevention and treatment of obesity and related complications: a role for protein?* Int J Obes (Lond), 2006. **30 Suppl 3**: p. S24-7.

64. Westerterp-Plantenga, M.S. and M.P. Lejeune, *Protein intake and body-weight regulation.* Appetite, 2005. **45**(2): p. 187-90.
65. Westerterp-Plantenga, M.S., et al., *Dietary protein, metabolism, and body-weight regulation: dose-response effects.* Int J Obes (Lond), 2006. **30 Suppl 3**: p. S16-23.
66. Pereira, M.A. and D.S. Ludwig, *Dietary fiber and body-weight regulation. Observations and mechanisms.* Pediatr Clin North Am, 2001. **48**(4): p. 969-80.
67. Warren, J.M., C.J. Henry, and V. Simonite, *Low glycemic index breakfasts and reduced food intake in preadolescent children.* Pediatrics, 2003. **112**(5): p. e414.
68. Roberts, S.B., *High-glycemic index foods, hunger, and obesity: is there a connection?* Nutr Rev, 2000. **58**(6): p. 163-9.
69. Bray, G.A., S.J. Nielsen, and B.M. Popkin, *Consumption of high-fructose corn syrup in beverages may play a role in the epidemic of obesity.* Am J Clin Nutr, 2004. **79**(4): p. 537-43.
70. Elliott, S.S., et al., *Fructose, weight gain, and the insulin resistance syndrome.* Am J Clin Nutr, 2002. **76**(5): p. 911-22.
71. Havel, P.J., *Dietary fructose: implications for dysregulation of energy homeostasis and lipid/carbohydrate metabolism.* Nutr Rev, 2005. **63**(5): p. 133-57.
72. Fowler, S., Williams, K etal. *Diet Soft Drink Consumption is Associated with Increased Incidence of Overweight and Obesity in the San Antonio Heart Study.* in *American Diabetic Association 65th Annual Assembly.* 2005.
73. Dhingra, R., et al, *Soft Drink Consumption and Risk of Developing Cardiometabolic Risk Factors and the Metabolic Syndrome in Middle-Aged Adults in the Community.* Circulation, 2007.
74. Davidson, T.L. and S.E. Swithers, *A Pavlovian approach to the problem of obesity.* Int J Obes Relat Metab Disord, 2004. **28**(7): p. 933-5.
75. Pierce, WD. *Overeating by Young Obese-prone and Lean Rats Caused by Tastes Associated with Low Energy Foods.* Obesity 2007: 15: 1969-79.
76. *Artificial Sweeteners May Damage Diet Efforts: Sugar Substitutes May Distort the Body's Natural Calorie Counter.* Web MD Medical News 2004 [cited 2007 Feb 25]; Available from: http://www.webmd.com/diet/news/20040630/artificial-sweeteners-damage-diet-efforts.

DIET AND INSULIN METABOLISM

Key concepts you should take away from this chapter:
• Loss of sensitivity to the hormone insulin is known as insulin resistance • Insulin resistance predisposes to development of the Big 7 U.S. diseases • The standard American diet promotes insulin resistance **Specifically**: • Excessive consumption of non-fiber carbohydrates (NFCs) and relative deficiency of fiber promotes insulin resistance • Excessive consumption of saturated fatty acids promotes insulin resistance • Consumption of trans fatty acids strongly promotes insulin resistance • Relative deficiency of monounsaturated and omega-3 polyunsaturated fatty acids promotes insulin resistance • Relative deficiency of protein contributes to insulin resistance • Excess abdominal fat tissue and other sources of inflammatory mediators promote insulin resistance

INSULIN IN HEALTH AND DISEASE

Insulin is a polypeptide hormone that regulates carbohydrate and energy metabolism. After a meal, starches and sugars are converted to glucose, which is absorbed by the small intestine, triggering specialized cells of the pancreas to secrete insulin. Insulin promotes uptake of glucose by muscle cells, fat cells, and other tissues [1]. Once inside the cell, glucose is converted to energy that powers cellular operations. In health, the efficiency of this system maintains blood glucose within the narrow range required to provide energy to tissues. However, certain factors cause muscle and fat cells to become insensitive to the effects of insulin, a process known as *insulin resistance*. Insulin resistance, or *pre*-diabetes, is an underlying metabolic abnormality involved in the development of the "metabolic syndrome," a constellation of abdominal fat tissue accumulation, hypertension, dysregulated cholesterol metabolism, and insulin resistance which affects nearly forty percent of U.S. adults [2, 3]!

The U.S. population has witnessed an explosion of insulin resistance and diabetes mellitus over the last 30 years to today's epidemic levels [4, 5]. Alarmingly, younger generations are developing pre-diabetes and diabetes at younger ages than ever before in human history, and rates are anticipated to increase [6]. Interestingly, westernization of dietary habits greatly increases the risk of developing insulin resistance and diabetes mellitus, and insulin resistance is virtually unheard of in current hunter-gatherer populations [7-11]. Taken together, these facts suggest that environmental factors, rather than genetic changes, are responsible for the recent epidemic of diabetes mellitus. In fact, environmental changes are thought to account for over 70% of the risk of developing diabetes mellitus [12].

Importantly, chronically elevated blood glucose levels promote inflammation, oxidative stress, thrombosis, and vascular damage, which helps explain the strong link between insulin resistance, diabetes, and cardiovascular disease [13-16]. In addition, insulin resistance can progress to full-fledged diabetes mellitus.

METABOLIC DETERMINANTS OF INSULIN RESISTANCE

Important metabolic processes that promote insulin resistance include fat accumulation, inflammation, membrane rigidity, and chronically elevated blood glucose, insulin, and free fatty acids.

FAT ACCUMULATION AND INFLAMMATION

Fat accumulation, inflammation, and insulin resistance are intimately related processes. In fact, excessive accumulation of fat tissue may be *the* most important determinant of insulin resistance, accounting for up to 75% of all cases of diabetes mellitus [17]. Fat tissue secretes large quantities of pro-inflammatory cytokines and other mediators which reduce insulin sensitivity [18-21]. These mediators likely account for the strong association between obesity, insulin resistance, and diabetes mellitus [22-24]. Interestingly, elevated levels of pro-inflammatory cytokines and acute phase proteins predict *future* development of diabetes mellitus, and precede overt diabetes mellitus by many years [25-28]. Of note, sources of inflammatory mediators unrelated to fat tissue also promote insulin resistance [16, 20].

MEMBRANE RIGIDITY

Both glucose and insulin receptors span the cellular membrane. In health, adequate fluidity of cell membranes allows receptors to efficiently bind circulating glucose and insulin, and transport glucose into the cell. To some extent, membrane fluidity is regulated by its fatty acid content. In general, the "kinked" structures of natural *un*saturated fatty acids prevent them from grouping together too tightly, thereby promoting membrane fluidity. On the other hand, the straight nature of saturated fats, trans fats, and cholesterol allows these fatty acids to pack tightly together, and increase membrane rigidity. Reduced membrane fluidity may account for the correlation between saturated and trans fat intake and insulin resistance and diabetes [29-33].

MEMBRANE RECEPTOR EFFICIENCY

Elevation of blood glucose, or hyperglycemia, leads to a compensatory elevation of blood insulin, also known as hyperinsulinemia. Chronic hyperglycemia and hyperinsulinemia desensitize glucose and insulin receptors, thereby promoting insulin resistance [34-36]. Similarly, chronically elevated free fatty acids reduce insulin receptor sensitivity and promote insulin resistance [37].

DIET AND INSULIN ACTION

INSULIN REGULATING PROPERTIES OF NUTRIENTS

SATURATED FATS

Saturated fats promote insulin resistance via multiple mechanisms including increased membrane rigidity and inefficient function of glucose and insulin receptors [29-32, 38, 39].

TRANS FATS

By reducing membrane fluidity *and* promoting inflammation, trans fats profoundly reduce glucose and insulin receptor sensitivity and promote insulin resistance [29, 30, 32, 40-42].

MONOUNSATURATED FATS

In contrast with saturated and trans fats, monounsaturated fats (MUFAs) increase membrane fluidity and improve insulin sensitivity [29-31, 39].

OMEGA-3 AND OMEGA-6 POLYUNSATURATED FATS

Like MUFAs, both classes of polyunsaturated fats (PUFAs) increase membrane fluidity and improve short-term insulin sensitivity [29-31, 43]. However, by promoting fat tissue expansion, long-term ω-6 to ω-3 imbalance *may* ultimately contribute to dysfunctional insulin metabolism [44, 45].

NON-FIBER CARBOHYDRATES (NFC)

High refined starch and glucose intake, especially in the absence of fiber, results in hyperglycemia and compensatory hyperinsulinemia [31, 46-50]. By reducing glucose and insulin receptor sensitivity, chronic hyperglycemia and hyperinsulinemia predispose to insulin resistance [34, 35]. Unlike dietary glucose and starches, dietary fructose only slightly raises short-term blood glucose levels [47]. For this reason, some dietary guidelines suggest that replacement of glucose with fructose may have beneficial metabolic effects. Importantly, however, dietary fructose promotes insulin resistance independently of raising blood glucose, and long-term fructose consumption appears to have similar adverse metabolic and health consequences as glucose and refined starches [51-55]. Failure to account for fructose's role in *long-term* promotion of insulin resistance is one of the crucial weaknesses of relying solely on glycemic index or glycemic load for food selections.

FIBER

By slowing and reducing glucose absorption, fibers attenuate blood glucose and insulin elevations after high-NFC meals, thereby helping maintain receptor sensitivity [56-58].

High-fiber diets reduce the risk of developing pre-diabetes and overt diabetes mellitus [24].

PROTEIN

Like fiber, protein attenuates blood glucose elevations [59-61]. In addition, protein consumption may favor formation and maintenance of lean body mass (muscle)[62]. Via these mechanisms, long-term protein consumption improves insulin sensitivity.

POLYCHLORINATED BIPHENYLS (PCBs)

Total body burden of PCBs is strongly associated with insulin resistance and diabetes mellitus in several epidemiological studies [63-65]. While further research is necessary to demonstrate a causal linkage, PCBs have been shown to disturb glucose metabolism in animal and metabolic studies [66, 67].

CONCLUSION

Many of the same dietary practices that predispose Americans to obesity and inflammatory diseases also promote insulin resistance and diabetes mellitus. The typical high NFC to fiber ratios, high intake of saturated and trans fats, and relatively low intakes of MUFAs and proteins, promote insulin resistance and predispose to diabetes mellitus. When combined with dietary strategies aimed at reducing fat accumulation and inflammation, replacement of saturated fats, trans fats, and non-fiber carbohydrates with fiber, protein, and monounsaturated fats can profoundly improve insulin sensitivity and protect against the "Big 7" diseases.

References:

1. Ducluzeau, P.H., et al., *Molecular mechanisms of insulin-stimulated glucose uptake in adipocytes.* Diabetes Metab, 2002. **28**(2): p. 85-92.
2. Ford, E.S., *Prevalence of the metabolic syndrome defined by the International Diabetes Federation among adults in the U.S.* Diabetes Care, 2005. **28**(11): p. 2745-9.
3. Reaven, G.M., *Pathophysiology of insulin resistance in human disease.* Physiol Rev, 1995. **75**(3): p. 473-86.
4. Fox, C.S., et al., *Trends in the incidence of type 2 diabetes mellitus from the 1970s to the 1990s: the Framingham Heart Study.* Circulation, 2006. **113**(25): p. 2914-8.
5. Satyanarayana, S., et al., *Antioxidant activity of the aqueous extracts of spicy food additives--evaluation and comparison with ascorbic acid in in-vitro systems.* J Herb Pharmacother, 2004. **4**(2): p. 1-10.
6. Babaoglu, K., et al., *Evaluation of glucose intolerance in adolescents relative to adults with type 2 diabetes mellitus.* J Pediatr Endocrinol Metab, 2006. **19**(11): p. 1319-26.
7. Cordain, L., et al., *Origins and evolution of the Western diet: health implications for the 21st century.* Am J Clin Nutr, 2005. **81**(2): p. 341-54.
8. Lieberman, L.S., *Dietary, evolutionary, and modernizing influences on the prevalence of type 2 diabetes.* Annu Rev Nutr, 2003. **23**: p. 345-77.
9. Collins, C., *Said another way: stroke, evolution, and the rainforests: an ancient approach to modern health care.* Nurs Forum, 2007. **42**(1): p. 39-44.
10. Eaton, S.B., M. Konner, and M. Shostak, *Stone agers in the fast lane: chronic degenerative diseases in evolutionary perspective.* Am J Med, 1988. **84**(4): p. 739-49.
11. Cordain, L., M.R. Eades, and M.D. Eades, *Hyperinsulinemic diseases of civilization: more than just Syndrome X.* Comp Biochem Physiol A Mol Integr Physiol, 2003. **136**(1): p. 95-112.
12. Hemminki, K., J. Lorenzo Bermejo, and A. Forsti, *The balance between heritable and environmental aetiology of human disease.* Nat Rev Genet, 2006. **7**(12): p. 958-65.
13. Dandona, P. and A. Aljada, *A rational approach to pathogenesis and treatment of type 2 diabetes mellitus, insulin resistance, inflammation, and atherosclerosis.* Am J Cardiol, 2002. **90**(5A): p. 27G-33G.
14. Biondi-Zoccai, G.G., et al., *Atherothrombosis, inflammation, and diabetes.* J Am Coll Cardiol, 2003. **41**(7): p. 1071-7.
15. Dandona, P., et al., *The potential influence of inflammation and insulin resistance on the pathogenesis and treatment of atherosclerosis-related complications in type 2 diabetes.* J Clin Endocrinol Metab, 2003. **88**(6): p. 2422-9.
16. Pradhan, A.D. and P.M. Ridker, *Do atherosclerosis and type 2 diabetes share a common inflammatory basis?* Eur Heart J, 2002. **23**(11): p. 831-4.
17. Costacou, T. and E.J. Mayer-Davis, *Nutrition and prevention of type 2 diabetes.* Annu Rev Nutr, 2003. **23**: p. 147-70.
18. Peraldi, P. and B. Spiegelman, *TNF-alpha and insulin resistance: summary and future prospects.* Mol Cell Biochem, 1998. **182**(1-2): p. 169-75.
19. Fernandez-Real, J.M. and W. Ricart, *Insulin resistance and chronic cardiovascular inflammatory syndrome.* Endocr Rev, 2003. **24**(3): p. 278-301.
20. Sjoholm, A. and T. Nystrom, *Inflammation and the etiology of type 2 diabetes.* Diabetes Metab Res Rev, 2006. **22**(1): p. 4-10.
21. Halvorsen, B.L., et al., *A systematic screening of total antioxidants in dietary plants.* J Nutr, 2002. **132**(3): p. 461-71.
22. Pickup, J.C. and M.A. Crook, *Is type II diabetes mellitus a disease of the innate immune system?* Diabetologia, 1998. **41**(10): p. 1241-8.
23. Xu, H., et al., *Chronic inflammation in fat plays a crucial role in the development of obesity-related insulin resistance.* J Clin Invest, 2003. **112**(12): p. 1821-30.
24. Schulze, M.B., et al., *Fiber and magnesium intake and incidence of type 2 diabetes: a prospective study and meta-analysis.* Arch Intern Med, 2007. **167**(9): p. 956-65.
25. Kolb, H. and T. Mandrup-Poulsen, *An immune origin of type 2 diabetes?* Diabetologia, 2005. **48**(6): p. 1038-50.
26. Pickup, J.C., *Inflammation and activated innate immunity in the pathogenesis of type 2 diabetes.* Diabetes Care, 2004. **27**(3): p. 813-23.
27. Pickup, J.C., et al., *NIDDM as a disease of the innate immune system: association of acute-phase reactants and interleukin-6 with metabolic syndrome X.* Diabetologia, 1997. **40**(11): p. 1286-92.
28. Thorand, B., et al., *C-reactive protein as a predictor for incident diabetes mellitus among middle-aged men: results from the MONICA Augsburg cohort study, 1984-1998.* Arch Intern Med, 2003. **163**(1): p. 93-9.
29. Storlien, L.H., et al., *Dietary fats and insulin action.* Diabetologia, 1996. **39**(6): p. 621-31.
30. Ludwig, D.S., *Symposium 2: Nutrition and Chronic Disease. Diet and development of the insulin resustence syndrome.* Proceedings of the Nutrition Society of Australia, 2003. **27**: p. S4.
31. Riccardi, G. and A.A. Rivellese, *Dietary treatment of the metabolic syndrome--the optimal diet.* Br J Nutr, 2000. **83 Suppl 1**: p. S143-8.
32. Christiansen, E., et al., *Intake of a diet high in trans monounsaturated fatty acids or saturated fatty acids. Effects on postprandial insulinemia and glycemia in obese patients with NIDDM.* Diabetes Care, 1997. **20**(5): p. 881-7.
33. Van Epps-Fung, M., et al., *Fatty acid-induced insulin resistance in adipocytes.* Endocrinology, 1997. **138**(10): p. 4338-45.
34. Del Prato, S., et al., *Effect of sustained physiologic hyperinsulinaemia and hyperglycaemia on insulin secretion and insulin sensitivity in man.* Diabetologia, 1994. **37**(10): p. 1025-35.
35. McClain, D.A., *Hexosamines as mediators of nutrient sensing and regulation in diabetes.* J Diabetes Complications, 2002. **16**(1): p. 72-80.

36.   Rose, G.A., W.B. Thomson, and R.T. Williams, *Corn Oil in Treatment of Ischaemic Heart Disease*. Br Med J, 1965. **1**(5449): p. 1531-3.

37.   Boden, G. and G.I. Shulman, *Free fatty acids in obesity and type 2 diabetes: defining their role in the development of insulin resistance and beta-cell dysfunction*. Eur J Clin Invest, 2002. **32 Suppl 3**: p. 14-23.

38.   Das, U.N., *A defect in the activity of Delta6 and Delta5 desaturases may be a factor predisposing to the development of insulin resistance syndrome*. Prostaglandins Leukot Essent Fatty Acids, 2005. **72**(5): p. 343-50.

39.   U.S. Department of Health and Human Services, U.S. Department of Agriculture: *Dietary Guidelines for Americans, 6th ed., Washington, D.C.* 2005 [cited 2006 August 15]; Available from: http://healthierus.gov/dietaryguidelines/

40.   Ibrahim, A., S. Natrajan, and R. Ghafoorunissa, *Dietary trans-fatty acids alter adipocyte plasma membrane fatty acid composition and insulin sensitivity in rats*. Metabolism, 2005. **54**(2): p. 240-6.

41.   Lopez-Garcia, E., et al., *Consumption of trans fatty acids is related to plasma biomarkers of inflammation and endothelial dysfunction*. J Nutr, 2005. **135**(3): p. 562-6.

42.   Mozaffarian, D., et al., *Dietary intake of trans fatty acids and systemic inflammation in women*. Am J Clin Nutr, 2004. **79**(4): p. 606-12.

43.   Gletsu, N.A. and M.T. Clandinin, *Impact of dietary fatty acid composition on insulin action at the nucleus*. Ann N Y Acad Sci, 1997. **827**: p. 188-99.

44.   Ailhaud, G., et al., *Temporal changes in dietary fats: role of n-6 polyunsaturated fatty acids in excessive adipose tissue development and relationship to obesity*. Prog Lipid Res, 2006. **45**(3): p. 203-36.

45.   Fickova, M., et al., *Dietary (n-3) and (n-6) polyunsaturated fatty acids rapidly modify fatty acid composition and insulin effects in rat adipocytes*. J Nutr, 1998. **128**(3): p. 512-9.

46.   Gross, L.S., et al., *Increased consumption of refined carbohydrates and the epidemic of type 2 diabetes in the United States: an ecologic assessment*. Am J Clin Nutr, 2004. **79**(5): p. 774-9.

47.   Bantle, J.P., *Is fructose the optimal low glycemic index sweetener?* Nestle Nutr Workshop Ser Clin Perform Programme, 2006. **11**: p. 83-91; discussion 92-5.

48.   Dahlqvist, A. and B. Borgstrom, *Digestion and absorption of disaccharides in man*. Biochem J, 1961. **81**: p. 411-8.

49.   Wahlqvist, M.L., E.G. Wilmshurst, and E.N. Richardson, *The effect of chain length on glucose absorption and the related metabolic response*. Am J Clin Nutr, 1978. **31**(11): p. 1998-2001.

50.   Holt, S.H., J.C. Miller, and P. Petocz, *An insulin index of foods: the insulin demand generated by 1000-kJ portions of common foods*. Am J Clin Nutr, 1997. **66**(5): p. 1264-76.

51.   Beck-Nielsen, H., O. Pedersen, and H.O. Lindskov, *Impaired cellular insulin binding and insulin sensitivity induced by high-fructose feeding in normal subjects*. Am J Clin Nutr, 1980. **33**(2): p. 273-8.

52.   Wu, T., et al., *Fructose, glycemic load, and quantity and quality of carbohydrate in relation to plasma C-peptide concentrations in US women*. Am J Clin Nutr, 2004. **80**(4): p. 1043-9.

53.   Reiser, S., et al., *Day-long glucose, insulin, and fructose responses of hyperinsulinemic and nonhyperinsulinemic men adapted to diets containing either fructose or high-amylose cornstarch*. Am J Clin Nutr, 1989. **50**(5): p. 1008-14.

54.   Dirlewanger, M., et al., *Effects of fructose on hepatic glucose metabolism in humans*. Am J Physiol Endocrinol Metab, 2000. **279**(4): p. E907-11.

55.   Elliott, S.S., et al., *Fructose, weight gain, and the insulin resistance syndrome*. Am J Clin Nutr, 2002. **76**(5): p. 911-22.

56.   Brennan, C.S., *Dietary fibre, glycaemic response, and diabetes*. Mol Nutr Food Res, 2005. **49**(6): p. 560-70.

57.   Chandalia, M., et al., *Beneficial effects of high dietary fiber intake in patients with type 2 diabetes mellitus*. N Engl J Med, 2000. **342**(19): p. 1392-8.

58.   Anderson, J.W., et al., *Carbohydrate and fiber recommendations for individuals with diabetes: a quantitative assessment and meta-analysis of the evidence*. J Am Coll Nutr, 2004. **23**(1): p. 5-17.

59.   Gannon, M.C. and F.Q. Nuttall, *Effect of a high-protein, low-carbohydrate diet on blood glucose control in people with type 2 diabetes*. Diabetes, 2004. **53**(9): p. 2375-82.

60.   Boden, G., et al., *Effect of a low-carbohydrate diet on appetite, blood glucose levels, and insulin resistance in obese patients with type 2 diabetes*. Ann Intern Med, 2005. **142**(6): p. 403-11.

61.   Blaak, E.E., *Prevention and treatment of obesity and related complications: a role for protein?* Int J Obes (Lond), 2006. **30 Suppl 3**: p. S24-7.

62.   Leidy, H.J., et al., *Higher Protein Intake Preserves Lean Mass and Satiety with Weight Loss in Pre-obese and Obese Women*. Obesity (Silver Spring), 2007. **15**(2): p. 421-9.

63.   Fierens, S., et al., *Dioxin/polychlorinated biphenyl body burden, diabetes and endometriosis: findings in a population-based study in Belgium*. Biomarkers, 2003. **8**(6): p. 529-34.

64.   Lee, D.H., et al., *Association between serum concentrations of persistent organic pollutants and insulin resistance among nondiabetic adults: results from the National Health and Nutrition Examination Survey 1999-2002*. Diabetes Care, 2007. **30**(3): p. 622-8.

65.   Lee, D.H., et al., *A strong dose-response relation between serum concentrations of persistent organic pollutants and diabetes: results from the National Health and Examination Survey 1999-2002*. Diabetes Care, 2006. **29**(7): p. 1638-44.

66.   Enan, E. and F. Matsumura, *2,3,7,8-Tetrachlorodibenzo-p-dioxin (TCDD)-induced changes in glucose transporting activity in guinea pigs, mice, and rats in vivo and in vitro*. J Biochem Toxicol, 1994. **9**(2): p. 97-106.

67.   Remillard, R.B. and N.J. Bunce, *Linking dioxins to diabetes: epidemiology and biologic plausibility*. Environ Health Perspect, 2002. **110**(9): p. 853-8.

DIET AND ANTIOXIDANT FUNCTION

Key concepts you should take away from this chapter:
• Oxidative stress, the term used to describe tissue damage caused by oxygen-derived free radicals, plays a key role in development of the Big 7 U.S. epidemic diseases • Free radicals are generated by normal metabolism, inflammation, environmental and dietary toxins, and mega-dose antioxidant supplements • Humans have an elaborate, coordinated anti-oxidant defense network to counter the harmful effects of free radicals • Mega-doses of single antioxidants can disrupt antioxidant network balance and may actually increase the risk of disease and death • Antioxidant network optimization requires *frequent* and *balanced* consumption of *diverse* antioxidant molecules • Network optimization can be achieved through frequent intake of antioxidant-rich fruits, vegetables, nuts, legumes, dark chocolate, spices, whole grains, teas, coffee, red wine, and ales

THE OXYGEN PARADOX

The fact that oxygen is both necessary for life and a potentially lethal toxin is considered a paradox of human life [1, 2]. A constant supply of oxygen is required for efficient conversion of dietary nutrients into life-giving energy. Within minutes, oxygen deprivation results in permanent injury and eventually death [3]. Yet, continuous exposure to oxygen is not without its costs. Oxygen metabolism invariably produces pro-oxidant free radicals, or reactive oxygen species [4, 5]. Reactive oxygen species, which contain highly-reactive unpaired electrons, react with and damage important biomolecules including DNA, proteins, and lipid membranes [6]. Left unchecked, free radical-mediated tissue damage leads to clinically apparent disease. Via these mechanisms, *persistent* oxidative stress has been implicated in the development and progression of cardiovascular disease, cancers, Alzheimer's dementia, and several other epidemic U.S. diseases [7-12]. Fortunately, humans have developed an elaborate, coordinated anti-oxidant defense network to counter the harmful effects of pro-oxidant molecules [1, 2, 5, 13]. However, in certain circumstances, excessive activity of oxygen-derived free radicals can overwhelm the antioxidant defense system, leading to *oxidative stress* [5].

One such example is chronic inflammation. During an inflammatory response, activated immune cells use oxygen-derived free radicals to destroy invading pathogens [14-16]. These free radicals can damage local lipid membranes, proteins, DNA, and other important biomolecules, triggering a vicious cycle of inflammation and oxidative stress [17]. *Persistent* inflammation overwhelms the antioxidant network and depletes antioxidant stores [18].

Other causes of oxidative stress include cigarette smoke, air pollution and other environmental toxins, polychlorinated biphenyls, heme iron, and other dietary toxins [19-24].

ANTIOXIDANTS

Antioxidants are a diverse group of molecules grouped together because they neutralize and deactivate oxygen-derived free radicals [25]. Antioxidants come in many shapes and sizes and have highly variable molecular properties [2, 5]. They are broadly classified as endogenous or exogenous; endogenous antioxidants are produced *by* the human body while exogenous antioxidants are supplied in the diet or via supplementation. In health, the combined efforts of both endogenous and exogenous antioxidants efficiently deactivate and clear free radicals, thereby limiting tissue damage [5].

DIETARY ANTIOXIDANTS

Dietary antioxidants can be classified according to solubility: **hydro**philic antioxidants such as vitamin C are water soluble, **lipo**philic antioxidants including vitamin E are fat soluble, and **amphi**philic antioxidants, such as hydroxytyrosol, are both water *and* fat soluble [5, 25-28]. The human body contains countless water-soluble regions, lipid-soluble regions, and water-lipid interfaces [27]. Hydrophilic antioxidants, which neutralize free radicals in water-rich environments such as the inside of cells, are unable to reach lipid-rich areas. Lipophilic antioxidants, which neutralize free radicals in lipid-rich environments such as cell membranes and lipoproteins, are ineffective in water-rich environments. Amphiphilic antioxidants function optimally at the water-lipid interface, areas where lipophilic and hydrophilic antioxidants have limited effectiveness [26]. Because oxygen-derived free radicals exist in all of these regions, adequate amounts of all three varieties of antioxidants are necessary to optimally neutralize free radicals throughout the human body [27].

Although vitamins C, E, and other vitamin antioxidants traditionally receive much of the attention, non-vitamin molecules known as polyphenolic antioxidants account for a larger percentage of free radical neutralizing ability in most foods [25, 29-32]. Dozens of polyphenolic antioxidants, also known as flavonoids, each with a unique molecular signature, exist in plant-derived foods and beverages available for human consumption [33]. Dietary polyphenolic and vitamin antioxidants interact with one another and endogenous antioxidants to regulate a complex antioxidant network [7, 12, 25, 29, 34-37].

THE ANTIOXIDANT NETWORK

Over the last two decades, fresh insight into the complexity of antioxidant interactions has generated a novel conceptual framework for limiting oxidative stress-induced tissue damage. The antioxidant network is under homeostatic control, and diet is the major contributor to body defenses against oxidative stress [5, 38]. *Optimal modulation requires frequent, diverse, and balanced antioxidant intake.*

FREQUENCY

Studies have clearly demonstrated that intake of antioxidant-rich foods including fruits, vegetables, tea, red wine, and chocolate can acutely raise plasma total antioxidant capacity (TAC) levels [39-44]. Peak elevations generally occur between one to six hours after consumption and may remain modestly elevated for up to twenty-four hours. Thus, maintenance of high blood antioxidant levels requires frequent intake of antioxidant-rich foods and/or beverages.

VARIETY

Different antioxidant compounds exhibit diverse beneficial properties: some scavenge free radicals most efficiently in water-soluble environments, others are fat-soluble, still others work at water-lipid interfaces. Some molecules are small, others larger [26-28]. Some increase expression of endogenous antioxidants, while others inhibit pro-inflammatory enzymes and transcription factors [13, 45, 46]. Different antioxidants interact on multiple levels, are capable of recharging one another, and improve function of the entire antioxidant network [5, 29, 30, 47-52]. Additive and synergistic effects of *combinations* of distinct antioxidants may be necessary for maximum health benefits [38].

BALANCE

The requirement of balanced intake of moderate doses of individual antioxidants is best exemplified by the lack of efficacy of antioxidant vitamin mega-supplementation [53]. By disrupting the delicate antioxidant balance, mega-dose supplements may paradoxically contribute to oxidative stress, inflammation, and tissue damage [37, 54-56]. Unlike mega-dose supplementation, which provides huge doses of a single molecule, antioxidant-rich foods and beverages provide *moderate* doses of many different antioxidant molecules with additive and synergistic properties. This balanced approach appears to be necessary for optimal function of the antioxidant network.

The requirements of frequency, variety, and balance for antioxidant network optimization can be met by consuming antioxidant-rich foods or beverages every few hours. This strategy provides additive and synergistic beneficial effects of a combination of different antioxidants *and* maintains a persistently elevated plasma total antioxidant capacity. These requirements for antioxidant network optimization help explain why both high intake of antioxidant-rich foods and beverages and high blood levels of antioxidants are closely associated with disease prevention and health, while individual antioxidant vitamins have failed to show beneficial effects [7, 12, 25, 29, 34-37]!

DIETARY TOTAL ANTIOXIDANT CAPACITY

Dietary total antioxidant capacity (TAC) reflects the cumulative capacity of dietary antioxidants to scavenge free radicals [25, 38]. The TACs of foods have important health implications and are associated with reduced markers of oxidative stress and inflammation [25]. Several assays have been created to quantify TAC of individual foods and beverages [38]. However, because different antioxidants work via different mechanisms, and each assay tests for slightly different chemical properties, no single assay can fully evaluate the TAC of food items [32, 38]. Although no single perfect assay exists, assessing an individual food item in multiple different assays can provide a more global picture of antioxidants *relative* to other food items. For example, Wu et al. combined two different assays, one lipophilic and the other hydrophilic, to estimate the TAC of over 100 commonly consumed U.S. food items as part of the USDA National Food and Nutrient Analysis Program [57]. Relative antioxidant scores for food items in this database are remarkably consistent with other published data using multiple assays [32, 57, 58].

Not all foods in the NQI are represented in the USDA database or other TAC databases using multiple assays. However, by supplementing USDA TAC values with multiple other antioxidant assays to fill in the gaps, TAC values for all food items rated in the NQI can be quantified with reasonable accuracy [31, 32, 44, 58-63]. These values, expressed as TAC per "true gram," form the foundation of points awarded to food items based on antioxidant content in the NQI. The NQI considers the antioxidant content of food items with >5 TAC per gram "exceptional," >3.5 TAC per gram "superior," >2.0 TAC per gram "noteworthy," >1.0 TAC per gram "moderate," > 0.5 TAC per gram "modest," and <0.5 TAC per gram "poor."

ANTIOXIDANT CONTENT OF SELECTED FOODS

Exceptional (>5 TAC/g)	Superior (>3.5 TAC/g)	Noteworthy (>2.0 TAC/g)	Moderate (>1.0 TAC/g)	Modest (>0.5 TAC/g)	Poor (<0.5 TAC/g)
Blueberry (W)	Blueberry (C)	Eggplant	Orange	Avocado	Banana
Cranberry	Blackberry	Olive (green)	Peach	Cauliflower	Cantaloupe
Artichoke	Raspberry	Apple*	Apple**	Pineapple	Honeydew
Black plum	Asparagus	Spinach	Onion	Tomato	Watermelon
Olive (black)	Strawberry	Red Cabbage	Bell Pepper***	Potato	Corn
Red currant	Plum	Beet	Pear	Kiwi	Cucumber

W= Wild, C = Cultivated. * = Red Delicious. ** = Gala, Golden Delicious, Granny Smith, Fuji. *** = Red or Green.

Other exceptional antioxidant-rich foods include dark chocolate, black and green teas, red wines, hot peppers, turmeric root, curry powder, ginger, and cinnamon [32, 33, 44, 58-61, 63, 64].

Importantly, the biological activities of antioxidants present in raw foods and beverages can be altered by food processing, cooking, or concurrent food consumption.
In comparison to plant-based foods in their natural forms, processed foods preserve only a small fraction of antioxidants. For example, nearly all of the antioxidant content of whole grains are found in the bran and germ, components generally removed during processing [65, 66]. Uncooked coffee beans have amongst the highest overall *quantity* of antioxidants of all food items [67, 68]. However, by changing the biologic properties, roasting appears to reduce the effectiveness of antioxidants in coffee. Lack of antioxidant effects may be responsible for the relative lack of health benefits of coffee compared to tea. Similarly, the addition of milk may reduce the antioxidant capacity of coffee and tea secondary to protein-antioxidant interactions [69, 70]. This suggests that concurrent consumption of certain protein and antioxidant-rich products, such as yogurt with fruit, may limit the usefulness of dietary antioxidants [70].

CONCLUSION

Fresh insight into optimal modulation of the antioxidant network has provided an unprecedented opportunity to prevent or attenuate oxidative stress–mediated disease. Prevention of oxidative stress induced tissue damage requires frequent, diverse, and balanced antioxidant intake. Habitual consumption of antioxidant-rich foods and beverages is an ideal means of achieving this goal.

References:

1. Benzie, I.F., *Evolution of antioxidant defence mechanisms*. Eur J Nutr, 2000. **39**(2): p. 53-61.
2. Davies, K.J., *Oxidative stress: the paradox of aerobic life*. Biochem Soc Symp, 1995. **61**: p. 1-31.
3. Grant, P.E. and D. Yu, *Acute injury to the immature brain with hypoxia with or without hypoperfusion*. Radiol Clin North Am, 2006. **44**(1): p. 63-77, viii.
4. Turrens, J.F., *Superoxide production by the mitochondrial respiratory chain*. Biosci Rep, 1997. **17**(1): p. 3-8.
5. Willcox, J.K., S.L. Ash, and G.L. Catignani, *Antioxidants and prevention of chronic disease*. Crit Rev Food Sci Nutr, 2004. **44**(4): p. 275-95.
6. Mateos, R. and L. Bravo, *Chromatographic and electrophoretic methods for the analysis of biomarkers of oxidative damage to macromolecules (DNA, lipids, and proteins)*. J Sep Sci, 2007. **30**(2): p. 175-91.
7. Mink, P.J., et al., *Flavonoid intake and cardiovascular disease mortality: a prospective study in postmenopausal women*. Am J Clin Nutr, 2007. **85**(3): p. 895-909.
8. Loft, S. and H.E. Poulsen, *Cancer risk and oxidative DNA damage in man*. J Mol Med, 1996. **74**(6): p. 297-312.
9. Valko, M., et al., *Free radicals, metals and antioxidants in oxidative stress-induced cancer*. Chem Biol Interact, 2006. **160**(1): p. 1-40.
10. Klaunig, J.E. and L.M. Kamendulis, *The role of oxidative stress in carcinogenesis*. Annu Rev Pharmacol Toxicol, 2004. **44**: p. 239-67.
11. Wang, J.Y., et al., *Dual effects of antioxidants in neurodegeneration: direct neuroprotection against oxidative stress and indirect protection via suppression of glia-mediated inflammation*. Curr Pharm Des, 2006. **12**(27): p. 3521-33.
12. Ceriello, A., et al., *Total plasma antioxidant capacity predicts thrombosis-prone status in NIDDM patients*. Diabetes Care, 1997. **20**(10): p. 1589-93.
13. Giovannini, C., et al., *[Polyphenols and endogenous antioxidant defences: effects on glutathione and glutathione related enzymes]*. Ann Ist Super Sanita, 2006. **42**(3): p. 336-47.
14. Conner, E.M. and M.B. Grisham, *Inflammation, free radicals, and antioxidants*. Nutrition, 1996. **12**(4): p. 274-7.
15. Quinn, M.T. and K.A. Gauss, *Structure and regulation of the neutrophil respiratory burst oxidase: comparison with nonphagocyte oxidases*. J Leukoc Biol, 2004. **76**(4): p. 760-81.
16. El-Benna, J., et al., *Phagocyte NADPH oxidase: a multicomponent enzyme essential for host defenses*. Arch Immunol Ther Exp (Warsz), 2005. **53**(3): p. 199-206.
17. Babior, B.M., *Phagocytes and oxidative stress*. Am J Med, 2000. **109**(1): p. 33-44.
18. McMillan, D.C., et al., *Changes in micronutrient concentrations following anti-inflammatory treatment in patients with gastrointestinal cancer*. Nutrition, 2000. **16**(6): p. 425-8.
19. Yamaguchi, Y., et al., *Oxidants in the gas phase of cigarette smoke pass through the lung alveolar wall and raise systemic oxidative stress*. J Pharmacol Sci, 2007. **103**(3): p. 275-82.
20. Lu, C.Y., et al., *Oxidative DNA damage estimated by urinary 8-hydroxydeoxyguanosine and indoor air pollution among non-smoking office employees*. Environ Res, 2007. **103**(3): p. 331-7.
21. Qi, L., et al., *Heme iron from diet as a risk factor for coronary heart disease in women with type 2 diabetes*. Diabetes Care, 2007. **30**(1): p. 101-6.
22. Tappel, A., *Heme of consumed red meat can act as a catalyst of oxidative damage and could initiate colon, breast and prostate cancers, heart disease and other diseases*. Med Hypotheses, 2007. **68**(3): p. 562-4.
23. Belanger, M.C., et al., *Dietary contaminants and oxidative stress in Inuit of Nunavik*. Metabolism, 2006. **55**(8): p. 989-95.
24. Lee, D.W., R.M. Gelein, and L.A. Opanashuk, *Heme-oxygenase-1 promotes polychlorinated biphenyl mixture aroclor 1254-induced oxidative stress and dopaminergic cell injury*. Toxicol Sci, 2006. **90**(1): p. 159-67.
25. Brighenti, F., et al., *Total antioxidant capacity of the diet is inversely and independently related to plasma concentration of high-sensitivity C-reactive protein in adult Italian subjects*. Br J Nutr, 2005. **93**(5): p. 619-25.
26. Rietjens, S., et al., *The olive oil antioxidant hydroxytyrosol efficiently protects against the oxidative stress induced impairment of the NO{middle dot} response of isolated rat aorta*. Am J Physiol Heart Circ Physiol, 2006.
27. Eastwood, M.A., *Interaction of dietary antioxidants in vivo: how fruit and vegetables prevent disease?* Qjm, 1999. **92**(9): p. 527-30.
28. Padayatty, S.J., et al., *Vitamin C as an antioxidant: evaluation of its role in disease prevention*. J Am Coll Nutr, 2003. **22**(1): p. 18-35.
29. Liu, R.H., *Health benefits of fruit and vegetables are from additive and synergistic combinations of phytochemicals*. Am J Clin Nutr, 2003. **78**(3 Suppl): p. 517S-520S.
30. Aldini, G., et al., *(-)-Epigallocatechin-3-gallate prevents oxidative damage in both the aqueous and lipid compartments of human plasma*. Biochem Biophys Res Commun, 2003. **302**(2): p. 409-14.
31. Vinson, J.A., et al., *Phenol antioxidant quantity and quality in foods: fruits*. J Agric Food Chem, 2001. **49**(11): p. 5315-21.
32. Pellegrini, N., et al., *Total antioxidant capacity of plant foods, beverages and oils consumed in Italy assessed by three different in vitro assays*. J Nutr, 2003. **133**(9): p. 2812-9.

33. *USDA Database for the Flavonoid Content of Selected Foods.* March 2003 [cited 2006 August 15]; Available from: http:/www.nal.usda.gov/fnic/foodcomp.

34. Terry, P., et al., *Fruit, vegetables, dietary fiber, and risk of colorectal cancer.* J Natl Cancer Inst, 2001. **93**(7): p. 525-33.

35. Cohen, J.H., A.R. Kristal, and J.L. Stanford, *Fruit and vegetable intakes and prostate cancer risk.* J Natl Cancer Inst, 2000. **92**(1): p. 61-8.

36. Steinmetz, K.A. and J.D. Potter, *Vegetables, fruit, and cancer prevention: a review.* J Am Diet Assoc, 1996. **96**(10): p. 1027-39.

37. Stanner, S.A., et al., *A review of the epidemiological evidence for the 'antioxidant hypothesis'.* Public Health Nutr, 2004. **7**(3): p. 407-22.

38. Serafini, M. and D. Del Rio, *Understanding the association between dietary antioxidants, redox status and disease: is the Total Antioxidant Capacity the right tool?* Redox Rep, 2004. **9**(3): p. 145-52.

39. Serafini, M., G. Maiani, and A. Ferro-Luzzi, *Alcohol-free red wine enhances plasma antioxidant capacity in humans.* J Nutr, 1998. **128**(6): p. 1003-7.

40. Maxwell, S., A. Cruickshank, and G. Thorpe, *Red wine and antioxidant activity in serum.* Lancet, 1994. **344**(8916): p. 193-4.

41. Serafini, M., et al., *Plasma antioxidants from chocolate.* Nature, 2003. **424**(6952): p. 1013.

42. McAnlis, G.T., et al., *Absorption and antioxidant effects of quercetin from onions, in man.* Eur J Clin Nutr, 1999. **53**(2): p. 92-6.

43. Serafini, M., et al., *Effect of acute ingestion of fresh and stored lettuce (Lactuca sativa) on plasma total antioxidant capacity and antioxidant levels in human subjects.* Br J Nutr, 2002. **88**(6): p. 615-23.

44. Serafini, M., A. Ghiselli, and A. Ferro-Luzzi, *In vivo antioxidant effect of green and black tea in man.* Eur J Clin Nutr, 1996. **50**(1): p. 28-32.

45. Moskaug, J.O., et al., *Polyphenols and glutathione synthesis regulation.* Am J Clin Nutr, 2005. **81**(1 Suppl): p. 277S-283S.

46. Bazan, N.G., *Cell survival matters: docosahexaenoic acid signaling, neuroprotection and photoreceptors.* Trends Neurosci, 2006. **29**(5): p. 263-71.

47. Liu, R.H., *Potential synergy of phytochemicals in cancer prevention: mechanism of action.* J Nutr, 2004. **134**(12 Suppl): p. 3479S-3485S.

48. Li, X., J. Huang, and J.M. May, *Ascorbic acid spares alpha-tocopherol and decreases lipid peroxidation in neuronal cells.* Biochem Biophys Res Commun, 2003. **305**(3): p. 656-61.

49. Kadoma, Y., M. Ishihara, and S. Fujisawa, *A quantitative approach to the free radical interaction between alpha-tocopherol and the coantioxidants eugenol, resveratrol or ascorbate.* In Vivo, 2006. **20**(1): p. 61-7.

50. Huang, J. and J.M. May, *Ascorbic acid spares alpha-tocopherol and prevents lipid peroxidation in cultured H4IIE liver cells.* Mol Cell Biochem, 2003. **247**(1-2): p. 171-6.

51. Ferns, G.A. and D.J. Lamb, *What does the lipoprotein oxidation phenomenon mean?* Biochem Soc Trans, 2004. **32**(Pt 1): p. 160-3.

52. Yeum, K.J., et al., *Biomarkers of antioxidant capacity in the hydrophilic and lipophilic compartments of human plasma.* Arch Biochem Biophys, 2004. **430**(1): p. 97-103.

53. Bjelakovic, G., et al., *Mortality in randomized trials of antioxidant supplements for primary and secondary prevention: systematic review and meta-analysis.* Jama, 2007. **297**(8): p. 842-57.

54. Podmore, I.D., et al., *Vitamin C exhibits pro-oxidant properties.* Nature, 1998. **392**(6676): p. 559.

55. Deiana, M., et al., *Inhibition of peroxynitrite dependent DNA base modification and tyrosine nitration by the extra virgin olive oil-derived antioxidant hydroxytyrosol.* Free Radic Biol Med, 1999. **26**(5-6): p. 762-9.

56. Rapola, J.M., et al., *Randomised trial of alpha-tocopherol and beta-carotene supplements on incidence of major coronary events in men with previous myocardial infarction.* Lancet, 1997. **349**(9067): p. 1715-20.

57. Wu, X., et al., *Lipophilic and hydrophilic antioxidant capacities of common foods in the United States.* J Agric Food Chem, 2004. **52**(12): p. 4026-37.

58. Pellegrini, N., et al., *Total antioxidant capacity of spices, dried fruits, nuts, pulses, cereals and sweets consumed in Italy assessed by three different in vitro assays.* Mol Nutr Food Res, 2006. **50**(11): p. 1030-8.

59. Halvorsen, B.L., et al., *A systematic screening of total antioxidants in dietary plants.* J Nutr, 2002. **132**(3): p. 461-71.

60. Proteggente, A.R., et al., *The antioxidant activity of regularly consumed fruit and vegetables reflects their phenolic and vitamin C composition.* Free Radic Res, 2002. **36**(2): p. 217-33.

61. Pellegrini, N., et al., *Polyphenol content and total antioxidant activity of vini novelli (young red wines).* J Agric Food Chem, 2000. **48**(3): p. 732-5.

62. Chu, Y.F., et al., *Antioxidant and antiproliferative activities of common vegetables.* J Agric Food Chem, 2002. **50**(23): p. 6910-6.

63. Satyanarayana, S., et al., *Antioxidant activity of the aqueous extracts of spicy food additives--evaluation and comparison with ascorbic acid in in-vitro systems.* J Herb Pharmacother, 2004. **4**(2): p. 1-10.

64. Tayyem, R.F., et al., *Curcumin content of turmeric and curry powders.* Nutr Cancer, 2006. **55**(2): p. 126-31.

65. Jones, J.M., et al., *Becoming Proactive With the Whole-Grains Message.* Nutr Today, 2004. **39**(1): p. 10-17.

66. Miller, H.E., et al., *Antioxidant content of whole grain breakfast cereals, fruits and vegetables.* J Am Coll Nutr, 2000. **19**(3 Suppl): p. 312S-319S.

67. Lee, K.W., et al., *Cocoa has more phenolic phytochemicals and a higher antioxidant capacity than teas and red wine.* J Agric Food Chem, 2003. **51**(25): p. 7292-5.

68. Vinson, J.A., J. Proch, and L. Zubik, *Phenol antioxidant quantity and quality in foods: cocoa, dark chocolate, and milk chocolate.* J Agric Food Chem, 1999. **47**(12): p. 4821-4.

69. Lorenz, M., et al., *Addition of milk prevents vascular protective effects of tea.* Eur Heart J, 2007. **28**(2): p. 219-23.

70. Arts, M.J., et al., *Interactions between flavonoids and proteins: effect on the total antioxidant capacity.* J Agric Food Chem, 2002. **50**(5): p. 1184-7.

DIET AND CANCER

Key concepts you should take away from this chapter:

- The term *cancer* refers to a group of diseases characterized by unrestrained cell growth and replication
- Cell growth and replication requires angiogenesis, or growth of new blood vessels, to supply vital nutrients and oxygen to rapidly dividing cells
- Through tissue invasion and metastases, cancer can eventually lead to organ failure and death
- The standard American diet promotes the molecular mechanisms involved in the development of cancer

Specifically:

- Excessive ω-6 LA and ArA intake, combined with inadequate ω-3 ALA, EPA and DHA intake, promotes the molecular mechanisms involved in the development of cancer
- Inadequate consumption of polyphenolic antioxidants promotes the molecular mechanisms involved in the development of cancer
- Dietary toxins including PCBs, heterocyclic amines, and nitrosamines promote the molecular mechanisms involved in the development of cancer
- Alcohol consumption promotes the development of certain cancers
- Excessive fat tissue accumulation promotes the molecular mechanisms involved in the development of cancer

BACKGROUND OF CANCER

The term *cancer* refers to a group of diseases characterized by uncontrolled growth and replication of cells. Hundreds of different types of cancer exist, representing nearly every kind of human cell. Although each type of cancer is technically a different disease, all cancers share features in common, including the molecular mechanisms that lead to disease. Collectively, these cancers account for over 500,000 U.S. deaths each year (nearly ¼ all U.S. deaths), making cancer the second leading cause of death [1].

THE MOST COMMON CANCERS

Men	Women
Prostate	Breast
Lung	Lung
Colorectal	Colorectal
Urinary tract*	Uterine

[1] * = Renal and Bladder

MOLECULAR MECHANISMS OF CANCER

Cancer results when a single cell develops the ability to grow and divide indefinitely. Once a cell has started on the path towards cancer, it may take ten years or longer to manifest as a clinically apparent disease. Cancerous *transformation* requires progression through a series of four integrated steps: genetic damage, cellular proliferation, angiogenesis, and tissue invasion/metastases [2].

STEP 1: GENETIC DAMAGE (MUTAGENESIS)

Human genes are regularly bombarded by stimuli capable of damaging DNA, known as mutagens. Examples include oxidative stress, toxins, ultraviolet light, and cosmic radiation [3, 4]. While cells contain elaborate molecular machinery capable of repairing *most* genetic mutations, some DNA mutations inevitably persist [5].

Mutations of two types of genes play especially important roles in the development of cancer: tumor suppresser genes and oncogenes. Tumor suppresser genes stimulate repair enzymes to mend damaged regions of DNA. When genetic damage is too extensive to be repaired, tumor suppressor genes signal for the cell to undergo apoptosis, or programmed cell death. Oncogenes are DNA sequences that stimulate the cellular machinery involved in cell growth and division. Genetic mutations that *inactivate* tumor-suppresser genes or *activate* oncogenes can promote unrestrained cell growth and division. Examples include "p53," a tumor suppressor gene mutated in over 50% of all cancers, and "RAS," an oncogene which plays a key role in many cancers [6, 7].

STEP 2: CELLULAR PROLIFERATION

The growth and replication of cells, known as cellular proliferation, is a tightly regulated process. Many adult cells divide infrequently. However, other cells, especially those of the immune system, skin cells, and those lining the gastrointestinal and urinary tracts must replicate frequently to replace lost cells. Similarly, after tissue injury, remaining cells must proliferate to replace lost or damaged tissue as part of a coordinated healing response. A variety of growth factors and inflammatory mediators, collectively known as mitogens, stimulate cellular proliferation. Excessive exposure to mitogens can lead to unrestrained cellular proliferation as part of a disproportionate "healing" response. Unrestrained cellular proliferation is a hallmark of all cancers.

STEP 3: ANGIOGENESIS

All human cells require continuous access to oxygen and vital nutrients in order to survive and function properly. Rapidly dividing cancer cells have amongst the highest metabolic requirements of *all* cells. Angiogenesis, or growth of new blood vessels, is necessary to keep up with the enormous metabolic demands of cancer cells. Many of the same mitogens involved in cellular proliferation also stimulate angiogenesis [8]. Because angiogenesis is essential for survival of all cancers, angiogenesis inhibition is considered one of the most promising cancer prevention strategies [9].

STEP 4: TISSUE INVASION AND METASTASIS

In order to continue growing, a tumor will eventually need to degrade surrounding tissues. Special enzymes that degrade collagen and other structural components allow tumors to break free from spatial constraints and gain access to the bloodstream. Access to the bloodstream and lymphatics allows cancer cells to spread, or metastasize, and begin growing at new sites far away from the original tumor. By damaging tissues, invasion and metastases can result in organ failure, and eventually, death.

Like all complex diseases, both genetic susceptibility and environmental factors determine which individuals will develop cancer. However, environmental and lifestyle factors are believed to play the dominant role, accounting for 75-90% of all cancer cases [10]. Perhaps the most convincing evidence for the leading role of environment are migration studies of individuals from areas with low incidence of cancer to areas of higher risk [11]. Cancer incidences vary as much as 12-fold to over 100-fold across populations [12]. While rates of prostate cancer in mainland China are very low, they are 5-fold higher for Chinese men living in Hong Kong and 16-fold higher for Chinese men living in the U.S. [13]. Importantly, the earlier the age of migration and longer duration of residence in the U.S., the higher the risk of prostate, breast, colorectal, and several other cancers [4, 14-19]. Similarly, westernization of diets in Asia and other areas of the world has coincided with a rapid rise in the rates of breast, colon, prostate, colorectal, renal, and other classically "western" cancers [14, 20, 21]. Studies comparing the incidence of cancer in identical twins further support the dominant role of environment. Despite sharing 100% of heritable genes, concordance rates among identical twins at age 75 were only 11% for colorectal cancer, 13% for breast cancer, and 18% for prostate cancer [22]. It is likely that shared *early* environmental experiences account for a significant portion of even these small percentages [10].

While 75-90% of cancers are thought to be the result of environmental factors, 30-40% of all cancers may be directly attributable to diet [23-25]. Accumulating evidence suggests that dietary nutrients and toxins regulate several key molecular mechanisms implicated in the development of cancer.

DIET AND CANCER

Some dietary components promote, and others inhibit, the molecular mechanisms that transform a previously healthy cell into a malignant tumor. Thus, excessive consumption of cancer-promoting compounds, and inadequate consumption of cancer-inhibiting compounds, predisposes to cancer [23, 26, 27].

Three of the molecular processes discussed in previous chapters: oxidative stress, inflammation, and fat accumulation, also play pivotal roles in the development of cancer through direct or indirect stimulation of mutagenesis, cellular proliferation, angiogenesis, tissue invasion, and metastasis. Not surprisingly then, several of the same dietary nutrients that regulate oxidative stress, inflammation, and fat accumulation also alter the risk of developing cancer.

DIET, OXIDATIVE STRESS, AND CANCER

When oxidative stress induced genetic damage activates oncogenes or inactivates tumor suppresser genes, uncontrolled cellular proliferation ensues. Thus, prevention of oxidative stress has the potential to reduce the risk of cancer [28]. By optimizing the antioxidant defense network, habitual consumption of a variety of antioxidant-rich foods and beverages limits oxidative stress induced mutations. Prevention of oxidative stress induced mutations helps explain the association between high intake of antioxidant-rich fruits and vegetables and reduced risk of several cancers [29, 30].

DIET, INFLAMMATION, AND CANCER

Inflammation, cellular proliferation, and angiogenesis are intimately related processes, and many pro-inflammatory mediators *also* promote cellular proliferation and angiogenesis [8, 31-34]. Interplay between inflammation, cellular proliferation, and angiogenesis allows for a coordinated, short-lived healing response after infection or injury, which terminates after inflammation resolves. However, *persistent* inflammation results in a continuous "healing" response. By stimulating cellular proliferation, angiogenesis, and tissue remodeling, chronic inflammation predisposes to the development of cancer [32, 34-36].

METABOLIC PATHWAYS LINKING INFLAMMATION TO CANCER

NF-kB

NF-kB is a transcription factor which regulates inflammatory responses to a wide variety of stressful stimuli [37, 38]. In short, NF-kB activation results in generation of a host of pro-inflammatory mediators, enzymes, and growth factors involved in inflammation, cellular proliferation, angiogenesis, tissue invasion, and metastases. Interruption of NF-kB signaling, through dietary or pharmaceutical means, is one of the most promising cancer prevention strategies [37, 39].

MEDIATORS GENERATED THROUGH NF-kB ACTIVATION

MEDIATORS	ACTIONS	ROLE IN CANCER DEVELOPMENT
COX-2, PLA2, 5-LOX, 12-LOX	Convert ω-6 Arachidonic acid to PGE2 and leukotrienes	Cell growth and division, angiogenesis, tissue invasion, and metastases
VEGF, EDGF	Stimulate growth of new blood vessels	Angiogenesis
MMP-1, MMP-2	Degrade collagen and other structural proteins	Tissue invasion and metastases

[37, 38, 40, 41]

ARACHIDONIC ACID METABOLISM

Arachidonic acid (ArA) is a twenty carbon ω-6 polyunsaturated fatty acid consumed in the diet or synthesized from its dietary precursor linoleic acid (LA) [42]. Enzymes generated through NF-kB activation, including phospholipases, cyclooxygenases (COX-2) and lipoxygenases (5-LOX and 12-LOX), convert ArA to hormone-like compounds known as eicosanoids [43].

Importantly, several ω-6 ArA-derived eicosanoids, especially PGE2, strongly promote cell growth and division, angiogenesis, tissue invasion, and metastases [44-54]. Multiple lines of evidence support the role of excessive COX-2 activity and PGE2 generation in many cancers, and COX-2 inhibition has shown promise in cancer prevention [55-58]. In fact, the molecular link between increased activity of this pathway, excessive generation of ω-6 ArA-derived eicosanoids, and cancer development is so strong that molecules which interfere with ArA metabolism are near the forefront of cancer drug discovery efforts [24, 59-62].

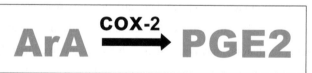

Figure 1: The COX-2 enzyme, upregulated in many cancers, boosts production of prostaglandin E2 (PGE2), which promotes cellular proliferation, angiogenesis, tissue invasion, and metastases.

"ARA OVERLOAD" AND CANCER

Typical American dietary practices, with excessive consumption of ω-6 LA and ArA, alongside inadequate ω-3 ALA, EPA, and DHA, result in blood and tissue ω-6 "ArA Overload" [42, 63-69].

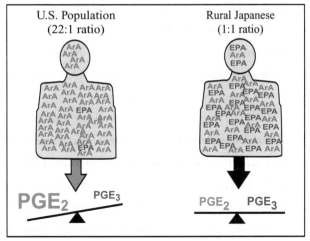

Figure 2: ArA Overload and cancer. Disparity between a U.S. population with a high incidence and a rural Japanese population with a low incidence of cancer. Accumulation of ω-6 ArA in plasma and tissues results in excessive formation of prostaglandins (PGE2) and leukotrienes (not shown) which favors the molecular mechanisms involved in cancer development.

Both animal and molecular evidence support the hypothesis that high ω-6 diets, which ultimately lead to excessive-ArA derived metabolite formation, play a role in cancer development, and populations with high consumption of ω-6 LA have amongst the highest rates of cancer in the world [24, 70-73]. While two interventional studies comparing high-LA to low-LA diets suggest that high LA intake *may* increase the risk of developing cancer, the results of other studies are inconsistent, and no firm conclusions can be drawn from them [70, 74-78].

Similarly, animal and molecular studies support the hypothesis that ω-3 ALA, by antagonizing conversion of ω-6 LA to ArA, and ultimately lowering PGE2 and LTB4 generation, inhibits the molecular mechanisms involved in cancer development [16, 37, 43, 70, 79, 80]. Mounting evidence suggests that the *ratio* of ω-6 LA to ω-3 ALA intake may be more important than the amounts, and a threshold of perhaps 5 to 1 exists, above which minimal benefit is seen [74, 76, 77]. The optimal ratio appears to be 1 or 2 to 1, similar to the ratio consumed by our ancestors [16, 80, 81]. Unfortunately, virtually the entire U.S. population consumes greater than a 7 to 1 ratio of ω-6 LA to ω-3 ALA (average >11:1), making this hypothesis difficult to prove without a strictly controlled interventional trial [74, 82].

Animal and molecular studies suggest that ω-3 EPA and DHA reduce the development of cancer by interfering with ω-6 ArA metabolism [45, 59, 83]. High intake of *fatty* fish, rich in ω-3 EPA and DHA, is associated with a dramatically reduced incidence of renal cancer [84]. Although some studies have suggested that fish consumption reduces the risk of developing colon and other cancers, a recent meta-analysis was unable to establish any consistent link [85-87]. These results are not surprising when put into context. ***Omega-6 ArA accumulation reflects a complex interaction of several different polyunsaturated fatty acids (PUFAs), rather than any individual PUFA*** [42, 68, 69, 88]. Simply increasing intake of short *or* long-chain ω-3 PUFAs in isolation, without simultaneously reducing both ω-6 LA and ArA intake, has a limited impact on ArA accumulation. Even high doses of ω-3 EPA and DHA may only reduce ω-6 ArA accumulation by 20% [89]. Rather, *long-term* increased intake of ω-3 ALA, EPA, and DHA, alongside reduced intake of both ω-6 LA and ArA, is required to cause a major reduction in plasma and tissue ω-6 ArA. To further complicate things, certain fish, especially farm-raised salmon, which account for the majority of U.S. salmon intake, actually contain massive amounts of ω-6 ArA acid, and thus may be expected to *promote*, rather than inhibit, the molecular processes involved in cancer development [59, 68, 90]. Farm-raised fish also contain high levels of PCBs, a known carcinogen [91, 92]. Certain cooking methods, especially grilling, smoking, and frying create other carcinogens which may counter beneficial effects of ω-3 EPA and DHA [93]. Although EPA and DHA likely play a role in cancer prevention, more comprehensive strategies aimed at reducing "ArA Overload" are needed to counter the molecular mechanisms involved in the development of cancer.

POLYPHENOLIC ANTIOXIDANTS AND CANCER

Polyphenolic antioxidants interfere with the development and progression of cancer via multiple mechanisms in addition to their antioxidant effects [94]. First, many polyphenolic antioxidants have direct COX-2 and 5-LOX inhibiting properties. By limiting PGE2 and leukotriene formation, COX-2 and lipoxygenase blockade reduces cellular proliferation, angiogenesis, tissue invasion, and metastases [44-48].

In addition to interfering with ω-6 ArA metabolism, polyphenolic antioxidant compounds, including resveratrol (grapes, red wine), gingerols (ginger), anthocyanins (berries), curcuminoids (turmeric, cumin), and EGCG (green tea), inhibit Nuclear Factor kappa B (NF-kB), thereby reducing the formation of growth factors, enzymes, and inflammatory mediators involved in cellular proliferation, angiogenesis, tissue invasion, and metastases [29, 95, 96].

DIET, FAT ACCUMULATION, AND CANCER

Excess fat accumulation dramatically increases the risk of developing cancer [97, 98]. Obesity alone accounts for an estimated 15-20% of all U.S. cancer-related deaths [99]. Fat cells, especially those surrounding abdominal organs, known as visceral fat, secrete estrogen, leptin, pro-inflammatory cytokines, and mitogens which promote cellular proliferation, angiogenesis, and tissue invasion [100, 101]. By limiting fat cell accumulation, strategies discussed in *Part 3: Diet and Fat Accumulation* (pages 131-141) may indirectly reduce the risk of cancer.

DIETARY TOXINS AND CANCER

Excess alcohol consumption increases the risk of developing cancer of the breast, liver, esophagus, and other sites [102]. Several other dietary toxins including PCBs (farm-raised fish), nitrates/nitrites (processed meats), and heterocyclic amines (grilled, fried meats) are associated with increased cancer risk [30, 92, 103, 104]. Avoidance of concentrated sources of these compounds has the potential to reduce the risk of developing cancer.

OTHER DIETARY CONSTITUENTS AND CANCER

Hundreds of other phytochemicals are believed to interfere with the molecular mechanisms involved in cancer development [29, 105-107]. Notable examples include polyphenolic antioxidants (discussed above) and isothiocyanates, found in broccoli, cabbage, and other cruciferous vegetables [95, 108]. Red meat consumption has been linked to a variety of cancers [109-112]. More research is necessary to determine if heme iron (pro-oxidant), ω-6 ArA (ArA Overload), heterocyclic amines (mutagen), or a combination of all three are responsible for this association [30, 59, 113, 114].

Fiber may reduce the risk of some cancers by improving insulin sensitivity, which may in turn lower levels of insulin-like growth factor, a molecule with cancer promoting properties [38, 97, 115, 116].

VITAMIN D AND CANCER

Mounting evidence suggests that high plasma levels of vitamin D3 (cholecalciferol) significantly reduce the risk of a variety of cancers [117]. The relationship is maintained whether vitamin D3 is attained through dietary means, supplementation, or sun exposure [118, 119]. Thus, consuming vitamin D3-rich foods (fish, fortified dairy, cod liver oil) or supplements during periods of sun deprivation may be beneficial.

SUMMARY

An estimated 30 to 40% of cancers are attributable to dietary practices. Improved understanding of the molecular mechanisms linking diet to cancer has allowed for a theoretical ideal diet for cancer prevention:

- Avoid ω-6 "ArA Overload" by reducing the ω-6 LA to ω-3 ALA ratio to less than 4:1, reducing ω-6 ArA intake, and increasing ω-3 EPA/DHA consumption.
- Optimize the antioxidant defense network through *habitual* intake of antioxidant-rich foods and beverages.
- Regularly consume cruciferous vegetables, fruits, and other concentrated sources of anti-cancer phytochemicals.
- Limit consumption of red meats and processed meats.
- Limit intake of PCBs, nitrates/nitrites, heterocyclic amines, alcohol, and other dietary toxins.
- Maintain *moderate* year-round sunlight exposure. During extended periods of sun deprivation, consume fish, cod liver oil, fortified dairy products, or a 600 to 1000 IU cholecalciferol (vitamin D3) supplement.
- Maintain a healthy weight.

References:
1. Jemal, A., et al., *Cancer statistics, 2003.* CA Cancer J Clin, 2003. **53**(1): p. 5-26.
2. Hanahan, D. and R.A. Weinberg, *The hallmarks of cancer.* Cell, 2000. **100**(1): p. 57-70.
3. Bartsch, H. and J. Nair, *Exocyclic DNA adducts as secondary markers for oxidative stress: applications in human cancer etiology and risk assessment.* Adv Exp Med Biol, 2001. **500**: p. 675-86.
4. Grover, P.L. and F.L. Martin, *The initiation of breast and prostate cancer.* Carcinogenesis, 2002. **23**(7): p. 1095-102.
5. Kasai, H., *Chemistry-based studies on oxidative DNA damage: formation, repair, and mutagenesis.* Free Radic Biol Med, 2002. **33**(4): p. 450-6.

6.   Strano, S., et al., *Mutant p53: an oncogenic transcription factor.* Oncogene, 2007. **26**(15): p. 2212-9.
7.   Schubbert, S., G. Bollag, and K. Shannon, *Deregulated Ras signaling in developmental disorders: new tricks for an old dog.* Curr Opin Genet Dev, 2007. **17**(1): p. 15-22.
8.   Costa, C., J. Incio, and R. Soares, *Angiogenesis and chronic inflammation: cause or consequence?* Angiogenesis, 2007.
9.   Tabruyn, S.P. and A.W. Griffioen, *Molecular pathways of angiogenesis inhibition.* Biochem Biophys Res Commun, 2007. **355**(1): p. 1-5.
10.   Hemminki, K., J. Lorenzo Bermejo, and A. Forsti, *The balance between heritable and environmental aetiology of human disease.* Nat Rev Genet, 2006. **7**(12): p. 958-65.
11.   Sim, H.G. and C.W. Cheng, *Changing demography of prostate cancer in Asia.* Eur J Cancer, 2005. **41**(6): p. 834-45.
12.   *IARC Cancer Incidence in Five Continents.* in *IARC.* 2002. Lyon.
13.   Muir, C.S., J. Nectoux, and J. Staszewski, *The epidemiology of prostatic cancer. Geographical distribution and time-trends.* Acta Oncol, 1991. **30**(2): p. 133-40.
14.   Yoo, K.Y., et al., *Lifestyle, genetic susceptibility and future trends of breast cancer in Korea.* Asian Pac J Cancer Prev, 2006. **7**(4): p. 679-82.
15.   Ziegler, R.G., et al., *Migration patterns and breast cancer risk in Asian-American women.* J Natl Cancer Inst, 1993. **85**(22): p. 1819-27.
16.   Brown, M.D., et al., *Promotion of prostatic metastatic migration towards human bone marrow stoma by Omega 6 and its inhibition by Omega 3 PUFAs.* Br J Cancer, 2006. **94**(6): p. 842-53.
17.   Doll, R. and R. Peto, *The causes of cancer: quantitative estimates of avoidable risks of cancer in the United States today.* J Natl Cancer Inst, 1981. **66**(6): p. 1191-308.
18.   Parkin, D.M. and M. Khlat, *Studies of cancer in migrants: rationale and methodology.* Eur J Cancer, 1996. **32A**(5): p. 761-71.
19.   McCredie, M., *Cancer epidemiology in migrant populations.* Recent Results Cancer Res, 1998. **154**: p. 298-305.
20.   Kodama, M., et al., *Nutrition and breast cancer risk in Japan.* Anticancer Res, 1991. **11**(2): p. 745-54.
21.   Wynder, E.L., et al., *Comparative epidemiology of cancer between the United States and Japan. A second look.* Cancer, 1991. **67**(3): p. 746-63.
22.   Lichtenstein, P., et al., *Environmental and heritable factors in the causation of cancer--analyses of cohorts of twins from Sweden, Denmark, and Finland.* N Engl J Med, 2000. **343**(2): p. 78-85.
23.   World Cancer Research Fund and American Institute for Cancer Research (1997). *Food, Nutrition, and the Prevention of Cancer, a Global Perspective.*, in *American Institute of Cancer Res.* 1997: Washington, DC.
24.   McEntee, M.F. and J. Whelan, *Dietary polyunsaturated fatty acids and colorectal neoplasia.* Biomed Pharmacother, 2002. **56**(8): p. 380-7.
25.   Lewis, C.J. and E.A. Yetley, *Health claims and observational human data: relation between dietary fat and cancer.* Am J Clin Nutr, 1999. **69**(6): p. 1357S-1364S.
26.   Willett, W.C., *Diet, nutrition, and avoidable cancer.* Environ Health Perspect, 1995. **103 Suppl 8**: p. 165-70.
27.   Willett, W.C., *Balancing life-style and genomics research for disease prevention.* Science, 2002. **296**(5568): p. 695-8.
28.   Wiseman, H. and B. Halliwell, *Damage to DNA by reactive oxygen and nitrogen species: role in inflammatory disease and progression to cancer.* Biochem J, 1996. **313** (Pt 1): p. 17-29.
29.   Liu, R.H., *Potential synergy of phytochemicals in cancer prevention: mechanism of action.* J Nutr, 2004. **134**(12 Suppl): p. 3479S-3485S.
30.   Steck, S.E., et al., *Cooked meat and risk of breast cancer--lifetime versus recent dietary intake.* Epidemiology, 2007. **18**(3): p. 373-82.
31.   Danese, S., E. Dejana, and C. Fiocchi, *Immune regulation by microvascular endothelial cells: directing innate and adaptive immunity, coagulation, and inflammation.* J Immunol, 2007. **178**(10): p. 6017-22.
32.   Ohshima, H., et al., *Prevention of human cancer by modulation of chronic inflammatory processes.* Mutat Res, 2005. **591**(1-2): p. 110-22.
33.   van Kempen, L.C., et al., *The tumor microenvironment: a critical determinant of neoplastic evolution.* Eur J Cell Biol, 2003. **82**(11): p. 539-48.
34.   Coussens, L.M. and Z. Werb, *Inflammatory cells and cancer: think different!* J Exp Med, 2001. **193**(6): p. F23-6.
35.   Balkwill, F. and A. Mantovani, *Inflammation and cancer: back to Virchow?* Lancet, 2001. **357**(9255): p. 539-45.
36.   Platz, E.A. and A.M. De Marzo, *Epidemiology of inflammation and prostate cancer.* J Urol, 2004. **171**(2 Pt 2): p. S36-40.
37.   Demark-Wahnefried, W. *Abstract 1510: Flaxseed slows prostate tumor growth.* in *American Society Clinical Oncology (ASCO).* 2007. Chicago, IL.
38.   Seow, A., et al., *Diabetes mellitus and risk of colorectal cancer in the Singapore Chinese Health Study.* J Natl Cancer Inst, 2006. **98**(2): p. 135-8.
39.   Garg, A. and B.B. Aggarwal, *Nuclear transcription factor-kappaB as a target for cancer drug development.* Leukemia, 2002. **16**(6): p. 1053-68.
40.   Leahy, K.M., A.T. Koki, and J.L. Masferrer, *Role of cyclooxygenases in angiogenesis.* Curr Med Chem, 2000. **7**(11): p. 1163-70.
41.   Denys, A., A. Hichami, and N.A. Khan, *n-3 PUFAs modulate T-cell activation via protein kinase C-alpha and -epsilon and the NF-kappaB signaling pathway.* J Lipid Res, 2005. **46**(4): p. 752-8.
42.   Hussein, N., et al., *Long-chain conversion of [13C]linoleic acid and alpha-linolenic acid in response to marked changes in their dietary intake in men.* J Lipid Res, 2005. **46**(2): p. 269-80.
43.   Rose, D.P. and J.M. Connolly, *Omega-3 fatty acids as cancer chemopreventive agents.* Pharmacol Ther, 1999. **83**(3): p. 217-44.
44.   Backlund, M.G., J.R. Mann, and R.N. Dubois, *Mechanisms for the prevention of gastrointestinal cancer: the role of prostaglandin E2.* Oncology, 2005. **69 Suppl 1**: p. 28-32.
45.   Furstenberger, G., et al., *What are cyclooxygenases and lipoxygenases doing in the driver's seat of carcinogenesis?* Int J Cancer, 2006. **119**(10): p. 2247-54.

46. Nie, D. and K.V. Honn, *Cyclooxygenase, lipoxygenase and tumor angiogenesis.* Cell Mol Life Sci, 2002. **59**(5): p. 799-807.

47. Williams, C.S., M. Mann, and R.N. DuBois, *The role of cyclooxygenases in inflammation, cancer, and development.* Oncogene, 1999. **18**(55): p. 7908-16.

48. Williams, C.S., et al., *Host cyclooxygenase-2 modulates carcinoma growth.* J Clin Invest, 2000. **105**(11): p. 1589-94.

49. Reddy, B.S. and H. Maruyama, *Effect of different levels of dietary corn oil and lard during the initiation phase of colon carcinogenesis in F344 rats.* J Natl Cancer Inst, 1986. **77**(3): p. 815-22.

50. Lipkin, M., et al., *Dietary factors in human colorectal cancer.* Annu Rev Nutr, 1999. **19**: p. 545-86.

51. Hansen-Petrik, M.B., et al., *Prostaglandin E(2) protects intestinal tumors from nonsteroidal anti-inflammatory drug-induced regression in Apc(Min/+) mice.* Cancer Res, 2002. **62**(2): p. 403-8.

52. Ghosh, J., *Rapid induction of apoptosis in prostate cancer cells by selenium: reversal by metabolites of arachidonate 5-lipoxygenase.* Biochem Biophys Res Commun, 2004. **315**(3): p. 624-35.

53. Ghosh, J. and C.E. Myers, *Inhibition of arachidonate 5-lipoxygenase triggers massive apoptosis in human prostate cancer cells.* Proc Natl Acad Sci U S A, 1998. **95**(22): p. 13182-7.

54. Nie, D., et al., *Role of eicosanoids in prostate cancer progression.* Cancer Metastasis Rev, 2001. **20**(3-4): p. 195-206.

55. Denkert, C., K.J. Winzer, and S. Hauptmann, *Prognostic impact of cyclooxygenase-2 in breast cancer.* Clin Breast Cancer, 2004. **4**(6): p. 428-33.

56. Singh, B. and A. Lucci, *Role of cyclooxygenase-2 in breast cancer.* J Surg Res, 2002. **108**(1): p. 173-9.

57. Steinbach, G., et al., *The effect of celecoxib, a cyclooxygenase-2 inhibitor, in familial adenomatous polyposis.* N Engl J Med, 2000. **342**(26): p. 1946-52.

58. Wallace, J.M., *Nutritional and botanical modulation of the inflammatory cascade--eicosanoids, cyclooxygenases, and lipoxygenases--as an adjunct in cancer therapy.* Integr Cancer Ther, 2002. **1**(1): p. 7-37; discussion 37.

59. Marks, F., K. Muller-Decker, and G. Furstenberger, *A causal relationship between unscheduled eicosanoid signaling and tumor development: cancer chemoprevention by inhibitors of arachidonic acid metabolism.* Toxicology, 2000. **153**(1-3): p. 11-26.

60. Masferrer, J.L., et al., *Antiangiogenic and antitumor activities of cyclooxygenase-2 inhibitors.* Cancer Res, 2000. **60**(5): p. 1306-11.

61. Claria, J. and M. Romano, *Pharmacological intervention of cyclooxygenase-2 and 5-lipoxygenase pathways. Impact on inflammation and cancer.* Curr Pharm Des, 2005. **11**(26): p. 3431-47.

62. Shureiqi, I. and S.M. Lippman, *Lipoxygenase modulation to reverse carcinogenesis.* Cancer Res, 2001. **61**(17): p. 6307-12.

63. Funk, C.D., *Prostaglandins and leukotrienes: advances in eicosanoid biology.* Science, 2001. **294**(5548): p. 1871-5.

64. Budowski, P. and M.A. Crawford, *a-Linolenic acid as a regulator of the metabolism of arachidonic acid: dietary implications of the ratio, n-6:n-3 fatty acids.* Proc Nutr Soc, 1985. **44**(2): p. 221-9.

65. Goyens, P.L., et al., *Conversion of alpha-linolenic acid in humans is influenced by the absolute amounts of alpha-linolenic acid and linoleic acid in the diet and not by their ratio.* Am J Clin Nutr, 2006. **84**(1): p. 44-53.

66. Emken, E.A., et al., *Effect of dietary docosahexaenoic acid on desaturation and uptake in vivo of isotope-labeled oleic, linoleic, and linolenic acids by male subjects.* Lipids, 1999. **34**(8): p. 785-91.

67. Schwab, U.S., et al., *Effects of hempseed and flaxseed oils on the profile of serum lipids, serum total and lipoprotein lipid concentrations and haemostatic factors.* Eur J Nutr, 2006. **45**(8): p. 470-7.

68. Whelan, J., B. Li, and C. Birdwell, *Dietary arachidonic acid increases eicosanoid production in the presence of equal amounts of dietary eicosapentaenoic acid.* Adv Exp Med Biol, 1997. **400B**: p. 897-904.

69. Garg, M.L., A.B. Thomson, and M.T. Clandinin, *Interactions of saturated, n-6 and n-3 polyunsaturated fatty acids to modulate arachidonic acid metabolism.* J Lipid Res, 1990. **31**(2): p. 271-7.

70. Ritch, C.R., et al., *Dietary fatty acids correlate with prostate cancer biopsy grade and volume in Jamaican men.* J Urol, 2007. **177**(1): p. 97-101; discussion 101.

71. Rose, D.P., et al., *Effects of dietary fish oil on fatty acids and eicosanoids in metastasizing human breast cancer cells.* Nutr Cancer, 1994. **22**(2): p. 131-41.

72. Okuyama, H., T. Kobayashi, and S. Watanabe, *Dietary fatty acids--the N-6/N-3 balance and chronic elderly diseases. Excess linoleic acid and relative N-3 deficiency syndrome seen in Japan.* Prog Lipid Res, 1996. **35**(4): p. 409-57.

73. Yam, D., A. Eliraz, and E.M. Berry, *Diet and disease--the Israeli paradox: possible dangers of a high omega-6 polyunsaturated fatty acid diet.* Isr J Med Sci, 1996. **32**(11): p. 1134-43.

74. de Lorgeril, M., et al., *Mediterranean dietary pattern in a randomized trial: prolonged survival and possible reduced cancer rate.* Arch Intern Med, 1998. **158**(11): p. 1181-7.

75. Dayton, S. and M.L. Pearce, *Prevention of coronary heart disease and other complications of arteriosclerosis by modified diet.* Am J Med, 1969. **46**(5): p. 751-62.

76. Dolecek, T.A., *Epidemiological evidence of relationships between dietary polyunsaturated fatty acids and mortality in the multiple risk factor intervention trial.* Proc Soc Exp Biol Med, 1992. **200**(2): p. 177-82.

77. Dolecek, T.A. and G. Granditis, *Dietary polyunsaturated fatty acids and mortality in the Multiple Risk Factor Intervention Trial (MRFIT).* World Rev Nutr Diet, 1991. **66**: p. 205-16.

78. Neuhouser, M.L., et al., *(n-6) PUFA Increase and Dairy Foods Decrease Prostate Cancer Risk in Heavy Smokers.* J Nutr, 2007. **137**(7): p. 1821-1827.

79. Hardman, W.E., *(n-3) fatty acids and cancer therapy.* J Nutr, 2004. **134**(12 Suppl): p. 3427S-3430S.

80. Cowing, B.E. and K.E. Saker, *Polyunsaturated fatty acids and epidermal growth factor receptor/mitogen-activated protein kinase signaling in mammary cancer.* J Nutr, 2001. **131**(4): p. 1125-8.

81. Kelavkar, U.P., et al., *Prostate tumor growth and recurrence can be modulated by the omega-6:omega-3 ratio in diet: athymic mouse xenograft model simulating radical prostatectomy.* Neoplasia, 2006. **8**(2): p. 112-24.

82. Ascherio, A., *Epidemiologic studies on dietary fats and coronary heart disease.* Am J Med, 2002. **113 Suppl 9B**: p. 9S-12S.

83. Phinney, S.D., *Metabolism of exogenous and endogenous arachidonic acid in cancer.* Adv Exp Med Biol, 1996. **399**: p. 87-94.

84. Wolk, A., et al., *Long-term fatty fish consumption and renal cell carcinoma incidence in women.* Jama, 2006. **296**(11): p. 1371-6.
85. Caygill, C.P., A. Charlett, and M.J. Hill, *Fat, fish, fish oil and cancer.* Br J Cancer, 1996. **74**(1): p. 159-64.
86. Larsson, S.C., et al., *Dietary long-chain n-3 fatty acids for the prevention of cancer: a review of potential mechanisms.* Am J Clin Nutr, 2004. **79**(6): p. 935-45.
87. MacLean, C.H., et al., *Effects of omega-3 fatty acids on cancer risk: a systematic review.* Jama, 2006. **295**(4): p. 403-15.
88. Brash, A.R., *Arachidonic acid as a bioactive molecule.* J Clin Invest, 2001. **107**(11): p. 1339-45.
89. Stark, K.D., et al., *Fatty acid compositions of serum phospholipids of postmenopausal women: a comparison between Greenland Inuit and Canadians before and after supplementation with fish oil.* Nutrition, 2002. **18**(7-8): p. 627-30.
90. U.S. Department of Agriculture, A.R.S. *USDA Nutrient Database for Standard Reference. Release 18, Nutrient Data Laboratory Home Page.* [cited Jan 1, 2006 Available from: http://www.nal.usda.gov/fnic/foodcomp.
91. *EWG report: PCBs in farmed salmon.* . [cited Aug 10 2006]; Available from: www.ewg.org/reports/farmedPCBs/printversion.php.
92. Knerr, S. and D. Schrenk, *Carcinogenicity of "non-dioxinlike" polychlorinated biphenyls.* Crit Rev Toxicol, 2006. **36**(9): p. 663-94.
93. Layton, D.W., et al., *Cancer risk of heterocyclic amines in cooked foods: an analysis and implications for research.* Carcinogenesis, 1995. **16**(1): p. 39-52.
94. Fresco, P., et al., *New insights on the anticancer properties of dietary polyphenols.* Med Res Rev, 2006. **26**(6): p. 747-66.
95. Zhang, Y., S. Yao, and J. Li, *Vegetable-derived isothiocyanates: anti-proliferative activity and mechanism of action.* Proc Nutr Soc, 2006. **65**(1): p. 68-75.
96. Brown, J.R. and R.N. DuBois, *Cyclooxygenase as a target in lung cancer.* Clin Cancer Res, 2004. **10**(12 Pt 2): p. 4266s-4269s.
97. Giovannucci, E. and D. Michaud, *The role of obesity and related metabolic disturbances in cancers of the colon, prostate, and pancreas.* Gastroenterology, 2007. **132**(6): p. 2208-25.
98. Silvera, S.A., et al., *Energy balance and breast cancer risk: a prospective cohort study.* Breast Cancer Res Treat, 2006. **97**(1): p. 97-106.
99. Calle, E.E., et al., *Overweight, obesity, and mortality from cancer in a prospectively studied cohort of U.S. adults.* N Engl J Med, 2003. **348**(17): p. 1625-38.
100. Mistry, T., et al., *Obesity and prostate cancer: a role for adipokines.* Eur Urol, 2007. **52**(1): p. 46-53.
101. Schaffler, A., J. Scholmerich, and C. Buechler, *Mechanisms of disease: adipokines and breast cancer - endocrine and paracrine mechanisms that connect adiposity and breast cancer.* Nat Clin Pract Endocrinol Metab, 2007. **3**(4): p. 345-54.
102. Pelucchi, C., et al., *Cancer risk associated with alcohol and tobacco use: focus on upper aero-digestive tract and liver.* Alcohol Res Health, 2006. **29**(3): p. 193-8.
103. Jakszyn, P. and C.A. Gonzalez, *Nitrosamine and related food intake and gastric and oesophageal cancer risk: a systematic review of the epidemiological evidence.* World J Gastroenterol, 2006. **12**(27): p. 4296-303.
104. Engel, L.S., Q. Lan, and N. Rothman, *Polychlorinated biphenyls and non-Hodgkin lymphoma.* Cancer Epidemiol Biomarkers Prev, 2007. **16**(3): p. 373-6.
105. Waladkhani, A.R. and M.R. Clemens, *Effect of dietary phytochemicals on cancer development (review).* Int J Mol Med, 1998. **1**(4): p. 747-53.
106. Nair, S., W. Li, and A.N. Kong, *Natural dietary anti-cancer chemopreventive compounds: redox-mediated differential signaling mechanisms in cytoprotection of normal cells versus cytotoxicity in tumor cells.* Acta Pharmacol Sin, 2007. **28**(4): p. 459-72.
107. Ding, H., et al., *Chemopreventive characteristics of avocado fruit.* Semin Cancer Biol, 2007.
108. Fowke, J.H., et al., *Urinary isothiocyanate levels, brassica, and human breast cancer.* Cancer Res, 2003. **63**(14): p. 3980-6.
109. Hsu, C.C., et al., *Dietary risk factors for kidney cancer in eastern and central europe.* Am J Epidemiol, 2007. **166**(1): p. 62-70.
110. Cho, E., et al., *Red meat intake and risk of breast cancer among premenopausal women.* Arch Intern Med, 2006. **166**(20): p. 2253-9.
111. Taylor, E.F., et al., *Meat consumption and risk of breast cancer in the UK Women's Cohort Study.* Br J Cancer, 2007. **96**(7): p. 1139-46.
112. Faramawi, M.F., et al., *Consumption of different types of meat and the risk of renal cancer: meta-analysis of case-control studies.* Cancer Causes Control, 2007. **18**(2): p. 125-33.
113. Tappel, A., *Heme of consumed red meat can act as a catalyst of oxidative damage and could initiate colon, breast and prostate cancers, heart disease and other diseases.* Med Hypotheses, 2007. **68**(3): p. 562-4.
114. Kabat, G.C., et al., *Dietary iron and heme iron intake and risk of breast cancer: a prospective cohort study.* Cancer Epidemiol Biomarkers Prev, 2007. **16**(6): p. 1306-8.
115. Cade, J.E., V.J. Burley, and D.C. Greenwood, *Dietary fibre and risk of breast cancer in the UK Women's Cohort Study.* Int J Epidemiol, 2007.
116. Wolk, A., *Diet, lifestyle and risk of prostate cancer.* Acta Oncol, 2005. **44**(3): p. 277-81.
117. Tuohimaa, P., et al., *Does solar exposure, as indicated by the non-melanoma skin cancers, protect from solid cancers: Vitamin D as a possible explanation.* Eur J Cancer, 2007.
118. Lappe, J.M., et al., *Vitamin D and calcium supplementation reduces cancer risk: results of a randomized trial.* Am J Clin Nutr, 2007. **85**(6): p. 1586-91.
119. Robien, K., G.J. Cutler, and D. Lazovich, *Vitamin D intake and breast cancer risk in postmenopausal women: the Iowa Women's Health Study.* Cancer Causes Control, 2007.

PART FOUR

EXPLAINING THE NQI RATING SYSTEM

THE NQI RATING SYSTEM

REVIEW OF KEY CONCEPTS

A healthy diet is capable of increasing longevity and maximizing quality of life, and is the common denominator among populations with low rates of chronic disease [1-15]. The human body expects to be nourished by certain molecules within genetically determined ranges [16-18]. However, recent changes in crop manipulation, animal rearing, and food processing have radically altered the content of the U.S. food supply, which now scarcely resembles that of our ancestors [16, 19-21]. Americans consume dramatically larger amounts of saturated fats, omega-6 fats, non-fiber carbohydrates, and sodium, and much lower amounts of omega-3 fats, monounsaturated fats, fibers, and polyphenolic antioxidants, than ever before in human history (Part 2, pages 27-88). In addition, considerable amounts of novel toxins, including trans fats, have entered the food supply with devastating consequences [22, 23]. These and other dietary components regulate inflammation, blood clotting, cholesterol metabolism, fat accumulation, insulin metabolism, oxidative stress, and cellular proliferation – metabolic processes that play key roles in the development of the Big 7 epidemic U.S. diseases. By initiating, amplifying, and perpetuating disturbances in *each* of these key metabolic processes, the "standard American diet" predisposes to the Big 7 epidemic U.S. diseases (Part 3, pages 89-174). In fact, poor diet is perhaps the most important reason for the recent explosion of chronic disease in the U.S. [16, 19, 24-32].

Despite widespread misperceptions, total *quantities* of fats and carbohydrates have little impact on health; wide ranges of these broadest categories of macronutrients can be consumed as part of a healthy diet (Part 1, pages 9-26). Rather, subsets of fats, carbohydrates, and other dietary components with distinct metabolic properties determine health impacts of individual foods. In some cases, individual molecules grouped into a single category (i.e. carbohydrates, polyunsaturated fats) have opposing metabolic and health effects. Therefore, *quality* is more important than the *total quantities* of fats and carbohydrates [23, 33-43].

Dietary patterns are more influential than single food choices, and multiple healthy dietary patterns (i.e. traditional Mediterranean, rural Japanese, Greenland Eskimo, etc.) have been identified [3, 6, 9, 12-14, 44-51]. However, each of these dietary patterns reflects specialized cultural traditions to which few modern Americans strictly adhere. Instead, most Americans make several dozen, more or less isolated food-related decisions each day [52]. Because the overall diet is determined by this series of individual selections, identification and habitual selection of high quality food items is a prerequisite of *any* healthy diet [52-54]. The ability to distinguish between high and low quality food items is particularly valuable in the U.S., where a seemingly endless variety of food items are available.

The potential of excellent dietary guidance to greatly improve public health has been appreciated for over a century [55-57]. In 1894, the federal government began publishing "official" dietary guidelines with the goal of helping Americans identify healthy foods [56]. Over the last few decades, several influential health promotion agencies have followed suit [58-62]. Traditional dietary advice has assumed two basic varieties: nutrient-based guidelines and food-based guidelines. While both provide some useful information, significant inadequacies have diminished their overall usefulness [56].

TRADITIONAL DIETARY GUIDELINES

Early nutrient-based guidelines focused almost exclusively on one-dimensional features of health (i.e. cholesterol reduction) and ignored other crucial health determinants [56, 58, 59, 61]. However, diets that target several key metabolic determinants profoundly outperform simplistic cholesterol reducing diets [4, 38, 63, 64]. Additionally, because nutrient-based guidelines fail to weigh the importance of each nutrient recommendation, consumers are forced to speculate, often erroneously, about the relative importance of different recommendations [65]. This lack of clarification leaves the consumer vulnerable to marketing campaigns using trendy "buzzwords." Importantly, the utility of nutrient-based guidelines is dependent upon accuracy and uniformity of serving sizes [66]. Unfortunately, serving sizes are far from uniform and rarely match actual amounts of foods consumed [56, 67, 68]. Precise implementation of nutrient-based dietary guidelines requires meticulous attention to detail regarding food labels, serving sizes, and servings consumed, as well as several complex mathematical calculations. Therefore, nutrient-based guidelines are difficult to apply to real-world situations [54, 56, 57, 69].

Food-based dietary guidelines, which advise consumption of a certain number of servings per day of specific food groups, are more easily applied to real-world situations [56, 57]. However, items with widely varied molecular contents often co-exist within the same food group (i.e. dairy, cooking oils, meats, breads, fish). Nevertheless, food-based guidelines imply that different items within the same group have similar health properties [54]. Like nutrient-based guidelines, the utility of food-based guidelines is dependent upon accuracy and uniformity of serving sizes [56]. Essentially, food-based guidelines sacrifice precision for ease-of-use. In light of the growing epidemics of the largely preventable Big 7 epidemic U.S. diseases, few would argue that nutrient-based or food-based dietary guidelines have achieved their goals.

NUTRITION FACTS LABELS

U.S. manufacturers are required to display a *Nutrition Facts* label containing basic nutritional information on most packaged food items. The *Nutrition Facts* label provides numerical values for serving size, calories, fat calories, total fat, saturated fat, trans fat, cholesterol, sodium, total carbohydrate, fiber, sugars, protein, vitamins A and C, calcium and iron, as well as percent daily values for each nutrient based on a 2000 calorie diet and the FDA recommended daily allowances (RDA) [70]. Listed weights and percentage daily values of all nutrients are dependent upon the listed serving size. These labels are intended to help consumers make quick, informed food choices that contribute to a healthy diet [70].

Nutrition Facts

Serving Size 2 slices (56g)
Servings per container 10

Calories 140
Calories from Fat 15

	Amount/serving	% Daily Value*	Amount/serving	% Daily Value*
Total Fat 1.5g		2%	Total Carbohydrate 26g	8%
Saturated Fat 0.5g		3%	Dietary Fiber 2g	8%
Trans Fat 0.5g			Sugars 1g	
Cholesterol 0mg		0%	Protein 4g	
Sodium 280mg		12%		

Vitamin A 0% • Vitamin C 0% • Calcium 6% • Iron 6%
Thiamin 15% • Riboflavin 8% • Niacin 10%

* Percent Daily Values are based on a 2,000 calorie diet. Your daily values may be higher or lower depending on your calorie needs:

		Calories:	2,000	2,500
Total Fat	Less than		65g	80g
Sat Fat	Less than		20g	25g
Cholesterol	Less than		300mg	300mg
Sodium	Less than		2,400mg	2,400mg
Total Carbohydrate			300g	375g
Dietary Fiber			25g	30g

Figure 1: *Nutrition Facts* label [71, 72]. **All nutrient amounts, calories, and percentage daily values are dependent upon listed serving sizes. Several critically important, metabolically active nutrients and nutrient categories, including short and long chain ω-3 and ω-6 fatty acids, are absent from food labels.**

While *Nutrition Facts* labeling does provide consumers with some useful information, several problems or inadequacies have been identified. Many consumers find the format of food labels difficult to understand [73]. In particular, consumers find serving sizes confusing and misleading, and their misapplication is a well-known source of error [66]. Because weights and percentage daily values of all nutrients and calories listed in the *Nutrition Facts* label are based on the listed serving size, accuracy and uniformity of serving size is of paramount importance [66, 70]. However, listed serving sizes are far from uniform, and actual amounts of food consumed *per serving* vary markedly among different individuals and may be radically different than the listed serving size [56, 67, 68]. ***Unfortunately, lack of uniformity and reliability of serving sizes plays a major role in compromising the accuracy and integrity of virtually all information listed in the Nutrition Facts label.***

Lack of uniform requirements may allow manufacturers to manipulate listed serving sizes in order to conceal the amount of undesirable nutrients present in food items or exaggerate the amount of a desirable nutrient. For example, the FDA requires manufacturers to acknowledge the presence of trans fats in any food item containing more than 500 mg (0.5 grams) *per serving* [74]. Items containing less than 500 mg per serving can list "0 grams" under trans fat and make claims of "no trans fat" or "0 grams of trans fat" on the packaging [71, 74, 75]. However, manufacturer-listed serving sizes for cereals range from 25 to over 60 grams. Consider an item with 880 mg of trans fatty acids per 50 grams. Simply listing the serving size as 28 grams allows the manufacturer to display "0 grams" in the trans fat section of the *Nutrition Facts* label and to market the food as "trans fat free," despite trans fats accounting for nearly 2% of the overall weight of the food item. Individuals who consume several "servings" at one sitting actually ingest significant quantities of trans fats from a "0 grams of trans fat" product. Similarly, it is theoretically possible to list unrealistically small serving sizes in an attempt to mislead the consumer into believing a food contains fewer calories, calories from fat, total fat, saturated fats, carbohydrates, sugar, sodium, or other nutrients than it actually does. In some instances, larger serving sizes can be used to provide the appearance of more fiber, protein, or vitamins [56, 68].

Perhaps more importantly, water and other essentially neutral components with minimal metabolic and health impacts account for a large percentage of the overall weight of many food items [76]. For example, water accounts for 0% of the weight of cooking oils, 40-50% of most cheeses, 50-85% of meats and fish, 65-85% of yogurts, and 70-90% of most fruits [76]. *Food items which contain less water are more concentrated sources of bioactive nutrients* [77]. No other dietary component plays a more important role than water in obscuring serving sizes. To illustrate this concept, consider two food items with identical nutrient contents aside from water, which accounts for 80% of the weight of food item # 1, and 40% of food item # 2. Expression of nutrient weights *per serving*, as on *Nutrition Facts* labels, results in *three-times* higher nutrient weights, percentage daily values, and calories *per serving* for food item # 2, despite similar metabolic and health effects. Therefore, water content can greatly obscure the nutrient content, caloric value, and health properties of foods [77].

Several key nutrients and nutrient categories are not included on *Nutrition Facts* labels. Notable examples of bioactive nutrients with central health properties not listed on labels are individual short and long chain ω-3 (ALA, EPA, and DHA) and ω-6 (LA and ArA) fatty acids, as well as monounsaturated fats. In fact, emerging evidence suggests that these unlisted fatty acids are amongst the most metabolically active and influential of all dietary components [2, 5, 10, 11, 20, 37, 50, 51, 78-81]! Under the carbohydrate section, total carbohydrates, dietary fiber, and sugars are quantified (per serving); starches must be calculated by subtracting fiber and sugars from total carbohydrates. This format may imply that sugars are less desirable than starches, despite mounting evidence suggesting that *pure* starches have essentially the same metabolic and overall health effects as sugars [35, 40, 82-84]. Furthermore, *Nutrition Facts* labels do not provide information about total antioxidant capacity, any minerals aside from sodium, calcium, and iron, or the content of various toxins (i.e. mercury, PCBs, nitrosamines).

Manufacturers often display health-related claims on food packaging (i.e. "low fat," "low in saturated fat," "low sodium," "zero grams of trans fat," "good" or "excellent" source of whole grains, or specific vitamins or minerals) based on FDA guidelines [72].

Marketing strategies based on nutrient claims may confuse consumers, making it difficult to distinguish between high and low quality food items upon first glance, or even after reading the *Nutrition Facts* label. Perhaps due to the complexity of interpreting information on food labels, and guessing the relative importance of different nutrients, consumers often make food choices based on a *single* nutrient or health claim [54]. However, because food items contain variable amounts of nutrients with both beneficial *and* adverse health properties, the health claim may be of limited importance. For example, a food that is labeled "no cholesterol," may contain large amounts of added sugar or other nutrients with potentially adverse health properties that outweigh any supposed benefits of having no cholesterol. Despite the claim, the food may have a negative overall effect on health.

While intended to help consumers "make quick, informed food choices that contribute to a healthy diet," crucial limitations of *Nutrition Facts* labels clearly limit their utility [53, 69, 70, 73]. Further, in their current format, *Nutrition Facts* labels do not provide, or claim to provide, an estimate of the *net* health consequences of consuming *individual* food items. Therefore, like conventional dietary guidelines, *Nutrition Facts* labels have failed to provide Americans with a simple and consistent way to distinguish between high and low quality foods.

FOOD RATING SYSTEMS

While several systems for assessing the quality of the *overall diet* have been presented, comparatively few have been designed to evaluate the quality of *individual* food items [44, 45]. Of those intended to measure the quality of individual foods, several provide a nutrient-by-nutrient analysis, rather than *overall* nutritional quality [85]. The remaining few systems designed to measure the *net* nutritional value of *individual* food items are primitive, outdated, and one-dimensional [54, 86-88]. None are comprehensive, and most ignore trans fats, short and long chain omega-3 and omega-6 fats, monounsaturated fats, and other key components [54, 86-88]. Further, most do not weigh different nutrients according to their *relative* metabolic and health impacts [54, 86, 88]. Despite limited evidence of health benefits, the inclusion of various vitamins and minerals (i.e. Vit C, Vit E, Vit A, iron), allows vitamin fortification to radically distort food quality ratings [85, 87, 89]. Components easily acquired through a standard multivitamin should not have a major impact on food ratings. Furthermore, each of these systems is dependent upon either serving size, calories, or both [54, 77, 85-89]. As discussed above, dependence upon the vagaries of serving sizes allows water-content and arbitrary manufacturer labeling choices to have major impacts on food quality ratings.

Consequently, there is an unmet need for a *comprehensive* food rating system that allows consumers to easily identify and select high quality food items and avoid low quality items. Such a system should provide a single, easily understood numerical value reflecting the aggregate nutritional quality of each item, and allow for *direct* comparison of food items both within and amongst food groups. Such a system should be based on global scientific evidence and have a broad focus on overall health, rather than just cholesterol metabolism. The system should appropriately weigh the relative importance of different desirable *and* undesirable components, and should not be skewed by vitamin fortification. Additionally, the system should be independent of the ambiguities of serving size, and should not be *directly* dependent on the important but narrow focus of caloric value.

INTRODUCING THE NQI

The Nutritional Quality Index (NQI) was designed to be that system. Individual food items are rated in terms of overall *quality* of nutrient content, which is expressed as an all-inclusive score between -10 and +10, with -10 signifying a food that will contribute to disease if consumed regularly, 0 signifying neutral health effects, and +10 signifying profound health benefits. The simplicity of this numerical ranking system allows busy consumers to easily and quickly distinguish between high and low quality food items. As a holistic system, ratings reflect predicted impacts on seven key metabolic processes as well as the Big 7 epidemic U.S. diseases, rather than simply cholesterol metabolism, glycemic response, or caloric value.

Based on a thorough review of nutritional, medical, and scientific literature, the NQI is the most comprehensive and versatile food rating system ever created. Unlike traditional guidelines and *Nutrition Facts* labeling, which require speculation about the significance of different nutrients, the NQI appropriately "weighs" both beneficial and deleterious nutrients according to *relative* importance. The comprehensive nature of the NQI makes it difficult for foods with adverse properties to receive unjustifiably positive ratings, and foods scores are not skewed by vitamin fortification.

Because the NQI is independent of serving size, water content and ambiguity of serving sizes do not compromise system integrity. Accurate determinations of net quality across a wide range of water contents are possible, which allows for direct comparison of food items in their natural states, as well as processed food items, dried items, and beverages. Additionally, the NQI system is not directly dependent upon caloric value. Instead, ratings are based on *net* health properties.

As such, the NQI allows consumers to compare the nutritional quality of food items, both within and amongst food groups, in order to identify and select items with maximum predicted health benefits. Additionally, the NQI allows consumers to identify and limit intake of foods with potentially deleterious metabolic and health properties, even in the face of incomplete or misleading nutritional information labeling and/or claims. By revealing health benefits or adverse health effects that may be caused by their products, the NQI system may motivate food manufacturers to design and produce foods of higher nutritional quality.

THE NQI SYSTEM AND FORMULA

The NQI system is dependent upon accurate values for each of the bioactive nutrients present in food items. Databases available to the public, including the USDA National Nutrient Database, contain the nutrient contents of thousands of food items [76]. These databases express the macronutrient and micronutrient content for a given weight of a food item, generally 100 grams of food including water and ash (the residue which remains after oxidation of a food item in a bomb calorimeter, which contains many of the minerals). With this information, one can determine the water-free and ash-free weight of a given food item by subtracting the weight of water and ash from 100 grams.

DETERMINING NUTRIENT PERCENTAGE VALUES (NPVs)

The NQI system breaks all food items into specific nutrients by weight. Each nutrient is expressed as a percentage of a food item's water-free and ash-free weight or "true grams," which is approximately equal to the sum of total fats, total carbohydrates, and total protein. For instance, consider this *simplified* example of a 100 gram sample of **wild sockeye salmon**. If water (70.0 grams) and ash (1.0 gram) combine to account for 71 grams out of 100 grams of total weight, then true grams are listed as 29.0 grams. Each respective bioactive nutrient's contribution to the 29 grams can then be quantified. A "nutrient percentage value" (NPV) is calculated for each nutrient by dividing the weight of each nutrient by 29.0 grams. For example, if 0.7 grams of ω-3 DHA are present in the sample, then DHA accounts for 2.4% of total water-free weight, or true grams. Analogous calculations are performed to determine NPVs for eleven nutrients or nutrient categories: eight categories of fats, two categories of carbohydrates, and one category of protein.

NUTRIENT PERCENTAGE VALUES of WILD SOCKEYE SALMON

NUTRIENT	NPV
Saturated fats (SFA)	5.2%
Monounsaturated fats (MUFA)	14.4%
ω-6 Linoleic acid (LA)	1.3%
ω-6 Arachidonic acid (ArA)	0.3%
ω-3 Alpha-linolenic acid (ALA)	0.3%
ω-3 EPA + DHA	4.1%
Trans fats	None
Dietary cholesterol	0.2%
Non-fiber carbohydrates (NFC)	None
Fiber	None
Protein	74.2%

[76]

NON-MACRONUTRIENT COMPONENTS

In addition to the eleven macronutrient categories listed above, the NQI quantifies three other important molecular categories: sodium, total antioxidant capacity (TAC), and toxins (i.e. mercury, PCBs). These *do not* contribute to the *true grams* of the food item. TAC, which is calculated by adding the lipophilic and hydrophilic antioxidant values obtained by Wu et al. as part of the USDA National Food and Nutrient Analysis Program, is expressed as TAC per true gram by the NQI [90]. For foods without listed USDA TAC values, other comparable assays are used to fill in the gaps [91-94]. Sodium, which accounts for a very small percentage of water-free weight (0.2% in this example) is expressed as a *relative* value or percentage, and does not contribute to the calculation of *true grams*.

CONTENT of WILD SOCKEYE SALMON
NUTRIENT and NON-NUTRIENT COMPONENTS

NUTRIENT CATEGORY	NPV
Saturated fats (SFA)	5.2%
Monounsaturated fats (MUFA)	14.4%
ω-6 Linoleic acid (LA)	1.3%
ω-6 Arachidonic acid (ArA)	0.3%
ω-3 Alpha-linolenic acid (ALA)	0.3%
ω-3 EPA + DHA	4.1%
Trans fats	None
Dietary cholesterol	0.2%
Non-fiber carbohydrates (NFC)	None
Fiber	None
Protein	74.2%
Sodium	0.2%
Total antioxidant capacity (TAC)	None
Toxins (Mercury and PCBs)	Mercury – 0.01 ppm PCBs – trace

Food items that consumers may consider similar or identical often contain radically different molecular contents. For example, calculated ω-6 ArA NPVs for wild sockeye and farmed Atlantic salmon are 0.3% and 3.9% respectively. Thus, ω-6 ArA concentrations vary up to 13-fold among different varieties of salmon! Similarly, although different varieties of fish are commonly grouped together, profound variations of ω-3 EPA/DHA, mercury, and PCBs often exist [76, 95-97].

Because manufacturers regularly change the chemical compositions of many food items, the USDA Nutrient Data Laboratory and other databases do not always provide accurate, up-to-date nutrient content for *name-brand* food items currently for sale. As discussed previously, *Nutrition Facts* labels on packaged foods provide a listing of the weights of some, but not all, important bioactive nutrients per serving. The weights attributable to total fat, total carbohydrate, and protein are listed, and *true grams* of macronutrients can be determined by simply adding these three components. Notably, the label does *not* include values for ω-3 ALA, EPA, or DHA, ω-6 LA and ArA, or monounsaturated fatty acids, despite growing recognition of their importance in health and disease. Estimates of the weights of these important but unlisted bioactive nutrients are required in order to accurately predict the *overall* metabolic and health consequence of consuming any given food item. Fortunately, information available from *Nutrient Facts* labels, ingredient lists, and the USDA Nutrient Data Laboratory database, combined with the current body of nutritional literature, allows for accurate estimations of compositions of name brand food items.

FATTY ACID CONTENTS OF VEGETABLE AND SEED OILS

OIL	SFA (%)	MUFA (%)	LA (%)	ALA (%)
CANOLA	8	60	24	8
COCONUT	94	6	0	0
CORN	14	25	60	1
COTTONSEED	27	19	54	0*
FLAXSEED	10	20	14	56
OLIVE (extra virgin)	15	75	9	1
OLIVE	15	75	9	1
PALM	50	40	10	0
PALM KERNEL	86	12	2	0
PEANUT	18	50	32	0
RICE BRAN	20	42	36	2
SAFFLOWER	7	15	78	0*
SAFFLOWER (high oleic)	6	79	15	0*
SESAME	15	42	43	0*
SOYBEAN	15	25	53	7
SUNFLOWER	10	20	70	0
SUNFLOWER (high oleic)	10	50	40	0
Partially hydrogenated Oils (see text for details)	Varies by type of oil and extent of hydrogenation- see text below			

[76, 98-100]* = trace (0.1-0.3%). Fatty acid content varies slightly by soil, climate, and season.

FATTY ACID CONTENTS OF DAIRY ITEMS

SFA	MUFA	LA	ALA
66	31	2	1

[76, 101]. Milkfat contains trace amounts of other fats including ω-6 EPA/DHA, ω-6 ArA, and cholesterol.

FATTY ACID CONTENTS OF CEREAL GRAINS

GRAIN	SFA %	MUFA %	LA %	ALA %
WHEAT	20	20	55	5
CORN	14	25	60	1
OATS	20	38	40	2
RICE	20	40	38	2
RYE	15	20	55	10
BARLEY	30	15	50	5
MILLET	20	20	57	3
AMARANTH	25	24	50	1
RANGES	14-30	15-40	38-60	1-10

[76]

The *per serving* weights of both total and saturated fatty acids (SFA) are listed in the *Nutrition Facts* label. Weights of ω-3 ALA, EPA, or DHA, ω-6 LA and ArA, and monounsaturated fats can be estimated from the information available in the *Nutrition Facts* label, the ingredient list, and knowledge of typical fatty acid profiles of vegetable oils, nuts and seeds, grains, dairy, and other foods via the following methods.

For name-brand food items which contain only one major source of fat, the typical individual fatty acid concentrations of that fat source can be multiplied by the total fat to estimate the amounts of individual fatty acids in a given food item. For example, the weights of individual fatty acids present in a cereal consisting solely of wheat and a sugar source (i.e. cane juice) with three listed grams of total fat can be assumed to be derived solely from the wheat, as cane juice contains no appreciable amount of fat. Thus, individual fatty acids are calculated by multiplying the typical percentages of fatty acids in wheat (SFA 20%, MUFA 20%, LA 55%, ALA 5%) by total fat as follows:

$$.20 \times 3g = 0.60 \text{ g SFA}$$
$$.20 \times 3g = 0.60 \text{ g MUFA}$$
$$.55 \times 3g = 1.65 \text{ g LA}$$
$$\underline{.05 \times 3g = 0.15 \text{ g ALA}}$$
Total fat = 3.00 grams

Alternatively, the weights of individual fatty acids provided by a cereal with *two* fat sources can be estimated as follows. Consider a cereal with a *true grams* weight of 40 grams, consisting of 4 total grams of fat, 30 total grams of carbohydrates, and 6 grams of protein. Wheat is the first ingredient listed, and can be assumed to provide some of the fat. However, one other appreciable fat source, soybean oil, is listed further down on the ingredient list. Given that water-free wheat contains approximately 2.5% fat, and the typical fatty acid profile of wheat is known (SFA 20%, MUFA 20%, LA 55%, ALA 5%), the weights of individual fatty acids attributable to wheat can be estimated via the following method. First, to determine the *total* amount of fat attributable to wheat, the typical percentage of total fat in wheat (2.5%) is multiplied by true grams (40).

$$\textbf{.025 x 40 g = 1.0 gram}$$

This 1.0 gram of wheat fat provides 0.20, 0.20, 0.55, and 0.05 grams of saturated fats, monounsaturated fats, ω-6 linoleic acid, and ω-3 alpha-linolenic acid respectively.

The remainder of the total fat, calculated by subtracting the wheat fat from total fat 4.0 – 1.0 g = 3.0 grams, is attributable to soybean oil, the only other fat source. The typical fatty acid profile of soybean oil (SFA 15%, MUFA 25%, LA 53%, and ALA 7%) is multiplied by the remaining 3.0 grams. Thus, 0.45, 0.75, 1.59, 0.21 grams are attributable to saturated, monounsaturated, linoleic, and alpha-linolenic fatty acids respectively from soybean oil.

By adding the weight of each fatty acid from both the wheat and soybean oil, the fatty acid profile of the cereal can be estimated as below:

$$0.20g + 0.45g = 0.65g \text{ SFA}$$
$$0.20g + 0.75g = 0.95g \text{ MUFA}$$
$$0.55g + 1.59g = 2.14g \text{ LA}$$
$$\underline{0.05g + 0.21g = 0.26g \text{ ALA}}$$
Total fat = 4.00 grams

Rarely, three or more fat sources are present in a single, highly processed food item. For instance, consider a wheat-based cereal that contains three fat sources on the ingredient list: wheat, soybean oil, and cottonseed oil. In order to calculate the fatty acids attributable to each fat source, one must first estimate the *relative* amounts of each fat source in the food item. The order of listed ingredients coincides with the amounts of each ingredient present in the food item. For instance, if soybean oil is ingredient number 2, and cottonseed oil is ingredient number 19, then it is apparent that a far greater percentage of the total fat is attributable to soybean oil than cottonseed oil. While one may estimate that less than 5% of fat content is supplied by cottonseed oil, calculations based on three or more fat sources are necessarily more subjective and less precise. However, because multi-ingredient packaged foods generally contain ingredients with similar characteristics (i.e. to maximize shelf-life), inaccuracies are often minimal.

FAT SOURCE	SFA (%)	MUFA (%)	LA (%)	ALA (%)
WHEAT	20	20	55	5
SOYBEAN	15	25	53	7
COTTONSEED	27	19	54	trace

ACCOUNTING FOR TRANS FATS

Mounting evidence suggests that even modest quantities of trans fats can have significant deleterious health consequences [23]. In anticipation of January 1, 2006 labeling requirements, manufacturers re-formulated products and/or adjusted listed serving sizes so trans fats would account for less than 500 mg per serving, in order to avoid listing trans fats in the *Nutrition Facts* label [71, 74]. As previously explained, under current FDA guidelines it is possible to consume significant quantities of trans fats from foods which appear to be "trans-fat free." In order to avoid underestimating the quantities of artificial trans fats in food items, the NQI assumes that items which contain partially hydrogenated soybean, cottonseed, peanut, and other predominantly *un*saturated oils contain 400 mg of trans fats per listed serving. Because hydrogenation of predominantly *saturated* oils produces fewer trans fats, foods containing partially hydrogenated palm, palm kernel, or coconut oils are assigned lower amounts per serving. Similarly, fully hydrogenated oils are assigned low amounts of trans fats.

DEALING WITH NON-SPECIFIC INGREDIENT LISTS

The ingredient lists of some processed food items contain two or more different oils in the same spot (i.e. soybean and/or cottonseed oil). Whenever this situation occurs, the NQI includes *only* the poorer quality oil in order to avoid overestimating the nutritional quality of these food items.

DETERMINATION OF INFLUENCE FACTORS

Once true grams and nutrient percentage values for each nutrient have been calculated, appropriate influence factors are assigned. Assignment of influence factors allows for the calculation of an accurate all-inclusive nutritional quality score for any given food item based on its precise molecular content, and allows this score to fall within a range easily understood by consumers. Criteria on which influence factor values are based include:

(1) relative beneficial or deleterious metabolic and health properties
(2) optimal ratios between nutrients with antagonistic or synergistic effects
(3) generating net scores within a predetermined range easily understood by consumers

RELATIVE BENEFICIAL AND DELETERIOUS METABOLIC AND HEALTH PROPERTIES

The NQI assigns influence factors to nutrients according to the *relative* potency of metabolic and health consequences of their ingestion. Different dietary nutrients have widely variable health consequences, ranging from profoundly deleterious, to profoundly beneficial and everywhere in between (see Parts 2 and 3). Deleterious nutrients are assigned negative influence factors commensurate with the potency of their adverse effects, neutral nutrients are assigned a zero influence factor, and beneficial nutrients are assigned positive influence factors proportionate to the potency of their beneficial effects. Sources of evidence of deleterious and beneficial properties of specific nutrients in the scientific literature include experimental, epidemiological, mechanistic, animal model, and other types of studies, generally published in peer-reviewed medical journals (see Parts 1-3).

For example, evidence suggests that each of the three ω-3 fatty acids have beneficial metabolic and health effects [5, 10, 50, 102-104]. However, this same evidence demonstrates that the longer-chain ω-3 EPA and DHA have significantly more profound beneficial health effects than the short-chain ω-3 ALA. Thus, in order to generate the most accurate net ratings of food items, EPA and DHA should be "weighted" more heavily, and assigned more positive influence factors than ALA, proportionate with their beneficial effects.

Similarly, saturated fats have widely recognized adverse effects on multiple metabolic pathways and their consumption raises the risk of developing coronary heart disease, diabetes, and other diseases [6, 105]. However, evidence suggests that adverse consequences of trans fats are several magnitudes more intense than saturated fats, and that on a gram for gram basis, trans fats may raise the risk of heart disease up to fifteen times as much as saturated fats [23, 106-108]. Thus, in order to generate the most accurate ratings of food items, trans fats are assigned a more negative influence factor than saturated fats, proportionate with their adverse health effects.

Like the examples above, *all* nutrients are assigned appropriate influence factors according to their *relative* metabolic and health effects. Whenever individual dietary molecules have established distinct health properties, they are listed separately. However, when evidence suggests that a group of molecules have equivalent health properties, they are grouped together. For example, stearic, palmitic, myristic, and lauric acid (which account for >90% of saturated fats) appear to have equivalent health effects. Thus, the entire group of saturated fats is assigned the same influence factor. Similarly, palmitoleic and oleic acid, the major monounsaturated fats, which appear to have equivalent health properties, are assigned equivalent influence factors. Likewise, *pure* starches and sugars containing glucose and fructose appear to have equivalent health properties - accompanying fiber, fatty acids, antioxidants, minerals, and other components account for the metabolic and health differences between grains and *pure* starches [35, 40, 41, 43, 109-112]. Therefore, the NQI groups sugars and starches together into non-fiber carbohydrates, and both are assigned equivalent influence factors.

The chart below reflects the current scientific evidence as detailed and referenced throughout Parts 1-3 of this book. Should evidence expand to indicate that *individual* nutrients or nutrient subsets within these groups have distinct net health effects, the rating system can be easily amended to reflect these changes.

Net Health Effects of Dietary Nutrients and other Dietary Components

Nutrient (or Molecular) Category	Metabolic and Health Effects
Saturated fats	Moderately deleterious
Monounsaturated fats	Modestly beneficial
ω-6 Linoleic acid	Modestly deleterious
ω-6 Arachidonic acid	Profoundly deleterious
ω-3 Alpha-linolenic acid	Moderately beneficial
ω-3 EPA and DHA	Profoundly beneficial
Trans fats	Profoundly deleterious
Cholesterol	Minimally deleterious
Non-fiber carbohydrates (NFC)	Modestly deleterious
Fiber	Moderately beneficial
Protein	Modestly beneficial
Total antioxidant content (TAC)	Moderately beneficial
Sodium	Moderately deleterious
Toxins (i.e. mercury, PCBs)	Moderately to profoundly deleterious

See Parts 1-3 for rationale and references.

OPTIMAL RATIOS BETWEEN NUTRIENTS WITH ANTAGONISTIC OR SYNERGISTIC EFFECTS

Relative *ratios* of consumption of some nutrients have important health consequences. For example, ω-6 LA and ω-3 ALA compete with one another in several critical metabolic pathways, and often have antagonistic effects [113-116]. However, as a result of recent radical changes in the food supply, Americans, on average, consume more than 10 times as much LA as ALA. Mounting evidence suggests that this excessive LA intake contributes to key metabolic abnormalities and increases the risk of developing several chronic diseases, and that reduction to a 4 to 1 ratio may dramatically reduce the risk of heart disease, cancer, and other illnesses [37, 38, 64, 102, 117-121]. Furthermore, roughly equal ratios of LA and ALA intake (1 to 1 ratio) consumed throughout millions of years of human history appears to provide even more health benefits and may be optimal [11, 120, 122-124].

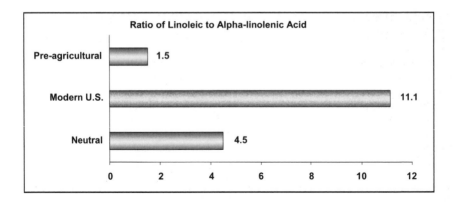

Based on this evidence, the NQI selects 4.5 to 1 as a "neutral" LA to ALA ratio, in which LA and ALA intake roughly cancel one another out. By assigning ALA a moderately positive influence factor proportionate with its health impact, and assigning LA a negative influence factor with 22.5% of the absolute value of ALA, food items with 4.5 times as much LA as ALA will receive zero net points, items containing more than a 4.5 to 1 ratio of LA to ALA will lose points, and items with less than 4.5 times as much LA as ALA will gain points from these two nutrients. Thus, the NQI rewards food items for containing more optimal ratios of these important nutrients. However, maximum points awarded for ω-3 ALA are capped, reflecting the possible (but unlikely) association between high ω-3 ALA intake and prostate cancer.

Likewise, radical changes in the U.S. food supply have stripped much of the fiber from U.S. carbohydrates, leaving purified sugars and starches [125]. Throughout millions of years of history, our human ancestors consumed at least 1 gram of fiber for every 5 grams of non-fiber carbohydrates (5 to 1 ratio) [18, 19, 24, 76, 126]. However, as a result of radical changes in food processing, this ratio has roughly tripled in recent years to more than 16 to 1 (see Part 2). A high ratio of non-fiber carbohydrates to fiber results in multiple metabolic disturbances and predisposes to obesity, diabetes, heart disease, and a variety of other illnesses (see Part 2). As a measure of carbohydrate quality, the NQI assigns non-fiber carbohydrates a modestly negative influence factor and fiber a moderately positive influence factor. By selecting a 5.8 to 1 ratio of non-fiber carbohydrates to fiber as "neutral," food items with higher ratios will lose points on these two nutrients and items with lower ratios will gain points commensurate with their health impacts.

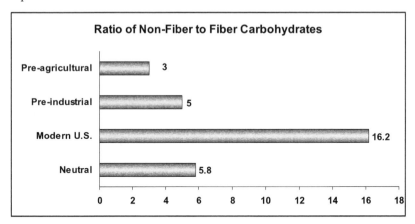

Similarly, recent changes in the U.S. food supply have increased saturated fat (SFA) intake and reduced intake of monounsaturated fats (MUFA) [19, 126]. The ratio of MUFA to SFA consumption has important metabolic and health consequences [127, 128]. Evidence suggests that throughout much of human history, humans consumed nearly three times as many MUFA as SFA [18, 24, 124, 129-131]. Today, however, Americans consume roughly equal amounts of SFA and MUFA (see Part 2). SFA promote and MUFA antagonize several metabolic disturbances which promote coronary heart disease, diabetes, dementia, and other illnesses [8, 127, 132-134]. Via these mechanisms, the high U.S. SFA consumption and low MUFA intake increases the risk of epidemic U.S. diseases. Evidence suggests that consuming at least twice as much MUFA as saturated fats may reduce the risk of several common U.S. diseases and that an even higher ratio may be optimal [1, 8, 13, 81, 135-138]. By selecting a 2 to 1 ratio of MUFA to SFA as "neutral," food items with higher ratios will receive points, and items with lower ratios will lose points commensurate with their health impacts.

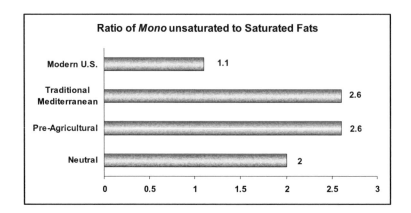

GENERATION OF SCORES WITHIN A PREDETERMINED RANGE

In order to generate useful *all-inclusive* numerical scores reflecting the net quality of food items, influence factors are weighted to keep the aggregate products of all *nutrient percentage values* and *influence factors* within a range easily understood by consumers. Scores range from -10 to 10, with -10 signifying a food item with profoundly deleterious health properties, 0 signifying neutral health attributes, and +10 signifying profound health benefits.

INFLUENCE FACTORS

Molecular Category	Metabolic and Health Effects	Influence Factor
Saturated fats	Moderately deleterious	-0.25
Monounsaturated fats	Modestly beneficial	+0.125
ω-6 Linoleic acid	Modestly deleterious	-0.18
ω-6 Arachidonic acid	Profoundly deleterious	-4.00
ω-3 Alpha-linolenic acid	Moderately beneficial	+0.80
ω-3 Eicosapentaenoic and Docosahexaenoic acids	Profoundly beneficial	+3.00
Trans fats	Profoundly deleterious	-3.60
Cholesterol	Minimally deleterious	-0.50
Non-fiber carbohydrates	Modestly deleterious	-0.07
Fiber	Moderately beneficial	+0.40
Protein	Modestly beneficial	+0.07
Total antioxidant content (TAC)	Moderately beneficial	+1.00 x TAC/gram
Sodium	Moderately deleterious	-0.50
Toxins (i.e. mercury, PCBs)	Moderately to profoundly deleterious	Mercury – 0 to -25 points PCBs – 0 to -6.6 points

EXPLANATION OF INFLUENCE FACTORS

Please refer to Parts 1-3, and Part 4 above for more detailed explanations of the underlying principles supporting the assignment of these influence factors. The explanations below are limited to concepts not previously discussed.

CALORIC VALUE: Influence factor assignments are *not directly* dependent on caloric value of nutrients. This is important as some fats have extraordinarily beneficial health properties, yet provide more than twice the calories per gram as carbohydrates and proteins. The caloric value, metabolic effects on fat accumulation, satiety, satiation, other features related to weight gain, and the Big 7 epidemic U.S. diseases are considered when determining influence factors.

DIETARY CHOLESTEROL versus SATURATED FATS: Despite the fact that dietary cholesterol has only "minimally deleterious" metabolic and health properties and saturated fats have "moderately deleterious" properties, cholesterol is assigned a *more* negative influence factor. This is because cholesterol, which accounts for less than 2% of the water-free weight of all foods, is present in comparatively small amounts in foods. Thus, cholesterol has only a modest impact on the overall score of even the most concentrated sources.

TOTAL ANTIOXIDANT CAPACITY (TAC): TAC is equal to the sum of water-soluble and fat-soluble antioxidants present in a given food item, expressed as TAC *per gram* of water-free weight, and added as a whole number to the net value of food items. While the maximum numerical adjustment assigned to any food item is +7 points (cranberries), most receive only a modest numerical boost.

MARINE TOXINS: Fish receive a numerical deduction according to average mercury and PCB concentrations. As mercury is considered "profoundly deleterious," fish contaminated with the highest amounts of mercury receive up to a 25-point deduction, while fish with trace amounts receive only a minimal deduction. Fish with the highest amounts of PCBs receive a moderate deduction of up to 6.6 points, commensurate with evidence of moderately deleterious properties. Therefore, the NQI weighs the beneficial nutrients supplied by fish against deleterious toxins to give an aggregate score reflecting *net* nutritional quality. In line with current evidence, in most situations, the benefits of fish consumption significantly outweigh the risks [139]. Exceptions include swordfish, king mackerel, orange roughy, and grouper.

NITRATES/NITRITES and RED MEATS: The NQI makes a modest negative adjustment to the net scores of processed meats and red meats, both of which have been linked to cancer and are considered "modestly deleterious."

POTASSIUM, MAGNESIUM, and CALCIUM: Unlike the USDA Nutrient Data Laboratory, *Nutrition Facts* labels do not include values for potassium or magnesium, and express calcium only as a percentage daily value (% DV). The NQI includes brand name food items without up-to-date USDA values. For consistency, these beneficial minerals are not *directly* scored. Rather, items rich in potassium, magnesium, and calcium receive a modest positive adjustment.

ARTIFICIAL SWEETENERS: Evidence that *long-term* substitution of artificially sweetened "diet" and "low-cal" foods for full calorie foods provides any health benefits is lacking. In fact, emerging evidence suggests that artificial sweeteners may actually *increase* the risk of obesity and metabolic syndrome [140, 141]. The NQI, which considers artificial sweeteners "modestly to moderately deleterious," automatically assigns a -3 *overall* rating to artificially sweetened foods.

By multiplying the above influence factors (IFs) by the nutrient percentage values (NPVs) for any given food item, a net positive or negative score proportionate to the predicted beneficial or adverse effects of consumption of that food item is generated.

COMPARISON OF TWO POPULAR "HEALTHY" CEREALS

EXAMPLE 1: To demonstrate the value of the NQI rating system, we will compare the net nutritional quality of two popular low fat, low saturated fat, and cholesterol-free breakfast cereals. Both are labeled "whole grain," and display a variety of other health claims. In addition, both meet the rudimentary and one-dimensional criteria necessary to

be labeled "heart healthy" [86]. However, upon closer inspection, their molecular
contents, metabolic properties, and health consequences are profoundly different.

CEREAL # 1

NUTRIENT CATEGORY	NPV	IFs	NPV x IF
Saturated fats (SFA)	1.1%	-0.25	-0.28
Monounsaturated fats (MUFA)	2.1%	+0.125	+0.26
ω-6 Linoleic acid (LA)	2.0%	-0.18	-0.36
ω-6 Arachidonic acid (ArA)	None	-4.00	-
ω-3 Alpha-linolenic acid (ALA)	0.1%	+0.80	+0.08
ω-3 EPA + DHA	None	+3.00	-
Trans fats	None	-3.60	-
Dietary cholesterol	None	-0.50	-
Non-fiber carbohydrates (NFC)	84.2%	-0.07	-5.89
Fiber	3.5%	+0.40	+1.40
Protein	7.0%	+0.07	+0.49
Sodium	0.4%	-0.50	-0.20
AGGREGATE SCORE			**-4.50**

CEREAL # 2

NUTRIENT CATEGORY	NPV	IFs	NPV x IF
Saturated fats (SFA)	1.0%	-0.25	-0.25
Monounsaturated fats (MUFA)	1.1%	+0.125	+0.14
ω-6 Linoleic acid (LA)	2.7%	-0.18	-0.49
ω-6 Arachidonic acid (ArA)	None	-4.00	-
ω-3 Alpha-linolenic acid (ALA)	0.7%	+0.80	+0.56
ω-3 EPA + DHA	None	+3.00	-
Trans fats	None	-3.60	-
Dietary cholesterol	None	-0.50	-
Non-fiber carbohydrates (NFC)	54.5%	-0.07	-3.82
Fiber	25.5%	+0.40	+10.20
Protein	14.5%	+0.07	+1.01
Sodium	0.7%	-0.50	-0.35
AGGREGATE SCORE			**+7.00**

ADJUSTMENTS

TOTAL ANTIOXIDANT CAPACITY (TAC): Unprocessed, uncooked, "whole" cereal grains
contain modest to moderate amounts of antioxidants, mostly located in the germ and bran. The refining
process, which removes most of the bran and germ, and the cooking process both significantly reduce
antioxidant content and activity. The customary practice of adding milk to cereal may further reduce
antioxidant activity through protein (casein)-antioxidant interactions [142]. Thus, breakfast cereals receive
no adjustments for TAC.

VITAMIN AND MINERAL FORTIFICATION: Many cereals, especially highly refined varieties,
are fortified with vitamins and minerals including vitamins A and C, B vitamins, zinc, iron, etc. Outside of
actual deficiencies, evidence that *added* vitamins and minerals have *any* beneficial health effects for people
already consuming a reasonably healthy diet is lacking, and high doses may actually have negative health
consequences [143-145]. Furthermore, Americans consuming low quality diets can easily obtain these and

other vitamins and minerals through an inexpensive multivitamin-mineral supplement. Thus, cereals receive no extra points for these fortified vitamins and minerals.

MINERALS: Unprocessed cereal grains contain modest to moderate amounts of potassium, magnesium, and calcium. Like TAC, these minerals are nearly absent from refined grains, which consist almost entirely of non-fiber carbohydrates. A modest positive numerical adjustment (+0.5 points), reflecting the presence of these minerals, is added to all cereals. Given the fact that refined cereals contain fewer beneficial minerals than whole grains, this adjustment may actually overestimate the health properties of processed foods.

After these modest adjustments, the net scores of cereal #1 and cereal #2 are -4.0, and +7.5, which are rounded to -4 and +8. These dramatic numerical differences reflect the fact that cereal #1 consists of little more than refined starches and sugars, which combine to account for over 84% of water-free weight! On a per gram basis, cereal #2 contains more than 7 times the fiber, twice the protein, and 7 times as much ω-3 ALA as cereal #1. Therefore, the NQI allows consumers to easily differentiate between high and low quality food items even in the face of inadequate nutritional information and/or misleading health claims.

EXAMPLE 2: As another demonstration of the value of the NQI system, we will compare the net nutritional quality of blackberries and grapes, two popular fruits widely believed to be beneficial for health. However, upon closer inspection, their molecular contents, metabolic properties, and health consequences are profoundly different.

Grape (green)

NUTRIENT CATEGORY	NPV	IFs	NPV x IF
Saturated fats (SFA)	0.5%	-0.25	-0.13
Monounsaturated fats (MUFA)	0.6%	+0.125	+0.08
ω-6 Linoleic acid (LA)	0.3%	-0.18	-0.05
ω-6 Arachidonic acid (ArA)	None	-4.00	-
ω-3 Alpha-linolenic acid (ALA)	0.1%	+0.80	+0.08
ω-3 EPA +DHA	None	+3.00	-
Trans fats	None	-3.60	-
Dietary cholesterol	None	-0.50	-
Non-fiber carbohydrates (NFC)	90.3%	-0.07	-6.32
Fiber	5.1%	+0.40	+2.04
Protein	3.7%	+0.07	+0.26
Sodium	0.0%	-0.50	**-0.00**
Total Antioxidant Capacity (TAC)	0.6	1.0	+0.60
AGGREGATE SCORE			-3.44
FINAL SCORE			-2

Blackberry

NUTRIENT CATEGORY	NPV	IFs	NPV x IF
Saturated fats (SFA)	0.1%	-0.25	-0.03
Monounsaturated fats (MUFA)	0.4%	+0.125	+0.05
ω-6 Linoleic acid (LA)	1.6%	-0.18	-0.29
ω-6 Arachidonic acid (ArA)	None	-4.00	-
ω-3 Alpha-linolenic acid (ALA)	0.8%	+0.80	+0.64
ω-3 EPA +DHA	None	+3.00	-
Trans fats	None	-3.60	-
Dietary cholesterol	None	-0.50	-
Non-fiber carbohydrates (NFC)	38.0%	-0.07	-2.66
Fiber	46.7%	+0.40	+18.70
Protein	12.3%	+0.07	+0.86
Sodium	0.0%	-0.50	-0.00
Total Antioxidant Capacity (TAC)	4.1	1.0	+4.10
AGGREGATE SCORE			+21.37
FINAL SCORE			+10

After modest positive adjustments are made for beneficial minerals (K+, Mg++, and Ca++), the final scores for green grapes and blackberries are -2, and +10 (maximum positive score), respectively. Scores reflect the high fiber, protein, antioxidant, and ω-3 ALA contents of blackberries, which rate among the highest of all foods in the NQI. The low score of green grapes, which score among the lowest of all *natural* foods in the NQI, reflects their high concentration of non-fiber carbohydrates (sugar equivalents), which account for more than 90% of water free weight!   In fact, green grapes are a considerably poorer source of fiber, protein, and ω-3 ALA than blackberries, and virtually all other fruits.

LIMITATIONS AND SOURCES OF ERROR

LIMITATIONS

It is important to understand the limitations of the NQI rating system. First, although the NQI allows consumers to easily identify the quality of *individual* food items, it says nothing about the *overall* diet. As an extreme example, an individual eating nothing but wild salmon would be deficient in fiber, antioxidants, and certain vitamins and minerals. Therefore, a variety of different foods should be consumed as part of any healthy diet.

To get the most out of the NQI system, simply select highly rated fruits, vegetables, nuts, fish, eggs, meats, legumes, cereals, breads, yogurts, oils, and other food items.

Similarly, the NQI purposefully does not include vitamins that can be and are commonly replaced by a multivitamin supplement. Except in special circumstances (i.e. Vit D3 in northern latitude winters and folic acid in early pregnancy), there is very little evidence that vitamin supplementation or food fortification provide *any* benefits for people consuming a high quality, varied diet. However, for those consuming a low quality or restricted diet, use of a **low-dose** multivitamin along with the NQI may be beneficial.

Because the NQI is not directly based on serving sizes or caloric value, one can theoretically overeat even exceptional foods. However, the nutrient compositions (i.e. high fiber, protein, low ω-6 to ω-3 ratios, etc.) of highly rated food-items tend to increase satiety and satiation, reduce concurrent and future caloric intake, and antagonize fat accumulation at the molecular level (see Part 3: Diet and Fat Accumulation). Essentially, if you select high quality food items, the rest will take care of itself.

Finally, because scores reflect *water-free* contents of food items, those following the NQI system need to ensure adequate hydration by alternative means. Simply consuming several glasses of water each day provides adequate hydration for most people. Fruits, vegetables, and other foods in their raw forms are also significant sources of water.

SOURCES OF ERROR

The integrity of the NQI rating system is dependent upon the accuracy of all compositional information used for calculations: the USDA National Nutrient Database, the *Nutrition Facts* labels of packaged food items, and a variety of other sources. The USDA National Nutrient Database, which periodically analyzes multiple samples of each food item and updates accordingly, is considered the gold standard of nutritional information.

However, even the USDA database may contain some errors. As explained in Part 2, recent changes in breeding and feeding practices have profoundly altered the fatty acid compositions of certain animal products. Because some composition data was collected before these agribusiness changes were implemented, fatty acid composition data may not entirely reflect modern nutrient contents. In particular, some scientists found consistently higher amounts of ω-6 ArA acid in U.S. meat than that reported by the USDA in 1998 [146]. It is unclear whether the USDA has since addressed these concerns.

Nutrient contents of brand name, packaged food items listed on *Nutrition Facts* labels are dependent upon the accuracy and integrity of manufacturer provided information. However, the FDA periodically collects "surveillance samples" for analysis to monitor the accuracy of listed nutrition information [147]. According to FDA reports, the vast majority (90%) of food samples correctly listed nutritional information [148]. In addition, rounding of nutrient content values on *Nutrition Facts* labels introduces another minor source of error. For example, the weights of total carbohydrates, proteins, and fats are rounded to the nearest whole numbers. Because these values are used to determine true grams, NPV values may not precisely reflect the content of foods.

Finally, the NQI system is based upon the author's interpretation of modern and historical collective nutritional, medical, and scientific evidence. Parts 1-4 provide ample foundation and a clear justification for the NQI system. However, as discussed in the *Introduction*, all scientific fields are dynamic, and nutrition science is no exception. Inevitably, as our understanding of the complex relationships between nutrition, health, and disease evolves, dietary guidance will continue to become more specific and comprehensive.

CONCLUSION

As an innovative, comprehensive, and versatile system for rating food items based on overall nutritional quality, the NQI provides consumers with a tool to easily identify and select foods likely to be beneficial for health.

References:

1. Knoops, K.T., et al., *Mediterranean diet, lifestyle factors, and 10-year mortality in elderly European men and women: the HALE project.* Jama, 2004. **292**(12): p. 1433-9.
2. Erkkila, A.T., et al., *n-3 Fatty acids and 5-y risks of death and cardiovascular disease events in patients with coronary artery disease.* Am J Clin Nutr, 2003. **78**(1): p. 65-71.
3. Fan, W.X., et al., *Erythrocyte fatty acids, plasma lipids, and cardiovascular disease in rural China.* Am J Clin Nutr, 1990. **52**(6): p. 1027-36.
4. Fung, T.T., et al., *Diet-quality scores and plasma concentrations of markers of inflammation and endothelial dysfunction.* Am J Clin Nutr, 2005. **82**(1): p. 163-73.
5. Iso, H., et al., *Intake of fish and n3 fatty acids and risk of coronary heart disease among Japanese: the Japan Public Health Center-Based (JPHC) Study Cohort I.* Circulation, 2006. **113**(2): p. 195-202.
6. Kromhout, D., et al., *Food consumption patterns in the 1960s in seven countries.* Am J Clin Nutr, 1989. **49**(5): p. 889-94.
7. McLaughlin, J., et al., *Adipose tissue triglyceride fatty acids and atherosclerosis in Alaska Natives and non-Natives.* Atherosclerosis, 2005. **181**(2): p. 353-62.
8. Menotti, A., et al., *Seven Countries Study. First 20-year mortality data in 12 cohorts of six countries.* Ann Med, 1989. **21**(3): p. 175-9.
9. Scarmeas, N., et al., *Mediterranean diet and risk for Alzheimer's disease.* Ann Neurol, 2006. **59**(6): p. 912-21.
10. Siscovick, D.S., et al., *Dietary intake and cell membrane levels of long-chain n-3 polyunsaturated fatty acids and the risk of primary cardiac arrest.* Jama, 1995. **274**(17): p. 1363-7.
11. Sugano, M. and F. Hirahara, *Polyunsaturated fatty acids in the food chain in Japan.* Am J Clin Nutr, 2000. **71**(1 Suppl): p. 189S-96S.
12. Tao, S.C., et al., *CHD and its risk factors in the People's Republic of China.* Int J Epidemiol, 1989. **18**(3 Suppl 1): p. S159-63.
13. Trichopoulou, A., et al., *Diet and survival of elderly Greeks: a link to the past.* Am J Clin Nutr, 1995. **61**(6 Suppl): p. 1346S-1350S.
14. Trichopoulou, A., et al., *Modified Mediterranean diet and survival: EPIC-elderly prospective cohort study.* Bmj, 2005. **330**(7498): p. 991.
15. Yamori, Y., A. Miura, and K. Taira, *Implications from and for food cultures for cardiovascular diseases: Japanese food, particularly Okinawan diets.* Asia Pac J Clin Nutr, 2001. **10**(2): p. 144-5.
16. O'Keefe, J.H., Jr. and L. Cordain, *Cardiovascular disease resulting from a diet and lifestyle at odds with our Paleolithic genome: how to become a 21st-century hunter-gatherer.* Mayo Clin Proc, 2004. **79**(1): p. 101-8.
17. Gowlett, J., *What actually was the Stone Age diet?* J Nutr Environ Med 2003. **13**: p. 143-7.
18. Eaton, S.B. and M. Konner, *Paleolithic nutrition. A consideration of its nature and current implications.* N Engl J Med, 1985. **312**(5): p. 283-9.
19. Cordain, L., et al., *Origins and evolution of the Western diet: health implications for the 21st century.* Am J Clin Nutr, 2005. **81**(2): p. 341-54.
20. Muskiet, F.A., et al., *Is docosahexaenoic acid (DHA) essential? Lessons from DHA status regulation, our ancient diet, epidemiology and randomized controlled trials.* J Nutr, 2004. **134**(1): p. 183-6.
21. Ghebremeskel, K. and M.A. Crawford, *Nutrition and health in relation to food production and processing.* Nutr Health, 1994. **9**(4): p. 237-53.
22. Emken, E.A., *Nutrition and biochemistry of trans and positional fatty acid isomers in hydrogenated oils.* Annu Rev Nutr, 1984. **4**: p. 339-76.
23. Willett, W.C., *Trans fatty acids and cardiovascular disease-epidemiological data.* Atheroscler Suppl, 2006. **7**(2): p. 5-8.
24. Eaton, S.B., M. Konner, and M. Shostak, *Stone agers in the fast lane: chronic degenerative diseases in evolutionary perspective.* Am J Med, 1988. **84**(4): p. 739-49.
25. Fox, C.S., et al., *Trends in the incidence of type 2 diabetes mellitus from the 1970s to the 1990s: the Framingham Heart Study.* Circulation, 2006. **113**(25): p. 2914-8.
26. Hemminki, K., J. Lorenzo Bermejo, and A. Forsti, *The balance between heritable and environmental aetiology of human disease.* Nat Rev Genet, 2006. **7**(12): p. 958-65.
27. Morrill, A.C. and C.D. Chinn, *The obesity epidemic in the United States.* J Public Health Policy, 2004. **25**(3-4): p. 353-66.
28. Narayan, K.M., et al., *Impact of recent increase in incidence on future diabetes burden: U.S., 2005-2050.* Diabetes Care, 2006. **29**(9): p. 2114-6.
29. Mooteri, S.N., et al., *Duration of residence in the United States as a new risk factor for coronary artery disease (The Konkani Heart Study).* Am J Cardiol, 2004. **93**(3): p. 359-61.
30. Goel, M.S., et al., *Obesity among US immigrant subgroups by duration of residence.* Jama, 2004. **292**(23): p. 2860-7.
31. Lauderdale, D.S. and P.J. Rathouz, *Body mass index in a US national sample of Asian Americans: effects of nativity, years since immigration and socioeconomic status.* Int J Obes Relat Metab Disord, 2000. **24**(9): p. 1188-94.
32. Ziegler, R.G., et al., *Migration patterns and breast cancer risk in Asian-American women.* J Natl Cancer Inst, 1993. **85**(22): p. 1819-27.
33. Khor, G.L., *Dietary fat quality: a nutritional epidemiologist's view.* Asia Pac J Clin Nutr, 2004. **13**(Suppl): p. S22.
34. Hu, F.B., J.E. Manson, and W.C. Willett, *Types of dietary fat and risk of coronary heart disease: a critical review.* J Am Coll Nutr, 2001. **20**(1): p. 5-19.
35. Pereira, M.A. and S. Liu, *Types of carbohydrates and risk of cardiovascular disease.* J Womens Health (Larchmt), 2003. **12**(2): p. 115-22.
36. Howard, B.V., et al., *Low-fat dietary pattern and risk of cardiovascular disease: the Women's Health Initiative Randomized Controlled Dietary Modification Trial.* Jama, 2006. **295**(6): p. 655-66.
37. de Lorgeril, M. and P. Salen, *Dietary prevention of coronary heart disease: focus on omega-6/omega-3 essential fatty acid balance.* World Rev Nutr Diet, 2003. **92**: p. 57-73.
38. de Lorgeril, M., et al., *Mediterranean diet, traditional risk factors, and the rate of cardiovascular complications after myocardial infarction: final report of the Lyon Diet Heart Study.* Circulation, 1999. **99**(6): p. 779-85.

39. *Dietary Fat-how much? What type? Consensus Statement from the Scientific Exchange.* Nutrition Today, 1998. **33-34**(173).

40. Liu, S., et al., *A prospective study of dietary glycemic load, carbohydrate intake, and risk of coronary heart disease in US women.* Am J Clin Nutr, 2000. **71**(6): p. 1455-61.

41. Griel, A.E., E.H. Ruder, and P.M. Kris-Etherton, *The changing roles of dietary carbohydrates: from simple to complex.* Arterioscler Thromb Vasc Biol, 2006. **26**(9): p. 1958-65.

42. Ludwig, D.S., *Symposium 2: Nutrition and Chronic Disease. Diet and development of the insulin resustence syndrome.* Proceedings of the Nutrition Society of Australia, 2003. **27**: p. S4.

43. Suter, P.M., *Carbohydrates and dietary fiber.* Handb Exp Pharmacol, 2005(170): p. 231-61.

44. Kant, A.K., *Indexes of overall diet quality: a review.* J Am Diet Assoc, 1996. **96**(8): p. 785-91.

45. Kennedy, E.T., et al., *The Healthy Eating Index: design and applications.* J Am Diet Assoc, 1995. **95**(10): p. 1103-8.

46. Baxter, A.J., T. Coyne, and C. McClintock, *Dietary patterns and metabolic syndrome--a review of epidemiologic evidence.* Asia Pac J Clin Nutr, 2006. **15**(2): p. 134-42.

47. Esmaillzadeh, A., et al., *Dietary patterns, insulin resistance, and prevalence of the metabolic syndrome in women.* Am J Clin Nutr, 2007. **85**(3): p. 910-8.

48. Suzuki, M., B.J. Wilcox, and C.D. Wilcox, *Implications from and for food cultures for cardiovascular disease: longevity.* Asia Pac J Clin Nutr, 2001. **10**(2): p. 165-71.

49. Bang, H.O., J. Dyerberg, and H.M. Sinclair, *The composition of the Eskimo food in north western Greenland.* Am J Clin Nutr, 1980. **33**(12): p. 2657-61.

50. Dyerberg, J. and H.O. Bang, *Dietary fat and thrombosis.* Lancet, 1978. **1**(8056): p. 152.

51. Dyerberg, J., H.O. Bang, and N. Hjorne, *Fatty acid composition of the plasma lipids in Greenland Eskimos.* Am J Clin Nutr, 1975. **28**(9): p. 958-66.

52. Wansink, B.e., *Mindless Eating: The 200 Daily Food Choices We Overlook.* Environment and Behavior, 2007. **39**: p. 106-23.

53. Lackey, C.J. and K.M. Kolasa, *Healthy Eating: Defining the Nutrient Quality of Foods.* Nutr Today, 2004. **39**(1): p. 26-29.

54. Scheidt, D.M. and E. Daniel, *Composite index for aggregating nutrient density using food labels: ratio of recommended to restricted food components.* J Nutr Educ Behav, 2004. **36**(1): p. 35-9.

55. Atwater, W.O., *Foods: Nutritive Value and Cost.* Washington, D.C.: U.S. Department of Agriculture, 1894. Farmer's Bulletin 23.

56. Gifford, K.D., *Dietary fats, eating guides, and public policy: history, critique, and recommendations.* Am J Med, 2002. **113 Suppl 9B**: p. 89S-106S.

57. Schneeman, B.O., *Evolution of dietary guidelines.* J Am Diet Assoc, 2003. **103**(12 Suppl 2): p. S5-9.

58. Grundy, S.M., et al., *Rationale of the diet-heart statement of the American Heart Association. Report of Nutrition Committee.* Circulation, 1982. **65**(4): p. 839A-854A.

59. *Dietary guidelines for healthy American adults. A statement for physicians and health professionals by the Nutrition Committee, American Heart Association.* Circulation, 1986. **74**(6): p. 1465A-1468A.

60. Ernst, N.D., et al., *The National Cholesterol Education Program: implications for dietetic practitioners from the Adult Treatment Panel recommendations.* J Am Diet Assoc, 1988. **88**(11): p. 1401-8, 1411.

61. *National Cholesterol Education Program. Report of the Expert Panel on Population Strategies for Blood Cholesterol Reduction: executive summary. National Heart, Lung and Blood Institute, National Institutes of Health.* Arch Intern Med, 1991. **151**(6): p. 1071-84.

62. Nixon, D.W., *Nutrition and cancer: American Cancer Society guidelines, programs, and initiatives.* CA Cancer J Clin, 1990. **40**(2): p. 71-5.

63. McCullough, M.L., et al., *Diet quality and major chronic disease risk in men and women: moving toward improved dietary guidance.* Am J Clin Nutr, 2002. **76**(6): p. 1261-71.

64. de Lorgeril, M., et al., *Mediterranean dietary pattern in a randomized trial: prolonged survival and possible reduced cancer rate.* Arch Intern Med, 1998. **158**(11): p. 1181-7.

65. *U.S. Department of Agricultural Research Service. 1997. Data Tables: Results from USDA's 1996 Continuing Survey of Food Intakes by Individuals and 1996 Diet and Health Knowledge Survey.* [cited 2006 August 10]; Available from: http:barc.usda.gov/bhnrc/foodsurvey/home.htm.

66. Rothman, R.L., et al., *Patient Understanding of Food Labels The Role of Literacy and Numeracy.* Am J Prev Med, 2006. **31**(5): p. 391-398.

67. *Food portions and servings: How do they differ?*, in *Nutrition Insights.* 1999, Center for Nutrition Policy and Promotion, USDA: Washington, DC.

68. *Food labeling: Serving sizes of products that can reasonably be consumed at one eating occasion; Udating of reference amounts customarily consumed; Approaches for recommending smaller portion sizes.* 2005 [cited 2006 December 19]; Federal register]. Available from: http://www.cfsan.fda.gov/~lrd/fr05404c.html.

69. Rothman, R.L., et al., *Patient understanding of food labels: the role of literacy and numeracy.* Am J Prev Med, 2006. **31**(5): p. 391-8.

70. *How to Understand and Use the Nutrition Facts Label. U.S. Food and Drug Administration, Center For Food Safety and Applied Nutrition.* . June 2000; Updated July 2003 and November 2004 [cited 2007 July 11]; Available from: http://www.cfsan.fda.gov/~dms/foodlab.html#compare.

71. *Trans Fat now Listed with Saturated Fat and Cholesterol on Nutrition Facts Label.* . Dept of Health and Human Services, U.S. FDA/CFSAN 2006 [cited 2007 July 15]; Available from: http://www.cfsan.fda.gov/~dms/foodlabs.gif.

72. *A Food Labeling Guide. U.S. Department of Health and Human services, U.S. FDA/CFSAN.* . 1994 (Editorial revisions June, 1999) [cited 2007 July 15]; Available from: http://www.cfsan.fda.gov/~dms/flg-6b.html.

73. Kristal, A.R., et al., *Trends in food label use associated with new nutrition labeling regulations.* Am J Public Health, 1998. **88**(8): p. 1212-5.

74. *Questions and Answers about Trans Fat Nutrition Labeling. U.S. Food and Drug Administration. CFSAN Office of Nutritional Products, Labeling, and Dietary Supplements.* 2003 [cited 2006 September 15]; Available from: http://www.cfsan.fda.gov/~dma/qatrans2.html.

75. *Food Labeling: Trans Fatty Acids in Nutrition Labeling, Nutrient Content Claims, and Health Claims. Final Rule.*, in *Food and Drug Administration, HHS. p. 1-74.* 2003, July 11.

76. *U.S. Department of Agriculture, Agricultural Research Service. 2006. USDA National Nutrient Database for Standard Reference, Release 19.* 2007 [cited 2007 July 15]; Available from: Nutrient Data Laboratory Home Page, http://www.ars.usda.gov/ba/bhnrc/ndl.

77. Drewnowski, A., *The role of energy density.* Lipids, 2003. **38**(2): p. 109-15.

78. Takase, B., et al., *Arachidonic acid metabolites in acute myocardial infarction.* Angiology, 1996. **47**(7): p. 649-61.

79. Simopoulos, A.P., *Genetics and nutrition: or what your genes can tell you about nutrition.* World Rev Nutr Diet, 1990. **63**: p. 25-34.

80. Dwyer, J.H., et al., *Arachidonate 5-lipoxygenase promoter genotype, dietary arachidonic acid, and atherosclerosis.* N Engl J Med, 2004. **350**(1): p. 29-37.

81. Stark, A.H. and Z. Madar, *Olive oil as a functional food: epidemiology and nutritional approaches.* Nutr Rev, 2002. **60**(6): p. 170-6.

82. Wahlqvist, M.L., E.G. Wilmshurst, and E.N. Richardson, *The effect of chain length on glucose absorption and the related metabolic response.* Am J Clin Nutr, 1978. **31**(11): p. 1998-2001.

83. Bantle, J.P., et al., *Postprandial glucose and insulin responses to meals containing different carbohydrates in normal and diabetic subjects.* N Engl J Med, 1983. **309**(1): p. 7-12.

84. Gross, L.S., et al., *Increased consumption of refined carbohydrates and the epidemic of type 2 diabetes in the United States: an ecologic assessment.* Am J Clin Nutr, 2004. **79**(5): p. 774-9.

85. Hansen, R.G., *An index of food quality.* Nutr Rev, 1973. **31**(1): p. 1-7.

86. *What Certification Means.* 2007 [cited 2007 July 17]; Available from: http://americanheart.org/presenter.jhtml?identifier=4973.

87. Kim H, P., DI., *Estimating the importance of individual nutrients from professionals' choices among food products. AFPC Policy Research Report 93-10.*, in *Agricultural and food Policy Center.* 1993, Texas A+M University: College Station, TX.

88. Mercer, N., *The M-Fit Grocery Shopping Guide Your Guide to Healthier Choices.* 1997.

89. Drewnowski, A., *Concept of a nutritious food: toward a nutrient density score.* Am J Clin Nutr, 2005. **82**(4): p. 721-32.

90. Wu, X., et al., *Lipophilic and hydrophilic antioxidant capacities of common foods in the United States.* J Agric Food Chem, 2004. **52**(12): p. 4026-37.

91. Pellegrini, N., et al., *Total antioxidant capacity of plant foods, beverages and oils consumed in Italy assessed by three different in vitro assays.* J Nutr, 2003. **133**(9): p. 2812-9.

92. Pellegrini, N., et al., *Total antioxidant capacity of spices, dried fruits, nuts, pulses, cereals and sweets consumed in Italy assessed by three different in vitro assays.* Mol Nutr Food Res, 2006. **50**(11): p. 1030-8.

93. Proteggente, A.R., et al., *The antioxidant activity of regularly consumed fruit and vegetables reflects their phenolic and vitamin C composition.* Free Radic Res, 2002. **36**(2): p. 217-33.

94. Halvorsen, B.L., et al., *A systematic screening of total antioxidants in dietary plants.* J Nutr, 2002. **132**(3): p. 461-71.

95. Hites, R.A., et al., *Global assessment of organic contaminants in farmed salmon.* Science, 2004. **303**(5655): p. 226-9.

96. Hamilton, M.C., et al., *Lipid composition and contaminants in farmed and wild salmon.* Environ Sci Technol, 2005. **39**(22): p. 8622-9.

97. *U.S. Department of Health and Human Services and EPA. Mercury Levels in Contaminated Fish and Shellfish.* [cited 2005 December 12]; Available from: http://www.cfsan.fda.gov/~frf/sea-mehg.html.

98. Kaput, J. and R.L. Rodriguez, *Nutritional genomics: the next frontier in the postgenomic era.* Physiol Genomics, 2004. **16**(2): p. 166-77.

99. Schiavone, A., et al., *Influence of dietary lipid source and strain on fatty acid composition of Muscovy duck meat.* J Anim Physiol Anim Nutr (Berl), 2004. **88**(3-4): p. 88-93.

100. Hu, X., et al., *Mapping of the loci controlling oleic and linolenic acid contents and development of fad2 and fad3 allele-specific markers in canola (Brassica napus L.).* Theor Appl Genet, 2006. **113**(3): p. 497-507.

101. Ellis, K.A., et al., *Comparing the fatty acid composition of organic and conventional milk.* J Dairy Sci, 2006. **89**(6): p. 1938-50.

102. Dolecek, T.A., *Epidemiological evidence of relationships between dietary polyunsaturated fatty acids and mortality in the multiple risk factor intervention trial.* Proc Soc Exp Biol Med, 1992. **200**(2): p. 177-82.

103. Hu, F.B., et al., *Dietary intake of alpha-linolenic acid and risk of fatal ischemic heart disease among women.* Am J Clin Nutr, 1999. **69**(5): p. 890-7.

104. Harris, W.S., *Alpha-linolenic acid: a gift from the land?* Circulation, 2005. **111**(22): p. 2872-4.

105. Kromhout, D., *Serum cholesterol in cross-cultural perspective. The Seven Countries Study.* Acta Cardiol, 1999. **54**(3): p. 155-8.

106. Hu, F.B., et al., *Dietary fat intake and the risk of coronary heart disease in women.* N Engl J Med, 1997. **337**(21): p. 1491-9.

107. Ascherio, A., *Epidemiologic studies on dietary fats and coronary heart disease.* Am J Med, 2002. **113 Suppl 9B**: p. 9S-12S.

108. Bendich, A.a.D., RJ., *Preventive Nutrition: the comprehensive guide for health professionals, 2nd edition.* 2001: Humana Press.

109. Bray, G.A., S.J. Nielsen, and B.M. Popkin, *Consumption of high-fructose corn syrup in beverages may play a role in the epidemic of obesity.* Am J Clin Nutr, 2004. **79**(4): p. 537-43.

110. Havel, P.J., *Dietary fructose: implications for dysregulation of energy homeostasis and lipid/carbohydrate metabolism.* Nutr Rev, 2005. **63**(5): p. 133-57.

111. Elliott, S.S., et al., *Fructose, weight gain, and the insulin resistance syndrome.* Am J Clin Nutr, 2002. **76**(5): p. 911-22.

112. Jones, J.M., et al., *Becoming Proactive With the Whole-Grains Message.* Nutr Today, 2004. **39**(1): p. 10-17.

113.   Hussein, N., et al., *Long-chain conversion of [13C]linoleic acid and alpha-linolenic acid in response to marked changes in their dietary intake in men.* J Lipid Res, 2005. **46**(2): p. 269-80.

114.   Budowski, P. and M.A. Crawford, *a-Linolenic acid as a regulator of the metabolism of arachidonic acid: dietary implications of the ratio, n-6:n-3 fatty acids.* Proc Nutr Soc, 1985. **44**(2): p. 221-9.

115.   Goyens, P.L., et al., *Conversion of alpha-linolenic acid in humans is influenced by the absolute amounts of alpha-linolenic acid and linoleic acid in the diet and not by their ratio.* Am J Clin Nutr, 2006. **84**(1): p. 44-53.

116.   Chan, J.K., et al., *Effect of dietary alpha-linolenic acid and its ratio to linoleic acid on platelet and plasma fatty acids and thrombogenesis.* Lipids, 1993. **28**(9): p. 811-7.

117.   Okuyama, H., T. Kobayashi, and S. Watanabe, *Dietary fatty acids--the N-6/N-3 balance and chronic elderly diseases. Excess linoleic acid and relative N-3 deficiency syndrome seen in Japan.* Prog Lipid Res, 1996. **35**(4): p. 409-57.

118.   Ailhaud, G., et al., *Temporal changes in dietary fats: role of n-6 polyunsaturated fatty acids in excessive adipose tissue development and relationship to obesity.* Prog Lipid Res, 2006. **45**(3): p. 203-36.

119.   Kiecolt-Glaser, J.K., et al., *Depressive symptoms, omega-6:omega-3 fatty acids, and inflammation in older adults.* Psychosom Med, 2007. **69**(3): p. 217-24.

120.   Simopoulos, A.P., A. Leaf, and N. Salem, Jr.,. *Workshop on the Essentiality of and Recommended Dietary Intakes for Omega-6 and Omega-3 Fatty Acids.* J Am Coll Nutr, 1999. *18(5): p. 487-9.* [cited.

121.   de Lorgeril, M. and P. Salen, *The Mediterranean diet in secondary prevention of coronary heart disease.* Clin Invest Med, 2006. **29**(3): p. 154-8.

122.   Simopoulos, A.P., *Evolutionary aspects of omega-3 fatty acids in the food supply.* Prostaglandins Leukot Essent Fatty Acids, 1999. **60**(5-6): p. 421-9.

123.   *Deutsche Gessellschaft fur Ernahrung. Referenzwerte fur die Nahrstoffzufuhr, Umschau Braus GmbH: Frankfurt am Main Germany.* 2000: p. 227pp.

124.   Eaton, S.B., et al., *Dietary intake of long-chain polyunsaturated fatty acids during the paleolithic.* World Rev Nutr Diet, 1998. **83**: p. 12-23.

125.   *U.S. Department of Agricultural Research Service. 1997. Data Tables: results from the USDA's 1994-1996 Continuing Survey of Food Intakes by Individuals and 1994-1996 Diet and Health Knowledge Survey [Online] ARS Food Surveys Research Group.* . [cited 2006 Aug 10]; Available from: http:barc.usda.gov/bhnrc/foodsurvey/home.htm.

126.   Cordain, L., *The Nutritional Characteristics of a Contemporary Diet.* JANA, 2002. **5**(3): p. 15-25.

127.   Mensink, R.P., et al., *Effects of dietary fatty acids and carbohydrates on the ratio of serum total to HDL cholesterol and on serum lipids and apolipoproteins: a meta-analysis of 60 controlled trials.* Am J Clin Nutr, 2003. **77**(5): p. 1146-55.

128.   Pacheco, Y.M., et al., *Ratio of oleic to palmitic acid is a dietary determinant of thrombogenic and fibrinolytic factors during the postprandial state in men.* Am J Clin Nutr, 2006. **84**(2): p. 342-9.

129.   Eaton, S.B., *Humans, lipids and evolution.* Lipids, 1992. **27**(10): p. 814-20.

130.   Cordain, L., et al., *The paradoxical nature of hunter-gatherer diets: meat-based, yet non-atherogenic.* Eur J Clin Nutr, 2002. **56 Suppl 1**: p. S42-52.

131.   Cordain, L., et al., *Fatty acid analysis of wild ruminant tissues: evolutionary implications for reducing diet-related chronic disease.* Eur J Clin Nutr, 2002. **56**(3): p. 181-91.

132.   Smith, R.D., et al., *Long-term monounsaturated fatty acid diets reduce platelet aggregation in healthy young subjects.* Br J Nutr, 2003. **90**(3): p. 597-606.

133.   Renaud, S.C., *What is the epidemiologic evidence for the thrombogenic potential of dietary long-chain fatty acids?* Am J Clin Nutr, 1992. **56**(4 Suppl): p. 823S-824S.

134.   Simon, J.A., et al., *Serum fatty acids and the risk of coronary heart disease.* Am J Epidemiol, 1995. **142**(5): p. 469-76.

135.   Trichopoulou, A., et al., *Adherence to a Mediterranean diet and survival in a Greek population.* N Engl J Med, 2003. **348**(26): p. 2599-608.

136.   Solfrizzi, V., et al., *Dietary intake of unsaturated fatty acids and age-related cognitive decline: a 8.5-year follow-up of the Italian Longitudinal Study on Aging.* Neurobiol Aging, 2006. **27**(11): p. 1694-704.

137.   Alvarez Leon, E.E., P. Henriquez, and L. Serra-Majem, *Mediterranean diet and metabolic syndrome: a cross-sectional study in the Canary Islands.* Public Health Nutr, 2006. **9**(8A): p. 1089-98.

138.   Stamatiou, K., D. Delakas, and F. Sofras, *Mediterranean diet, monounsaturated: saturated fat ratio and low prostate cancer risk. A myth or a reality?* Minerva Urol Nefrol, 2007. **59**(1): p. 59-66.

139.   Mozaffarian, D. and E.B. Rimm, *Fish intake, contaminants, and human health: evaluating the risks and the benefits.* Jama, 2006. **296**(15): p. 1885-99.

140.   Dhingra, R., et al., *Soft Drink Consumption and Risk of Developing Cardiometabolic Risk Factors and the Metabolic Syndrome in Middle-Aged Adults in the Community.* Circulation, 2007.

141.   Fowler, S., Williams, K et al. . *Diet Soft Drink Consumption is Associated with Increased Incidence of Overweight and Obesity in the San Antonio Heart Study.* . in *American Diabetic Association 65th Annual Assembly.* . 2005.

142.   Lorenz, M., et al., *Addition of milk prevents vascular protective effects of tea.* Eur Heart J, 2007. **28**(2): p. 219-23.

143.   Meltzer, H.M., et al., *Risk analysis applied to food fortification.* Public Health Nutr, 2003. **6**(3): p. 281-91.

144.   Prentice, R.L., *Clinical trials and observational studies to assess the chronic disease benefits and risks of multivitamin-multimineral supplements.* Am J Clin Nutr, 2007. **85**(1): p. 308S-313S.

145.   Bjelakovic, G., et al., *Mortality in randomized trials of antioxidant supplements for primary and secondary prevention: systematic review and meta-analysis.* Jama, 2007. **297**(8): p. 842-57.

146.   Taber, L., C.H. Chiu, and J. Whelan, *Assessment of the arachidonic acid content in foods commonly consumed in the American diet.* Lipids, 1998. **33**(12): p. 1151-7.

147.   *Food Labeling Questions and Answers.* 1993 [cited 2007; Available from: http://www.cfsan.fda.gov/~lrd/qa2.html

148.   *Nutrition Facts Labels Getting It Right.* K-State Research and Extension 1996 [cited 2007 Dec 31, 1996]; Available from: http://www.oznet.k-state.edu/humannutrition/_timely/nutrition.htm.

PART FIVE

THE NQI RATINGS

The NQI Ratings

The NQI assigns all-inclusive numerical scores to more than 600 food items based on *overall* nutritional quality. Scores range from -10 to +10, with -10 signifying a food that will contribute to disease if consumed regularly, 0 signifying neutral health effects, and +10 signifying profound health benefits. Rated foods are separated into the following twelve categories:

1. Breakfast Cereals

2. Breads

3. Yogurts

4. Fats & Oils

5. Finfish

6. Shellfish

7. Animal Meats
   Chicken, Turkey, Duck, Ostrich, Beef, Veal, Pork, Lamb, Game

8. Eggs

9. Fruits

10. Vegetables

11. Nuts & Seeds

12. Legumes

The introduction to each section clarifies common misconceptions, advises how to identify high quality selections, and explains how to integrate each food category into a healthy diet. Next, top-rated *NQI Superior Selections* are revealed. For example, the 24 highest rated cereals, all of which score +5 or higher, are listed separately in descending order. Finally, the scores and nutritional compositions of *all rated* food items in each section are provided. For instance, the overall scores and nutrient compositions of all 233 rated breakfast cereals are listed in alphabetical order, according to manufacturer. Nutrients are expressed as a percentage of water free-weight, or true grams, as described in Part 4. See the tables below for the formatting and abbreviations used to depict each nutrient category.

FORMAT FOR DISPLAYING NUTRITIONAL INFORMATION

NET SCORE*	SFA	MUFA	LA	ArA	ALA	EPA DHA	TFA	Chol	NFC	Fiber	Protein	Na	AOX	TOX

*Positive scores = BLUE, neutral scores = BLACK, negative scores = RED.

ABBREVIATIONS

SFA	Total Saturated fats
MUFA	Total Monounsaturated fats
LA	Omega-6 Linoleic acid
ArA	Omega-6 Arachidonic acid
ALA	Omega-3 Alpha linolenic acid
EPA + DHA	Omega-3 Eicosapentaenoic and Docosahexaenoic acids
TFA	Total Trans fats
Chol	Dietary cholesterol
NFC	Non-fiber carbohydrates (total sugar equivalents)
Fiber	Total Fiber
Protein	Total Protein
Na	Sodium
AOX	Total antioxidant capacity
TOX	Mercury, PCBs, and other toxins

HOW TO USE THE NQI

By translating the precise nutritional composition of each food item into an all-inclusive score between -10 to +10, the NQI allows you to easily distinguish between high and low quality foods in order to effortlessly improve dietary selections. *The work is done for you!*

SUGGESTED USES

Perhaps the simplest way to use the NQI is to identify food items within your current diet with the lowest NQI scores (the biggest "offenders") and replace those items with higher quality choices. Alternatively, you may seek to consume more foods with outstanding health properties from the top-rated *NQI Superior Selections.* In lieu of a conventional "diet," health enthusiasts can select *only* food items that score +3 or higher.

Author's Note: *Although designed to rate foods based on overall health properties, the NQI can be adapted for more specific goals. For example, as explained in Part 3: Diet and Fat Accumulation, food items likely to promote weight loss contain high concentrations of fiber and protein, low NFC to fiber and omega-6 to omega-3 ratios, and no artificial sweeteners. Savvy users can identify suitable foods from the nutritional information supplied in Part 5. Similar strategies can be used to identify foods likely to combat the development of cancer, inflammatory diseases, and other specific health concerns.*

As a versatile and all-inclusive instrument designed to improve dietary choices, the NQI will empower Americans to apply recent advances in nutritional biochemistry and preventative medicine to their everyday lives. Whatever your specific goals, our hope is that the NQI will serve as a useful tool to guide your food consumption and optimize your health.

Breakfast Cereals

The NQI rates 233 breakfast cereals based on *overall* nutritional quality. Scores range from -10 (toxic) to +10 (exceptional) reflecting the dramatic variation in molecular contents and predicted metabolic and health consequences of different cereals.

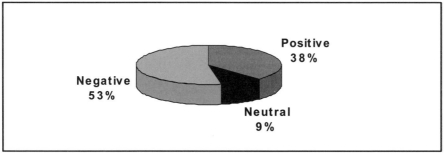

Figure 1: Breakfast Cereals. Only 38% of cereals evaluated by the NQI receive favorable ratings. Twenty-four cereals (10%) score +5 or higher, reflecting superior nutritional quality.

Most cereal health claims focus attention on their low quantities of total fat, saturated fat, and cholesterol. Some even receive "heart healthy" approval by meeting these one-dimensional criteria. However, as high carbohydrate grain-based foods, *all* breakfast cereals are low in total fat, saturated fat, and cholesterol, making these claims nearly meaningless! ***Despite health claims to the contrary, most available cereals are low quality foods.*** Habitual consumption of low quality cereals can significantly increase your risk of developing the Big 7 epidemic U.S. diseases.

The NQI easily distinguishes between high and low quality cereals.
Because cereals are high carbohydrate foods, NQI scores reflect carbohydrate *quality*. Cereals receiving low scores, including some labeled as "heart healthy" and "whole grain," contain little more than refined grains (sugar equivalents), added sugar, and added vitamins. A few still contain small but significant amounts of trans fats, despite listing "0 grams" on *Nutrition Facts* labels. The highest rated cereals contain significant amounts of fiber and low non-fiber carbohydrate to fiber ratios. Other beneficial attributes include comparatively

high concentrations of protein and omega-3 fats. As part of a healthy diet, regular consumption of these high quality cereals will optimize your metabolism and reduce your risk of developing the Big 7 epidemic U.S. diseases.

NQI SUPERIOR SELECTIONS
TOP 24 SUPER CEREALS

+10	Kellogg's	All-Bran Original
+10	Post	100% Bran
+9	Barbara's Bakery	Organic Grain Shop
+9	Kashi	Go Lean
+8	Back to Nature	Heart Basics Hi-Fiber Multibran
+8	Nature's Path	Flax Plus Flakes 0-3
+7	Kashi	Good Friends
+7	Peace	Essential 10 – Organic
+7	Weight Watchers	Banana Almond Medley
+6	Back to Nature	Heart Basics – Banana Nut Multibran
+6	Back to Nature	Heart Basics – Flax & Fiber Crunch
+6	Kashi	Vive – Probiotic Digestive Wellness
+6	Nature's Path	FlaxPlus Raisin Bran
+6	Nature's Path	Heritage Heirloom – Whole Grains
+6	Nature's Path	Optimum Slim
+6	U.S. Mills	Uncle Sam – Original
+6	U.S. Mills	Uncle Sam with Mixed Berries
+6	Zoe's	Cinnamon
+6	Zoe's	Flax & Soy Granola – Cranberries Currants
+6	Zoe's	Flax & Soy Granola – Honey Almond
+6	Zoe's	Natural
+5	Nature's Path	Optimum Power Breakfast
+5	Barbara's Bakery	Organic Wheatabix – Crispy Flakes & Fiber
+5	Weight Watchers	Cinnamon Cluster Crunch

CEREALS		Score	SFA	MUFA	LA	ALA	TFA	NFC	Fiber	Protein	Na
ARROWHEAD MILLS	Amaranth Flakes	0	1.3%	2.4%	2.5%	0.1%	0.0%	71.9%	9.4%	12.5%	0.0%
ARROWHEAD MILLS	Corn Flakes	-2	0.2%	0.3%	0.8%	0.0%	0.0%	85.0%	6.8%	6.8%	0.2%
ARROWHEAD MILLS	Kamut Flakes	-1	0.7%	0.7%	1.8%	0.2%	0.0%	76.7%	6.7%	13.3%	0.2%
ARROWHEAD MILLS	Multigrain Flakes	-1	1.0%	2.0%	1.9%	0.1%	0.0%	75.0%	7.5%	12.5%	0.5%
ARROWHEAD MILLS	Organic Nature O's	-1	1.3%	2.5%	2.6%	0.1%	0.0%	74.2%	6.5%	12.9%	0.0%
ARROWHEAD MILLS	Puffed Millet	-1	0.7%	0.7%	2.2%	0.0%	0.0%	74.1%	7.4%	14.8%	0.0%
ARROWHEAD MILLS	Rice Flakes Sweetened	-4	0.5%	0.9%	0.9%	0.0%	0.0%	88.6%	2.3%	6.8%	0.4%
ARROWHEAD MILLS	Shredded Wheat	+2	0.4%	0.4%	1.2%	0.1%	0.0%	71.1%	13.3%	13.3%	0.0%
ARROWHEAD MILLS	Spelt Flakes	+1	0.7%	0.7%	1.9%	0.2%	0.0%	72.4%	10.3%	13.8%	0.3%
ARROWHEAD MILLS	Sweetened Shredded Wheat	0	0.4%	0.4%	1.1%	0.1%	0.0%	77.1%	10.4%	10.4%	0.0%
BACK TO NATURE	Energy Start Hi-Protein Crunch	+2	0.7%	0.7%	1.9%	0.2%	0.0%	56.2%	6.7%	33.7%	0.3%
BACK TO NATURE	Heart Basics Organic Apple Cinnamon	+4	0.6%	0.6%	1.6%	0.2%	0.0%	69.3%	19.8%	7.9%	0.2%
BACK TO NATURE	Heart Basics Banana Nut Multibran	+6	0.6%	0.7%	1.4%	0.2%	0.0%	64.8%	22.9%	9.5%	0.2%
BACK TO NATURE	Heart Basics Flax & Fiber Crunch	+6	0.9%	1.1%	2.5%	0.7%	0.0%	57.7%	18.6%	18.6%	0.2%
BACK TO NATURE	Heart Basics Hi-Fiber Multibran	+8	0.4%	0.4%	1.2%	0.1%	0.0%	60.9%	26.1%	10.9%	0.2%
BARBARA'S BAKERY	Alpen	-1	0.9%	2.4%	2.6%	0.1%	0.0%	74.0%	8.0%	12.0%	0.1%
BARBARA'S BAKERY	Organic Breakfast O's	+1	1.4%	2.7%	2.9%	0.1%	0.0%	67.9%	10.7%	14.3%	0.5%
BARBARA'S BAKERY	Organic Brown Rice Crisps	-3	0.7%	1.4%	1.4%	0.1%	0.0%	85.7%	3.6%	7.1%	0.5%
BARBARA'S BAKERY	Organic Grain Shop	+9	0.7%	0.7%	2.0%	0.2%	0.0%	57.1%	28.6%	10.7%	0.4%
BARBARA'S BAKERY	Organic Honey Crunch 'n Oats	0	0.6%	1.6%	3.0%	0.0%	0.0%	77.2%	10.5%	7.0%	0.4%
BARBARA'S BAKERY	Organic Honey Nut O's	-2	1.0%	2.2%	3.8%	0.1%	0.0%	75.9%	6.9%	10.3%	0.3%
BARBARA'S BAKERY	Organic Soy Essence	+4	0.3%	0.3%	1.0%	0.1%	0.0%	69.0%	17.2%	12.1%	0.4%
BARBARA'S BAKERY	Organic Weetabix	+1	0.5%	0.5%	1.5%	0.1%	0.0%	64.9%	10.8%	10.8%	0.4%
BARBARA'S BAKERY	Organic Weetabix Crispy Flakes & Fiber	+5	0.6%	0.6%	1.6%	0.2%	0.0%	64.1%	21.4%	11.7%	0.6%
BARBARA'S BAKERY	Organic Wild Puffs - Cocoa	-4	0.5%	0.9%	2.1%	0.0%	0.0%	85.7%	3.6%	7.1%	0.7%
BARBARA'S BAKERY	Organic Wild Puffs - Original	-4	0.4%	0.4%	1.1%	0.1%	0.0%	88.2%	2.0%	7.8%	0.2%
BARBARA'S BAKERY	Puffins - Cinnamon	+4	0.4%	0.7%	2.3%	0.0%	0.0%	69.0%	20.7%	6.9%	0.8%

CEREALS		Score	SFA	MUFA	LA	ALA	TFA	NFC	Fiber	Protein	Na
BARBARA'S BAKERY	Puffins - Peanut Butter	-1	1.0%	1.8%	4.3%	0.1%	0.0%	75.0%	7.1%	10.7%	0.2%
BARBARA'S BAKERY	Shredded Oats	0	0.9%	1.7%	1.8%	0.1%	0.0%	75.2%	9.2%	11.0%	0.5%
BARBARA'S BAKERY	Shredded Wheat	+2	0.6%	0.6%	1.5%	0.1%	0.0%	72.2%	13.9%	11.1%	0.0%
BREADSHOP'S	Original Crunchy Granola - Honey Gone Nuts	+2	2.0%	10.8%	5.7%	1.5%	0.0%	58.0%	8.0%	14.0%	0.0%
BREADSHOP'S	SuperNatural with Almonds & Raisins	+1	2.0%	11.3%	5.3%	1.4%	0.0%	62.2%	6.7%	11.1%	0.0%
CASCADIUM FARM	Cinnamon Raisin Granola	-2	0.9%	1.7%	3.3%	0.1%	0.0%	78.0%	6.0%	10.0%	0.4%
CASCADIUM FARM	Clifford Crunch	+3	0.7%	1.4%	1.4%	0.1%	0.0%	71.4%	6.0%	7.1%	0.6%
CASCADIUM FARM	Hearty Morning	+2	0.8%	1.0%	3.0%	0.2%	0.0%	69.3%	17.9%	9.9%	0.7%
CASCADIUM FARM	Multi Grain Squares	-1	0.4%	0.4%	1.0%	0.1%	0.0%	80.7%	15.8%	10.5%	0.4%
CASCADIUM FARM	Purely O's	0	1.5%	2.8%	3.0%	0.1%	0.0%	70.4%	7.0%	11.1%	1.0%
CASCADIUM FARM	Raisin Bran	+1	0.6%	0.6%	1.7%	0.2%	0.0%	74.7%	12.1%	10.1%	0.7%
FAMILIA	Swiss Muesli - Original Recipe	0	1.2%	2.3%	2.4%	0.1%	0.0%	74.0%	8.0%	12.0%	0.0%
FAMILIA	Swiss Muesli - No Sugar added	0	1.2%	2.3%	2.4%	0.1%	0.0%	74.0%	8.0%	12.0%	0.0%
FOOD FOR LIFE	Ezekiel 4:9 Sprouted Grain - Almond	+2	1.0%	1.4%	3.4%	0.3%	0.0%	65.3%	12.2%	16.3%	0.4%
FOOD FOR LIFE	Ezekiel 4:9 Sprouted Grain - Cinnamon Raisin	+1	0.4%	0.4%	1.1%	0.1%	0.0%	73.5%	10.2%	14.3%	0.3%
FOOD FOR LIFE	Ezekiel 4:9 Sprouted Grain - Golden Flax	+3	0.9%	1.1%	2.4%	0.9%	0.0%	65.3%	12.6%	16.8%	0.4%
FOOD FOR LIFE	Ezekiel 4:9 Sprouted Grain - Original	+2	0.4%	0.4%	1.1%	0.1%	0.0%	69.4%	12.2%	16.3%	0.4%
GENERAL MILLS	Apple Cinnamon Cheerios	-3	1.1%	2.1%	2.0%	0.1%	0.0%	84.2%	3.5%	7.0%	0.4%
GENERAL MILLS	Basic 4	-5	1.0%	1.2%	2.9%	0.0%	0.8%	80.4%	5.9%	7.8%	0.6%
GENERAL MILLS	Berry Burst Cheerios	-1	1.1%	2.2%	2.3%	0.1%	0.0%	75.5%	7.5%	11.3%	0.6%
GENERAL MILLS	Cheerios	0	1.5%	2.8%	3.0%	0.1%	0.0%	70.4%	11.1%	11.1%	0.8%
GENERAL MILLS	Chex - Corn	-4	0.2%	0.5%	1.1%	0.0%	0.0%	87.7%	3.5%	7.0%	1.0%
GENERAL MILLS	Chex - Multi Bran	+1	0.4%	0.7%	1.7%	0.0%	0.0%	75.7%	13.6%	7.8%	0.0%
GENERAL MILLS	Chex - Rice	-4	0.4%	0.7%	0.7%	0.0%	0.0%	87.7%	3.5%	7.0%	1.0%
GENERAL MILLS	Chex - Wheat	0	0.7%	0.7%	1.9%	0.2%	0.0%	75.0%	11.4%	11.4%	0.9%
GENERAL MILLS	Cinnamon Toast Crunch	-4	2.5%	5.5%	4.0%	0.3%	0.0%	80.7%	3.5%	3.5%	0.7%
GENERAL MILLS	Cinnamon Toast Crunch - Reduced Sugar	-3	Contains Artificial Sweetener								

CEREALS		Score	SFA	MUFA	LA	ALA	TFA	NFC	Fiber	Protein	Na
GENERAL MILLS	Cocoa Puffs	-4	1.0%	2.0%	2.8%	0.1%	0.0%	86.3%	3.9%	3.92%	0.59%
GENERAL MILLS	Cookie Crisp	-4	0.9%	1.7%	2.6%	0.1%	0.0%	87.7%	3.5%	3.5%	0.6%
GENERAL MILLS	Country Corn Flakes	-4	0.2%	0.4%	1.0%	0.0%	0.0%	88.5%	3.3%	6.6%	1.0%
GENERAL MILLS	Fiber One	-3			Contains Artificial Sweetener						
GENERAL MILLS	Frosted Cheerios	-3	0.8%	1.5%	1.5%	0.1%	0.0%	84.6%	3.8%	7.7%	0.8%
GENERAL MILLS	Golden Grahams	-4	0.7%	0.7%	1.9%	0.2%	0.0%	86.2%	3.4%	6.9%	0.9%
GENERAL MILLS	Honey Nut Cheerios	-1	1.1%	2.2%	2.3%	0.1%	0.0%	75.5%	7.5%	11.3%	0.7%
GENERAL MILLS	Honey Nut Clusters	-2	0.9%	1.5%	2.0%	0.2%	0.0%	82.2%	5.6%	7.5%	0.6%
GENERAL MILLS	Kaboom	-4	0.7%	1.4%	1.6%	0.0%	0.0%	88.9%	3.7%	3.7%	0.7%
GENERAL MILLS	Kix	0	0.5%	0.9%	2.1%	0.0%	0.0%	78.6%	10.7%	7.1%	0.8%
GENERAL MILLS	Lucky Charms	-4	0.8%	1.6%	1.7%	0.1%	0.0%	87.5%	4.2%	8.3%	0.8%
GENERAL MILLS	Milk 'n Cereal Bars - Cinnamon Toast Crunch	-3			Contains Artificial Sweetener						
GENERAL MILLS	Multi Grain Cheerios	0	0.8%	1.5%	1.5%	0.1%	0.0%	76.9%	11.5%	7.7%	0.8%
GENERAL MILLS	Oatmeal Crisp - Crunchy Almond	-1	1.8%	3.7%	3.2%	0.2%	0.0%	73.7%	7.0%	10.5%	0.2%
GENERAL MILLS	Oatmeal Crisp - Hearty Raisin	-2	0.9%	1.6%	1.7%	0.1%	0.0%	80.3%	6.8%	8.5%	0.2%
GENERAL MILLS	Para Su Familia Raisin Bran	+1	0.4%	0.4%	1.2%	0.1%	0.0%	76.1%	13.0%	8.7%	0.7%
GENERAL MILLS	Raisin Nut Bran	-3	1.5%	1.5%	3.1%	0.1%	0.0%	74.7%	10.1%	8.1%	0.5%
GENERAL MILLS	Reese's Puffs	-3	2.4%	4.8%	5.3%	0.2%	0.0%	76.4%	3.6%	7.3%	0.7%
GENERAL MILLS	Team Cheerios	-2	0.8%	1.5%	1.5%	0.1%	0.0%	80.8%	7.7%	7.7%	0.7%
GENERAL MILLS	Total	0	0.4%	0.4%	1.1%	0.1%	0.0%	78.4%	11.8%	7.8%	0.8%
GENERAL MILLS	Total Raisin Bran	0	0.4%	0.4%	1.2%	0.1%	0.0%	80.4%	10.9%	6.5%	0.5%
GENERAL MILLS	Total - Vanilla Yogurt	-2	2.4%	0.8%	1.7%	0.1%	0.0%	78.8%	8.1%	6.1%	0.6%
GENERAL MILLS	Total with Strawberries	-1	0.4%	0.4%	1.2%	0.1%	0.0%	82.6%	8.7%	6.5%	0.6%
GENERAL MILLS	Trix	-4	0.5%	1.0%	2.0%	0.0%	0.0%	89.3%	3.6%	3.6%	0.7%
GENERAL MILLS	Wheaties	+1	0.4%	0.6%	0.9%	0.1%	0.0%	74.5%	11.8%	11.8%	0.8%
GENERAL MILLS	Yogurt Burst Cheerios - Strawberry	-2	4.2%	1.6%	1.3%	0.1%	0.0%	78.6%	7.1%	7.1%	0.6%
HEALTH VALLEY	Banana Gone Nuts !	+1	0.1%	0.7%	0.3%	0.1%	0.0%	78.5%	11.6%	8.7%	0.1%

CEREALS		Score	SFA	MUFA	LA	ALA	TFA	NFC	Fiber	Protein	Na
HEALTH VALLEY	Blueberry Bliss	0	0.8%	2.5%	2.4%	0.4%	0.0%	75.5%	8.2%	10.2%	0.2%
HEALTH VALLEY	Empower	+2	0.9%	2.5%	1.8%	0.7%	0.0%	70.6%	11.8%	11.8%	0.3%
HEALTH VALLEY	Heart Wise	+2	0.9%	2.0%	2.2%	0.8%	0.0%	62.7%	9.8%	21.6%	0.3%
HEALTH VALLEY	Granola Date Almond	+1	0.4%	0.8%	0.8%	0.0%	0.0%	75.5%	12.2%	10.2%	0.2%
HEALTH VALLEY	Organic Fiber 7 Multigrain	+3	0.5%	0.5%	1.3%	0.1%	0.0%	68.2%	15.9%	13.6%	0.2%
HEALTH VALLEY	Organic Golden Flax	+4	0.9%	1.3%	2.0%	2.3%	0.0%	68.1%	12.8%	12.8%	0.2%
HEALTH VALLEY	Organic Healthy Fiber Multigrain	+3	0.3%	0.3%	0.8%	0.1%	0.0%	72.0%	15.2%	11.4%	0.1%
HEALTH VALLEY	Organic Oat Bran O's	+1	0.3%	0.6%	0.6%	0.0%	0.0%	75.8%	11.4%	11.4%	0.4%
HEALTH VALLEY	Slender	+1	0.6%	0.6%	1.7%	0.2%	0.0%	68.0%	8.2%	20.6%	0.3%
HEARTLAND GRANOLA	Lowfat Raisin	-1	0.9%	3.1%	2.0%	0.3%	0.0%	77.1%	6.3%	10.4%	0.2%
KASHI	Go Lean	+9	0.3%	0.6%	1.4%	0.0%	0.0%	45.5%	22.7%	29.5%	0.2%
KASHI	Go Lean Crunch	+4	1.3%	2.4%	2.5%	0.1%	0.0%	58.3%	16.7%	18.8%	0.2%
KASHI	Heart to Heart - Honey Toasted Oat	+3	1.0%	1.9%	2.0%	0.1%	0.0%	65.6%	16.4%	13.1%	0.3%
KASHI	Heart to Heart - Oat Flakes & Blueberry Clusters	-1	1.0%	1.9%	2.0%	0.1%	0.0%	75.2%	7.9%	11.9%	0.3%
KASHI	Organic Promise - Autumn Wheat	+1	0.4%	0.4%	1.1%	0.1%	0.0%	78.0%	12.0%	10.0%	0.0%
KASHI	Organic Promise - Strawberry Fields	-4	0.2%	0.5%	0.5%	0.0%	0.0%	83.3%	3.1%	6.2%	0.6%
KASHI	Good Friends	+7	0.7%	1.2%	1.9%	0.2%	0.0%	62.0%	24.0%	10.0%	0.3%
KASHI	7 Whole Grain Flakes	+1	0.4%	0.4%	1.1%	0.1%	0.0%	72.9%	12.5%	12.5%	0.3%
KASHI	7 Whole Grain Nuggets	+1	0.5%	0.5%	1.5%	0.1%	0.0%	72.1%	12.6%	12.6%	0.5%
KASHI	Mighty Bites - Cinnamon	+1	0.8%	2.4%	1.7%	0.2%	0.0%	67.8%	10.2%	16.9%	0.5%
KASHI	Mighty Bites - Honey Crunch	+1	0.8%	2.4%	1.7%	0.2%	0.0%	67.8%	10.2%	16.9%	0.5%
KASHI	Vive - Probiotic Digestive Wellness	+6	2.4%	0.8%	1.7%	0.1%	0.0%	62.6%	24.2%	8.1%	0.2%
KELLOGG'S	All-Bran Extra Fiber	-3	Contains Artificial Sweetener								
KELLOGG'S	All-Bran Original	+10	0.7%	0.7%	2.0%	0.2%	0.0%	46.4%	35.7%	14.3%	0.3%
KELLOGG'S	Apple Jacks	-4	0.2%	0.4%	1.0%	0.0%	0.0%	92.1%	3.2%	3.2%	0.5%
KELLOGG'S	Berry Krispies	-5	0.3%	0.5%	0.5%	0.0%	0.0%	91.8%	0.0%	6.8%	0.8%
KELLOGG'S	Cocoa Krispies	-9	0.4%	0.8%	0.8%	0.0%	1.4%	89.7%	3.4%	3.4%	0.7%

CEREALS		Score	SFA	MUFA	LA	ALA	TFA	NFC	Fiber	Protein	Na
KELLOGG'S	Complete All Bran - Oat Bran	+2	0.7%	1.4%	1.5%	0.1%	0.0%	70.4%	14.8%	11.1%	0.8%
KELLOGG'S	Corn Pops	-7	0.3%	0.0%	0.3%	0.0%	0.7%	93.5%	1.7%	3.4%	0.4%
KELLOGG'S	Cracklin' Oat Bran	+1	7.4%	6.6%	2.5%	0.1%	0.0%	69.0%	14.3%	9.5%	0.4%
KELLOGG'S	Crispix	-5	0.2%	0.4%	0.9%	0.0%	0.0%	89.4%	1.8%	7.3%	0.8%
KELLOGG'S	Eggo Cereal - Maple Syrup	-7	0.9%	0.8%	1.7%	0.2%	1.3%	82.0%	6.6%	6.6%	0.5%
KELLOGG'S	Froot Loops	-9	1.1%	0.3%	0.6%	0.0%	1.3%	90.0%	3.3%	3.3%	0.5%
KELLOGG'S	Fruit Harvest - Strawberry Blueberry	-4	0.3%	0.3%	0.8%	0.1%	0.0%	87.6%	3.6%	7.3%	0.5%
KELLOGG'S	Honey Smacks	-6	0.8%	0.0%	0.4%	0.0%	0.8%	86.8%	3.8%	7.5%	0.2%
KELLOGG'S	Just Right	-2	0.8%	0.8%	2.2%	0.2%	0.0%	81.6%	6.1%	8.2%	0.5%
KELLOGG'S	Kellogg's Corn Flakes	-4	0.2%	0.4%	0.9%	0.0%	0.0%	87.1%	3.8%	7.6%	0.8%
KELLOGG'S	Kellogg's Frosted Flakes	-4	0.2%	0.3%	0.8%	0.0%	0.0%	91.8%	3.4%	3.4%	0.5%
KELLOGG'S	Kellogg's Frosted Flakes - 1/3 less sugar	-5	0.2%	0.3%	0.8%	0.0%	0.0%	93.5%	1.7%	3.4%	0.6%
KELLOGG'S	Kellogg's Raisin Bran	+1	0.6%	0.6%	1.6%	0.2%	0.0%	73.8%	13.6%	9.7%	0.7%
KELLOGG'S	Low Fat Granola with Raisins	-3	1.8%	2.1%	1.4%	0.1%	0.0%	82.1%	5.4%	7.1%	0.3%
KELLOGG'S	Mini Swirlz - Cinnamon Bun	-8	0.8%	1.4%	3.0%	0.3%	1.4%	82.8%	3.4%	6.9%	0.4%
KELLOGG'S	Mini-Wheats Frosted - Bite Size	+1	0.4%	0.4%	1.0%	0.1%	0.0%	76.4%	10.9%	10.9%	0.0%
KELLOGG'S	Mini-Wheats Frosted - Original	0	0.4%	0.4%	1.2%	0.1%	0.0%	76.6%	10.6%	10.6%	0.0%
KELLOGG'S	Mini-Wheats Frosted - Strawberry Delight	-3	Contains Artificial Sweetener								
KELLOGG'S	Mueslix with Raisins, Dates & Almonds	-4	1.3%	1.1%	2.8%	0.3%	0.8%	75.0%	8.3%	10.4%	0.4%
KELLOGG'S	Organic Mini-Wheats Frosted - Bite Size	0	0.4%	0.4%	1.1%	0.1%	0.0%	79.6%	10.2%	8.2%	0.0%
KELLOGG'S	Organic Raisin Bran	+2	0.4%	0.4%	1.1%	0.1%	0.0%	73.1%	15.4%	9.6%	0.7%
KELLOGG'S	Product 19	-4	0.2%	0.4%	0.9%	0.0%	0.0%	87.6%	3.6%	7.3%	0.8%
KELLOGG'S	Raisin Bran Crunch	-4	0.2%	0.5%	0.5%	0.0%	0.8%	83.7%	8.2%	6.1%	0.4%
KELLOGG'S	Rice Krispies	-6	0.3%	0.5%	0.5%	0.0%	0.0%	92.4%	0.0%	6.4%	1.0%
KELLOGG'S	Smart Start - Antioxidants	-5	0.0%	0.1%	0.1%	0.0%	0.9%	86.0%	6.5%	6.5%	0.6%
KELLOGG'S	Smart Start- Healthy Heart	-3	0.9%	1.6%	2.1%	0.2%	0.7%	73.2%	8.9%	12.5%	0.3%
KELLOGG'S	Special K	-2	0.3%	0.5%	0.5%	0.0%	0.0%	73.1%	1.7%	23.8%	0.8%

CEREALS		Score	SFA	MUFA	LA	ALA	TFA	NFC	Fiber	Protein	Na
KELLOGG'S	Special K - Fruit & Yogurt	-6	0.4%	0.7%	1.4%	0.2%	0.7%	86.7%	3.3%	6.7%	1.2%
KELLOGG'S	Special K - Low Carb Lifestyle Protein Plus	-3	Contains Artificial Sweetener								
KELLOGG'S	Special K - Vanilla Almond	-4	1.1%	2.1%	2.0%	0.1%	0.0%	84.2%	3.5%	7.0%	0.6%
KELLOGG'S	Toasted Honey Crunch	-6	0.4%	0.8%	0.8%	0.0%	0.7%	88.1%	3.7%	5.5%	0.6%
MALT-O-MEAL	Balance	-9	0.4%	0.8%	2.6%	0.0%	1.4%	84.2%	3.5%	7.0%	0.7%
MALT-O-MEAL	Cinnamon Toasters	-9	1.8%	2.6%	5.8%	0.7%	1.4%	80.7%	3.5%	3.5%	0.5%
MALT-O-MEAL	Frosted Flakes	-4	0.2%	0.3%	0.8%	0.0%	0.0%	88.8%	3.3%	6.6%	0.6%
MALT-O-MEAL	Frosted Mini Spooners	-3	Contains Artificial Sweetener								
MALT-O-MEAL	Golden Puffs	-8	0.4%	0.0%	0.4%	0.0%	0.8%	90.9%	0.0%	7.6%	0.3%
MALT-O-MEAL	Honey Nut Toasty O's	-2	1.1%	2.1%	2.2%	0.1%	0.0%	80.0%	7.3%	7.3%	0.8%
MALT-O-MEAL	Marshmellow Mateys	-4	0.7%	1.4%	1.4%	0.1%	0.0%	85.7%	3.6%	7.1%	0.7%
MALT-O-MEAL	Tootie Fruities	-8	0.4%	0.5%	1.1%	0.0%	1.3%	87.1%	3.2%	6.5%	0.5%
MALT-O-MEAL	Honey & Oat Blenders	-9	0.7%	1.3%	1.8%	0.1%	1.4%	84.2%	3.5%	7.0%	0.5%
MOTHER'S NATURAL FOOD	Peanut Butter Bumpers	-4	1.1%	2.9%	3.9%	0.1%	0.0%	79.4%	3.2%	9.5%	0.9%
MOTHER'S NATURAL FOOD	Cocoa Bumpers	-4	0.2%	0.4%	1.0%	0.0%	0.0%	88.9%	3.2%	6.3%	0.6%
MOTHER'S NATURAL FOOD	Cinnamon Oat Crunch	-1	1.1%	2.1%	2.2%	0.1%	0.0%	78.2%	9.1%	10.9%	0.5%
MOTHER'S NATURAL FOOD	Toasted Oat Bran	0	1.0%	1.9%	2.0%	0.1%	0.0%	71.2%	10.2%	13.6%	0.7%
NATURE'S PATH	Pumpkin FlaxPlus Granola	+2	2.6%	4.6%	7.8%	2.3%	0.0%	62.1%	10.3%	10.3%	0.1%
NATURE'S PATH	Raspberry Heritage Granola	+2	1.2%	5.8%	3.1%	0.7%	0.0%	67.9%	10.7%	10.7%	0.2%
NATURE'S PATH	Soy Plus Granola	-1	1.8%	3.1%	5.3%	0.6%	0.0%	71.4%	7.1%	10.7%	0.1%
NATURE'S PATH	Spelt Flakes	+1	0.4%	0.4%	1.2%	0.1%	0.0%	72.3%	12.8%	12.8%	0.6%
NATURE'S PATH	Synergy 8 Whole Grain	+4	0.7%	0.7%	2.0%	0.2%	0.0%	67.9%	17.9%	10.7%	0.0%
NATURE'S PATH	Blueberry Muesli	+2	0.9%	3.4%	2.1%	0.4%	0.0%	68.0%	13.6%	11.7%	0.3%
NATURE'S PATH	EnviroKidz - Amazon Frosted Flakes	-2	0.2%	0.4%	0.8%	0.0%	0.0%	84.5%	7.0%	7.0%	0.4%
NATURE'S PATH	EnviroKidz - Cheetah Chomps	-2	1.4%	1.4%	3.8%	0.3%	0.0%	75.9%	6.9%	10.3%	0.2%
NATURE'S PATH	EnviroKidz - Panda Puffs	-2	1.2%	2.1%	4.7%	0.4%	0.0%	74.6%	6.8%	10.2%	0.5%
NATURE'S PATH	FlaxPlus Flakes O-3	+8	1.0%	1.1%	2.7%	0.7%	0.0%	54.5%	25.5%	14.5%	0.7%

CEREALS		Score	SFA	MUFA	LA	ALA	TFA	NFC	Fiber	Protein	Na
NATURE'S PATH	Blueberry Muesli	+2	0.9%	3.4%	2.1%	0.4%	0.0%	68.0%	13.6%	11.7%	0.3%
NATURE'S PATH	EnviroKidz - Amazon Frosted Flakes	-2	0.2%	0.4%	0.8%	0.0%	0.0%	84.5%	7.0%	7.0%	0.4%
NATURE'S PATH	EnviroKidz - Cheetah Chomps	-2	1.4%	1.4%	3.8%	0.3%	0.0%	75.9%	6.9%	10.3%	0.2%
NATURE'S PATH	EnviroKidz - Panda Puffs	-2	1.2%	2.1%	4.7%	0.4%	0.0%	74.6%	6.8%	10.2%	0.5%
NATURE'S PATH	FlaxPlus Flakes O-3	+8	1.0%	1.1%	2.7%	0.7%	0.0%	54.5%	25.5%	14.5%	0.7%
NATURE'S PATH	FlaxPlus Raisin Bran	+6	0.9%	1.0%	2.5%	0.6%	0.0%	60.6%	22.2%	12.1%	0.6%
NATURE'S PATH	Ginger Zing Granola	-1	2.7%	4.7%	8.8%	1.1%	0.0%	65.5%	6.9%	10.3%	0.1%
NATURE'S PATH	HempPlus Granola	+2	2.8%	4.8%	8.0%	2.4%	0.0%	60.7%	10.7%	10.7%	0.1%
NATURE'S PATH	Heritage Heirloom - Whole Grains	+6	0.7%	0.7%	2.0%	0.2%	0.0%	60.7%	21.4%	14.3%	0.5%
NATURE'S PATH	Heritage O's	+1	0.7%	1.3%	1.4%	0.1%	0.0%	72.4%	10.3%	13.8%	0.4%
NATURE'S PATH	Kamut Puffs	+3	0.4%	0.7%	1.8%	0.0%	0.0%	67.2%	14.9%	14.9%	0.0%
NATURE'S PATH	Mesa Sunrise	0	0.7%	1.3%	2.8%	0.5%	0.0%	73.7%	10.5%	10.5%	0.5%
NATURE'S PATH	Multigrain Oatbran with Raisins	+2	0.6%	1.2%	1.2%	0.1%	0.0%	72.2%	14.4%	10.3%	0.3%
NATURE'S PATH	Oaty Bites	-2	0.7%	1.4%	1.4%	0.1%	0.0%	82.1%	7.1%	7.1%	0.5%
NATURE'S PATH	Optimum Power Breakfast	+5	1.2%	1.2%	3.2%	0.3%	0.0%	58.8%	19.6%	15.7%	0.4%
NATURE'S PATH	Optimum ReBound	+3	1.8%	2.7%	5.6%	1.6%	0.0%	56.9%	11.8%	19.6%	0.3%
NATURE'S PATH	Optimum Slim	+7	1.2%	1.2%	3.3%	0.3%	0.0%	54.0%	22.0%	18.0%	0.5%
PEACE	Apple Cinnamon Low Fat Crisp	-3	0.4%	0.7%	2.9%	0.0%	0.0%	84.0%	4.0%	8.0%	0.5%
PEACE	Banana Nut Rainforest Crisp	-1	1.5%	8.1%	4.0%	1.0%	0.0%	70.8%	4.2%	10.4%	0.4%
PEACE	Essential 10 - Organic	+7	1.1%	1.4%	3.1%	0.9%	0.0%	54.3%	21.7%	17.4%	0.8%
PEACE	Heart Goodness - Organic	+4	1.1%	2.0%	2.1%	0.1%	0.0%	66.7%	17.5%	10.5%	0.3%
PEACE	Hearty Raisin Bran - Organic	+3	0.8%	0.9%	2.2%	0.2%	0.0%	71.4%	16.3%	8.2%	0.5%
PEACE	Mango Passion Low Fat Crisp	-5	0.3%	0.6%	2.1%	0.0%	0.0%	87.1%	2.0%	7.9%	0.8%
PEACE	Maple Raisin Low Fat Crisp	-4	0.7%	1.3%	2.1%	0.1%	0.0%	86.6%	4.1%	6.2%	0.6%
POST	Alpha-Bits	-5	0.7%	1.4%	1.4%	0.1%	0.0%	89.3%	0.0%	7.1%	0.7%
POST	Cocoa Pebbles	-5	2.8%	0.7%	0.7%	0.1%	1.1%	80.7%	10.5%	3.5%	0.7%
POST	Fruit & Bran	-2	0.8%	1.0%	3.3%	0.1%	0.8%	73.5%	12.2%	8.2%	0.0%

CEREALS		Score	SFA	MUFA	LA	ALA	TFA	NFC	Fiber	Protein	Na
POST	Honey Bunches of Oats with Almonds	-7	0.7%	1.5%	4.9%	0.0%	1.4%	78.0%	6.8%	6.8%	0.5%
POST	Honey Bunches of Oats with Real Strawberries	-9	0.6%	1.1%	3.6%	0.0%	1.3%	83.3%	3.3%	6.7%	0.5%
POST	Honeycomb	-1	0.5%	0.8%	1.9%	0.0%	0.0%	80.6%	9.7%	6.5%	0.6%
POST	Post Bran Flakes	+4	0.4%	0.4%	1.0%	0.1%	0.0%	69.1%	18.2%	10.9%	0.8%
POST	Post 100% Bran	+10	0.7%	0.7%	2.0%	0.2%	0.0%	48.1%	33.3%	14.8%	0.5%
POST	Post Selects - Cranberry Almond Crunch	-5	0.8%	1.0%	3.1%	0.2%	0.8%	80.4%	5.9%	7.8%	0.4%
POST	Post Selects - Great Grains - Crunchy Pecans	-1	1.5%	4.1%	6.5%	0.1%	0.0%	69.4%	8.2%	10.2%	0.3%
POST	Post Selects -Great Grains - Raisins, Dates, Pecan	-2	1.2%	1.9%	6.1%	0.1%	0.0%	74.2%	8.2%	8.2%	0.3%
POST	Post Selects - Blueberry Morning	-3	0.7%	1.2%	3.5%	0.0%	0.0%	81.8%	5.5%	7.3%	0.5%
POST	Post Shredded Wheat	+2	0.5%	0.5%	1.3%	0.1%	0.0%	72.1%	14.0%	11.6%	0.0%
POST	Post Shredded Wheat - Frosted	0	0.4%	0.4%	1.1%	0.1%	0.0%	79.2%	10.4%	8.3%	0.0%
POST	Post Shredded Wheat - Honey Nut	-4	1.0%	0.8%	0.4%	0.0%	0.8%	78.8%	8.1%	10.1%	0.1%
POST	Post Shredded Wheat & Bran - Spoon Size	+2	0.4%	0.4%	1.2%	0.1%	0.0%	72.3%	12.8%	12.8%	0.0%
POST	Post Toasties Corn Flakes	-4	0.2%	0.4%	0.9%	0.0%	0.0%	87.1%	3.8%	7.6%	1.0%
POST	Post Raisin Bran	+2	0.4%	0.4%	1.1%	0.1%	0.0%	74.5%	15.7%	7.8%	0.6%
QUAKER	Cap'n Crunch - Original	-5	4.8%	0.6%	0.6%	0.0%	0.0%	86.3%	3.9%	3.9%	0.8%
QUAKER	Cap'n Crunch - Crunchberries	-10	3.5%	0.4%	0.6%	0.0%	1.6%	85.7%	4.1%	4.1%	0.7%
QUAKER	Cap'n Crunch - Peanut Butter Crunch	-10	5.5%	2.2%	0.6%	0.0%	1.6%	78.4%	3.9%	7.8%	0.8%
QUAKER	Life	-2	1.0%	1.9%	2.0%	0.1%	0.0%	78.0%	6.8%	10.2%	0.5%
QUAKER	Life - Cinnamon	-2	1.0%	1.9%	2.0%	0.1%	0.0%	78.0%	6.8%	10.2%	0.5%
QUAKER	Life - Honey Graham	-2	1.0%	1.9%	2.0%	0.1%	0.0%	78.0%	6.8%	10.2%	0.5%
QUAKER	Essentials Oat Bran	+1	1.1%	1.19%	2.5%	0.2%	0.0%	69.8%	11.3%	13.2%	0.4%
QUAKER	Quaker's 100% Natural Granola, Oats & Honey	-3	9.3%	1.7%	1.2%	0.1%	0.0%	71.4%	6.1%	10.2%	0.1%
U.S. MILLS	Erewhon Crispy Brown Rice - Original	-4	0.3%	0.6%	0.5%	0.0%	0.0%	87.6%	3.6%	7.3%	0.7%
U.S. MILLS	Erewhon Crispy Brown Rice - No Salt Added	-3	0.3%	0.6%	0.5%	0.0%	0.0%	87.6%	3.6%	7.3%	0.0%
U.S. MILLS	Erewhon Crispy Brown Rice w/ Mixed Berries	-4	0.3%	0.7%	0.6%	0.0%	0.0%	88.1%	3.4%	6.8%	0.3%
U.S. MILLS	Erewhon Rice Twice	-5	0.3%	0.6%	0.5%	0.0%	0.0%	91.5%	0.0%	7.0%	0.2%

CEREALS		Score	SFA	MUFA	LA	ALA	TFA	NFC	Fiber	Protein	Na
U.S. MILLS	Erewhon Raisin Bran	+2	0.4%	0.4%	1.2%	0.1%	0.0%	73.9%	13.0%	10.9%	0.2%
U.S. MILLS	Erewhon Kamut Flakes	+2	0.3%	0.3%	0.7%	0.1%	0.0%	69.1%	13.2%	16.4%	0.3%
U.S. MILLS	New Morning - Oatios - Original	+1	1.4%	2.6%	2.8%	0.1%	0.0%	65.5%	10.3%	17.2%	0.4%
U.S. MILLS	New Morning - Oatios - Honey Almond	0	1.0%	1.8%	1.9%	0.1%	0.0%	71.4%	9.5%	14.3%	0.2%
U.S. MILLS	New Morning - Fruit-e-O's	-2	0.7%	1.3%	3.1%	0.1%	0.0%	78.0%	6.8%	10.2%	0.3%
U.S. MILLS	New Morning - Cocoa Crispy Rice	-4	0.4%	0.7%	0.7%	0.0%	0.0%	87.7%	3.5%	7.0%	0.4%
U.S. MILLS	Skinner's Raisin Bran	+2	0.4%	0.4%	1.1%	0.1%	0.0%	70.8%	14.6%	12.5%	0.2%
U.S. MILLS	Uncle Sam - Original	+6	1.9%	2.0%	4.9%	1.3%	0.0%	56.0%	20.0%	14.0%	0.3%
U.S. MILLS	Uncle Sam with Mixed Berries	+6	1.6%	1.8%	4.3%	1.1%	0.0%	56.3%	19.4%	15.5%	0.2%
WEIGHT WATCHER'S	Banana Almond Medley	+7	0.7%	1.4%	4.7%	0.0%	0.0%	47.7%	22.7%	22.7%	0.3%
WEIGHT WATCHER'S	Cinnamon Cluster Crunch	+5	0.5%	0.9%	1.0%	0.0%	0.0%	61.0%	17.1%	19.5%	0.4%
WEIGHT WATCHER'S	Flakes 'n Fiber with Oats	-3	Contains Artificial Sweetener								
WEIGHT WATCHER'S	Honey Almond Crisp w/ Real Blueberries	+1	1.0%	2.5%	2.9%	0.4%	0.0%	74.0%	11.0%	8.2%	0.2%
ZOE'S	Cinnamon	+6	0.5%	1.0%	0.9%	2.6%	0.0%	65.6%	16.4%	13.1%	0.5%
ZOE'S	Natural	+6	0.9%	1.4%	1.7%	2.7%	0.0%	60.0%	16.7%	16.7%	0.6%
ZOE'S	Flax & Soy Granola - Cranberries Currants	+6	1.4%	3.6%	3.4%	3.0%	0.0%	56.8%	15.9%	15.9%	0.2%
ZOE'S	Flax & Soy Granola - Honey Almond	+6	1.4%	3.6%	3.3%	2.9%	0.0%	55.6%	15.6%	17.8%	0.2%

Breads

The NQI rates 89 breads based on *overall* nutritional quality. Scores range from
-10 (toxic) to +10 (exceptional) reflecting the dramatic variation in molecular
contents and predicted metabolic and health consequences of different breads.

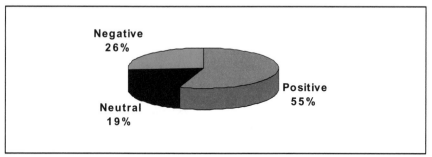

**Figure 2: Breads. Fifty-five percent of breads evaluated by the NQI receive favorable
ratings. Fourteen breads (16%) score +5 or higher, reflecting superior nutritional quality.**

Like cereals, most bread health claims focus attention on their low quantities of
total fat, saturated fat, and cholesterol. Some even receive "heart healthy"
approval by meeting these one-dimensional criteria. However, as high
carbohydrate grain-based foods, *all* breads are low in total fat, saturated fat, and
cholesterol, making these claims nearly meaningless! *Despite health claims to
the contrary, many available breads are low quality foods.* Habitual
consumption of low quality breads can significantly increase your risk of
developing the Big 7 epidemic U.S. diseases.

The NQI easily distinguishes between high and low quality breads.
Because breads are high carbohydrate foods, NQI scores reflect carbohydrate
quality. Breads receiving low scores, including some labeled as "heart healthy"
and "whole grain," contain little more than refined grains (sugar equivalents).
The highest rated breads contain significant amounts of fiber and low non-fiber
carbohydrate to fiber ratios. Some also contain moderate amounts of protein,
omega-3 fats, and other beneficial components. As part of a healthy diet, regular

consumption of these high quality breads will optimize your metabolism and reduce your risk of developing the Big 7 epidemic U.S. diseases.

NQI SUPERIOR SELECTIONS

TOP 14 BEST BREADS

+10	French Meadow	Men's Bread
+10	Nature's Own	Double Fiber Wheat
+9	French Meadow	Women's Bread
+7	Food For Life	Bran for Life – Organic 100% Whole Grain
+6	Masada	Fiber Rich
+6	Nature's Own	Light Wheat
+6	Sara Lee	Heart Healthy Plus -100% Multi-Grain
+6	Sara Lee	Heart Healthy Plus -100% Whole Wheat
+5	Earthgrains	100% Multi-Grain
+5	Earthgrains	100% Whole Wheat with Fiber
+5	Nature's Path	Fruit and Nut Manna
+5	Nature's Path	Sun Seed Manna
+5	Weight Watchers	Multigrain
+5	Weight Watchers	Whole Wheat

Brand	Product										
ALVARADO STREET	Sprouted Whole Wheat	+2	0.4%	0.4%	1.2%	0.1%	0.0%	68.1%	12.8%	17.0%	0.7%
ALVARADO STREET	Sprouted California Style	+2	0.5%	0.5%	1.4%	0.1%	0.0%	63.4%	9.8%	24.4%	0.8%
ALVARADO STREET	Sprouted Soy Crunch	+2	0.5%	0.5%	1.4%	0.1%	0.0%	63.4%	9.8%	24.4%	0.8%
ALVARADO STREET	Ultimate Kids	+1	0.5%	0.5%	1.4%	0.1%	0.0%	68.3%	9.8%	19.5%	0.8%
ARNOLD	100% Whole Wheat - Whole Grain Classics	+2	0.8%	1.0%	2.3%	0.2%	0.0%	65.2%	13.0%	17.4%	0.8%
ARNOLD	12 Grain - Whole Grain Classics	0	1.4%	1.8%	4.3%	0.5%	0.0%	68.0%	8.0%	16.0%	0.7%
ARNOLD	Healthy Multi-Grain - Whole Grain Classics	-3	Contains Artificial Sweetener								
ARNOLD	7 Grain - 100% Whole Grain Classics	0	0.8%	0.8%	2.2%	0.2%	0.0%	72.0%	8.0%	16.0%	0.7%
ARNOLD	Oatnut - 100% Whole Grain Classics	0	1.4%	1.8%	4.3%	0.5%	0.0%	68.0%	8.0%	16.0%	0.8%
ARNOLD	Health Nut - 100% Whole Grain Classics	0	1.4%	1.8%	4.3%	0.5%	0.0%	68.0%	8.0%	16.0%	0.8%
ARNOLD	100% Whole Wheat - Stone Ground	+2	1.2%	1.4%	3.4%	0.4%	0.0%	62.5%	12.5%	18.8%	0.8%
ARNOLD	Country White - Country Classics	-3	1.1%	1.4%	3.3%	0.4%	0.0%	77.6%	4.1%	12.2%	0.9%
ARNOLD	Honey Wheat - Dutch Country	0	0.8%	1.0%	2.3%	0.2%	0.0%	73.9%	8.7%	13.0%	0.7%
ARNOLD	100% Whole Wheat - Dutch Country	+2	0.8%	1.0%	2.3%	0.2%	0.0%	65.2%	13.0%	17.4%	0.8%
BROWNBERRY	Natural Wheat	0	1.2%	1.6%	3.6%	0.4%	0.0%	71.1%	8.9%	13.3%	1.1%
BROWNBERRY	Natural Healthnut	0	1.7%	2.5%	5.7%	0.7%	0.0%	68.1%	8.5%	12.8%	0.9%
COBBLESTONE MILL	Cinnamon Swirl	-10	1.8%	1.5%	1.9%	0.1%	2.0%	80.5%	2.4%	9.8%	0.5%
COBBLESTONE MILL	German Pumpernickel	-2	0.9%	1.1%	2.7%	0.3%	0.0%	75.0%	5.0%	15.0%	1.0%
COBBLESTONE MILL	New York Style Jewish Rye	-2	0.9%	1.2%	2.8%	0.3%	0.0%	73.7%	5.3%	15.8%	1.3%
COBBLESTONE MILL	San Francisco Sourdough	-3	0.4%	0.6%	1.4%	0.2%	0.0%	79.5%	2.6%	15.4%	0.9%
COLONIAL	Wheat	-1	0.9%	0.4%	1.6%	0.1%	0.0%	72.7%	6.1%	18.2%	0.8%
COLONIAL	Light Wheat	+4	0.3%	0.3%	0.9%	0.1%	0.0%	63.0%	15.7%	19.7%	1.0%
COLONIAL	Light White	+3	0.6%	0.3%	1.0%	0.1%	0.0%	66.7%	15.7%	15.7%	1.0%
EARTHGRAINS	100% Multi-Grain	+5	1.4%	1.1%	3.2%	0.2%	0.0%	54.9%	19.6%	19.6%	0.7%
EARTHGRAINS	100% Whole Wheat with Fiber	+5	1.3%	1.1%	3.1%	0.2%	0.0%	56.6%	18.9%	18.9%	0.7%
EARTHGRAINS	Oat & Nut	-2	3.2%	3.8%	2.3%	0.2%	0.0%	71.7%	3.8%	15.1%	0.8%
EARTHGRAINS	Wheat Berry	-2	0.5%	0.4%	1.1%	0.0%	0.0%	77.6%	4.1%	16.3%	0.9%

BREAD		Score	SFA	MUFA	LA	ALA	TFA	NFC	Fiber	Protein	Na
EARTHGRAINS	Whole Grain	0	1.4%	1.1%	3.2%	0.2%	0.0%	66.7%	7.8%	19.6%	0.6%
EARTHGRAINS	Whole Wheat	0	0.9%	0.8%	2.3%	0.2%	0.0%	70.8%	8.3%	16.7%	0.7%
FOOD FOR LIFE	7 Organic Sprouted 100% Whole Grain Flourless	+4	0.5%	0.5%	1.4%	0.2%	0.0%	61.5%	15.4%	20.5%	0.4%
FOOD FOR LIFE	Bran for Life - Organic 100% Whole Grain	+7	0.7%	0.8%	2.9%	0.1%	0.0%	54.5%	22.7%	18.2%	0.6%
FOOD FOR LIFE	Cinn Raisin-7 Organic Sprout 100% Whole Grain Flourless	0	0.4%	0.4%	1.2%	0.1%	0.0%	75.6%	8.9%	13.3%	0.3%
FOOD FOR LIFE	Ezekiel 4:9-Organic Sprout 100% Whole Grain Flourless	+4	0.5%	0.5%	1.4%	0.2%	0.0%	61.5%	15.4%	20.5%	0.4%
FOOD FOR LIFE	Ezekiel 4:19-Organic Sprout 100% Flourless-Low Sodium	+4	0.5%	0.5%	1.4%	0.2%	0.0%	61.5%	15.4%	20.5%	0.0%
FRENCH MEADOW	Cinnamon Raisin Spelt	+2	0.4%	0.4%	1.2%	0.1%	0.0%	72.3%	12.8%	12.8%	0.5%
FRENCH MEADOW	Flax & Sunflower Seed	+3	1.5%	1.7%	4.1%	1.1%	0.0%	62.5%	12.5%	16.7%	0.4%
FRENCH MEADOW	Men's Bread	+10	3.1%	3.3%	8.1%	2.1%	0.0%	27.8%	22.2%	33.3%	0.7%
FRENCH MEADOW	Spelt	+2	0.2%	0.2%	0.6%	0.1%	0.0%	65.9%	11.0%	22.0%	0.6%
FRENCH MEADOW	Women's Bread	+9	1.9%	2.1%	5.2%	1.4%	0.0%	36.8%	21.1%	31.6%	0.6%
MASADA	Fiber Rich	+6	0.9%	0.9%	2.4%	0.2%	0.0%	56.5%	21.7%	17.4%	0.7%
MASADA	Honey Whole Wheat	0	1.0%	1.0%	2.6%	0.2%	0.0%	71.4%	9.5%	14.3%	0.7%
MASADA	Multi-Grain	0	0.7%	0.8%	1.9%	0.5%	0.0%	73.1%	7.7%	15.4%	0.7%
NATURE'S OWN	100% Honey Wheat with Organic Flour - Specialty Bread	+1	0.7%	0.7%	2.1%	0.1%	0.0%	70.4%	11.1%	14.8%	0.7%
NATURE'S OWN	100% Whole Grain Wheat - Sugar Free	+3	1.1%	1.5%	3.6%	0.4%	0.0%	60.0%	13.3%	20.0%	0.7%
NATURE'S OWN	100% Whole Wheat	+4	1.3%	1.3%	3.7%	0.3%	0.0%	53.3%	13.3%	26.7%	0.8%
NATURE'S OWN	100% Whole Wheat - Specialty Bread	+1	1.0%	1.2%	3.0%	0.3%	0.0%	65.5%	10.9%	18.2%	0.9%
NATURE'S OWN	9 Grain - Specialty Bread	-1	1.2%	1.5%	3.6%	0.4%	0.0%	70.0%	6.7%	16.7%	0.8%
NATURE'S OWN	12 Grain - Specialty Bread	+2	0.7%	0.8%	2.1%	0.2%	0.0%	65.4%	11.5%	19.2%	0.9%
NATURE'S OWN	Butterbread	-2	2.1%	1.0%	0.6%	0.0%	0.0%	71.0%	6.5%	19.4%	0.9%
NATURE'S OWN	Double Fiber Wheat	+10	1.1%	1.5%	3.6%	0.4%	0.0%	33.3%	33.3%	26.7%	1.0%
NATURE'S OWN	Hearty Oatmeal - Specialty Bread	+2	1.1%	1.4%	3.3%	0.4%	0.0%	61.2%	12.2%	20.4%	0.7%
NATURE'S OWN	Honey Wheat	-1	1.1%	1.4%	3.5%	0.4%	0.0%	71.0%	6.5%	19.4%	0.8%
NATURE'S OWN	Light Wheat	+6	0.8%	0.8%	2.2%	0.2%	0.0%	56.0%	20.0%	20.0%	0.8%
NATURE'S OWN	Whitewheat	+4	1.2%	1.5%	3.6%	0.4%	0.0%	60.0%	16.7%	20.0%	0.8%

BREAD		Score									
NATURE'S PATH	Carrot Raisin Manna	+3	0.2%	0.2%	0.7%	0.0%	0.1%	67.9%	15.4%	15.4%	0.0%
NATURE'S PATH	Fruit & Nut Manna	+5	0.6%	0.6%	1.6%	0.0%	0.1%	61.8%	17.6%	17.6%	0.0%
NATURE'S PATH	MultiGrain Manna	+2	0.2%	0.2%	0.6%	0.0%	0.2%	67.9%	12.3%	18.5%	0.0%
NATURE'S PATH	Sun Seed Manna	+6	1.0%	1.1%	2.6%	0.0%	0.7%	59.5%	18.9%	16.2%	0.0%
PEPPERIDGE FARM	Farmhouse - 12 Grain	+1	1.3%	1.7%	4.0%	0.0%	0.4%	66.7%	11.1%	14.8%	0.7%
PEPPERIDGE FARM	Farmhouse - Sourdough	-3	1.0%	1.2%	3.0%	0.0%	0.3%	76.4%	3.6%	14.5%	0.8%
PEPPERIDGE FARM	Italian with Sesame Seeds	-3	0.3%	0.7%	1.3%	0.0%	0.1%	80.5%	2.4%	14.6%	0.9%
PEPPERIDGE FARM	Natural - Whole Grain - 9 Grain	+1	1.3%	1.8%	4.2%	0.0%	0.5%	65.4%	11.5%	15.4%	0.7%
PEPPERIDGE FARM	Natural - Whole Grain - German Dark Wheat	+1	1.0%	1.3%	3.2%	0.0%	0.4%	66.7%	11.8%	15.7%	0.8%
PEPPERIDGE FARM	Natural - Whole Grain - Multi-Grain	+1	1.3%	1.8%	4.2%	0.0%	0.5%	65.4%	11.5%	15.4%	0.8%
PEPPERIDGE FARM	Natural - Whole Wheat - Whole Grain	+1	1.3%	1.8%	4.2%	0.0%	0.5%	65.4%	11.5%	15.4%	0.7%
PEPPERIDGE FARM	Oatmeal	-1	1.1%	1.5%	3.6%	0.0%	0.4%	73.3%	6.7%	13.3%	0.9%
PEPPERIDGE FARM	White Original	-2	1.6%	1.8%	2.6%	0.0%	0.3%	75.0%	6.3%	12.5%	0.6%
PEPPERIDGE FARM	Whole Grain - 100% Whole Wheat	+1	1.0%	1.3%	3.2%	0.0%	0.4%	66.7%	11.8%	15.7%	0.6%
PEPPERIDGE FARM	Whole Grain - 15 Grain - Hearty Texture	+1	1.3%	1.8%	4.2%	0.0%	0.5%	65.4%	11.5%	15.4%	0.7%
PEPPERIDGE FARM	Whole Grain - Honey Oat - Soft Texture	+1	0.9%	1.0%	2.5%	0.0%	0.3%	39.5%	7.0%	9.3%	0.4%
PEPPERIDGE FARM	Whole Grain - Honey Oat Wheat	+1	1.3%	1.8%	4.2%	0.0%	0.5%	65.4%	11.5%	15.4%	0.7%
ROMAN MEAL	Natural Whole Grain	-1	1.0%	1.3%	3.2%	0.0%	0.4%	70.6%	5.9%	17.6%	0.8%
RUDI'S ORGANIC BAKERY	Colorado Cracked Wheat	-1	0.9%	1.9%	2.7%	0.0%	0.2%	71.7%	7.5%	15.1%	0.6%
RUDI'S ORGANIC BAKERY	Country Morning White	-1	0.7%	1.0%	2.0%	0.0%	0.1%	74.1%	7.4%	14.8%	0.7%
RUDI'S ORGANIC BAKERY	Honey Sweet Whole Wheat	+2	0.7%	1.1%	2.0%	0.0%	0.2%	64.0%	12.0%	20.0%	0.7%
RUDI'S ORGANIC BAKERY	Jewish Light Rye	-2	0.7%	1.1%	2.0%	0.0%	0.2%	76.0%	4.0%	16.0%	0.9%
RUDI'S ORGANIC BAKERY	Spelt Ancient Grain	0	1.4%	4.1%	4.5%	0.0%	1.1%	66.7%	7.4%	14.8%	0.6%
RUDI'S ORGANIC BAKERY	Wheat & Oat	+4	0.7%	1.4%	2.3%	0.0%	0.1%	63.6%	18.2%	13.6%	0.9%
SARA LEE	Delightful Wheat	-3	Contains Artificial Sweetener								
SARA LEE	Heart Healthy - 100% Whole Wheat - Classic	+1	1.4%	1.1%	3.2%	0.0%	0.2%	64.7%	11.8%	17.6%	0.8%
SARA LEE	Heart Healthy - 100% Whole Wheat - Homestyle	0	1.3%	1.1%	3.1%	0.0%	0.2%	67.9%	7.5%	18.9%	0.7%

BREAD		Score	SFA	MUFA	LA	ALA	TFA	NFC	Fiber	Protein	Na
SARA LEE	Heart Healthy - Multi-Grain	0	0.8%	0.9%	2.0%	0.5%	0.0%	70.8%	8.3%	16.7%	0.8%
SARA LEE	Heart Healthy Plus - 100% Multi-Grain	+6	1.2%	1.0%	2.8%	0.2%	0.0%	52.6%	21.1%	21.1%	0.7%
SARA LEE	Heart Healthy Plus - 100% Whole Wheat	+6	1.2%	1.0%	2.8%	0.2%	0.0%	52.6%	21.1%	21.1%	0.7%
SARA LEE	Iron Kids	-1	0.7%	0.7%	1.9%	0.1%	0.0%	75.9%	6.9%	13.8%	0.8%
SUNBEAM	Giant	-3	0.7%	0.8%	2.0%	0.2%	0.0%	76.4%	3.6%	14.5%	1.0%
SUNBEAM	Old Fashioned	-1	1.1%	1.4%	3.4%	0.4%	0.0%	75.0%	6.3%	12.5%	0.0%
SUNBEAM	Thin	-2	0.7%	0.8%	2.2%	0.2%	0.0%	74.5%	3.9%	15.7%	1.0%
WEIGHT WATCHERS	Multigrain	+5	0.8%	0.9%	2.3%	0.3%	0.0%	54.2%	16.7%	25.0%	0.8%
WEIGHT WATCHERS	Whole Wheat	+5	0.8%	0.9%	2.3%	0.2%	0.0%	55.3%	17.0%	21.3%	0.8%

Yogurts

The NQI rates 82 yogurts based on *overall* nutritional quality. On a scale of -10 (toxic) to +10 (exceptional), scores range from -8 to +8 reflecting the dramatic variation in molecular contents and predicted metabolic and health consequences of different yogurts.

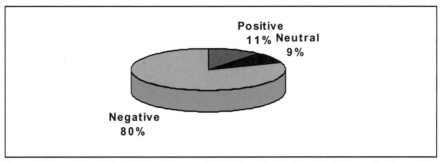

Figure 3: Yogurts. Only 9 of the 82 yogurts (11%) evaluated by the NQI receive favorable ratings. Only one yogurt (1%) receives a score of +5 or higher, reflecting superior nutritional quality.

Approximately four out of every five yogurts receive negative scores, signifying poor nutritional quality. The high saturated fat content of dairy products is partially responsible for these negative scores. However, even *low-fat* and *fat-free* yogurts score poorly due to vast amounts of added and natural sugars. In fact, the majority of commercial yogurts have similar compositions as desserts: very high sugar, low protein, and no fiber. Habitual consumption of low quality yogurts can significantly increase your risk of developing the Big 7 epidemic U.S. diseases.

The NQI easily distinguishes between high and low quality yogurts. The few highly rated yogurts, including one rated +8, contain high amounts of protein, moderate amounts of fiber, and relatively low non-fiber carbohydrate to fiber ratios. As part of a healthy diet, regular consumption of these high quality yogurts will optimize your metabolism and reduce your risk of developing the Big 7 epidemic U.S. diseases.

NQI SUPERIOR SELECTION

THE TOP RATED YOGURT

+8	Woodstock Water Buffalo	Plain

QUALITY CHOICES

+4	Fage (Greek)	Total 0%
+4	Stonyfield	Plain – All Natural Fat Free
+4	Weight Watchers	Blueberry
+3	Stonyfield	Plain – Organic Lowfat
+2	Fage (Greek)	Total 2%
+1	Cascade Fresh	Plain – Fat Free
+1	Stonyfield	Blueberry – Light – All Natural Fat Free
+1	Stonyfield	Plain – Organic Whole Milk

Author's Notes

- As milk-based products, yogurts contain a protein (casein) that limits activity of accompanying antioxidants. Thus, the addition of different fruits to yogurts is likely to have similar, yet limited, health benefits.

- For consistency, most fruit-based yogurts evaluated by the NQI contain blueberry. In general, the scores of equivalent brands containing strawberry, peach, banana, and other fruits are nearly identical.

- **Strategy for improving the nutritional quality of store-bought yogurt:** Select a highly rated yogurt. Add a tablespoon of ground flaxseed. Flaxseed, rich in fiber and omega-3 ALA, will not ruin the taste or texture. If necessary, add a modest amount of honey to taste.

YOGURT		Score	SFA	MUFA	LA	ALA	Chol	NFC	Fiber	Protein	Na
BREYERS	Blueberry - Fruit on the Bottom - Lowfat	-3	2.4%	1.1%	0.1%	0.0%	0.0%	80.0%	1.8%	14.5%	0.3%
BREYERS	Strawberry - Smooth & Creamy	-4	2.4%	1.1%	0.1%	0.0%	0.0%	83.6%	0.0%	12.7%	0.2%
BREYERS	Blueberries & Creme - Creme Savers	-4	4.2%	2.0%	0.1%	0.1%	0.0%	81.1%	0.0%	12.6%	0.2%
BREYERS	Raspberries 'N Cream - Smooth & Creamy	-4	2.3%	1.1%	0.1%	0.0%	0.0%	84.2%	0.0%	12.3%	0.2%
BREYERS	Vanilla - All Natural Lowfat	-4	2.9%	1.4%	0.1%	0.1%	0.0%	80.9%	0.9%	13.9%	0.3%
BREYERS	Blueberries 'N Crème - Light - with Probiotics Plus	-3	Contains Artificial Sweetener								
BROWN COW	Blueberry - Cream Top	-5	10.4%	4.9%	0.3%	0.2%	0.1%	71.1%	0.0%	13.2%	0.2%
BROWN COW	Plain - Cream Top	-4	21.0%	9.9%	0.6%	0.3%	0.1%	40.9%	0.0%	27.3%	0.4%
BROWN COW	Blueberry - Low Fat	-4	3.9%	1.8%	0.1%	0.1%	0.1%	76.5%	0.0%	17.6%	0.3%
BROWN COW	Plain - Low Fat	-1	7.1%	3.3%	0.2%	0.1%	0.0%	53.6%	0.0%	35.7%	0.6%
BROWN COW	Blueberry - Nonfat	-3	0.0%	0.0%	0.0%	0.0%	0.0%	78.8%	0.0%	21.2%	0.4%
BROWN COW	Plain - Nonfat	-3	0.0%	0.0%	0.0%	0.0%	0.0%	79.1%	0.0%	20.9%	0.3%
BROWN COW	Blueberry & Grains - Low Fat Fruit & Grains	-2	4.6%	2.2%	0.1%	0.1%	0.0%	70.4%	2.8%	19.7%	0.3%
CASCADE FRESH	Plain - Fat Free	+1	0.0%	0.0%	0.0%	0.0%	0.0%	55.2%	0.0%	44.8%	0.5%
CASCADE FRESH	Blueberry - Fat Free	-2	0.0%	0.0%	0.0%	0.0%	0.0%	74.1%	0.0%	25.9%	0.3%
CASCADE FRESH	Strawberry - Low Fat	-3	4.0%	1.9%	0.1%	0.1%	0.0%	69.7%	0.0%	24.2%	0.3%
CASCADE FRESH	Plain - Whole Milk	-1	16.0%	7.5%	0.5%	0.2%	0.1%	36.4%	0.0%	39.4%	0.3%
CASCADE FRESH	Orange Cream - Whole Milk	-4	11.8%	5.6%	0.4%	0.2%	0.1%	61.5%	0.0%	20.5%	0.2%
CASCADE FRESH	Greek-Style	-6	34.5%	16.2%	1.0%	0.5%	0.1%	27.3%	0.0%	20.5%	0.3%
CASCADE FRESH	Mediterranean-Style	-8	44.0%	20.7%	1.3%	0.7%	0.2%	22.2%	0.0%	11.1%	0.2%
DANNON	Plain - All Natural	-3	18.2%	8.6%	0.6%	0.3%	0.1%	41.4%	0.0%	31.0%	0.4%
DANNON	Plain - All Natural Lowfat	-1	7.3%	3.5%	0.2%	0.1%	0.0%	53.3%	0.0%	35.6%	0.5%
DANNON	Plain - All Natural Nonfat	0	0.0%	0.0%	0.0%	0.0%	0.0%	57.1%	0.0%	42.9%	0.6%
DANNON	Blueberry - Creamy Fruit Blends	-3	2.4%	1.1%	0.1%	0.0%	0.0%	79.5%	0.0%	16.9%	0.3%
DANNON	Blueberry - Activia	-3	5.1%	2.4%	0.2%	0.1%	0.0%	73.1%	0.0%	19.2%	0.3%

YOGURT		Score	SFA	MUFA	LA	ALA	Chol	NFC	Fiber	Protein	Na
DANNON	Blueberry - Fruit on the Bottom	-3	3.0%	1.4%	0.1%	0.1%	0.0%	76.1%	1.5%	17.9%	0.4%
DANNON	Raspberry - Activia Light	-3	Contains Artificial Sweetener								
DANNON	Strawberry - La Crème Mousse	-5	15.0%	7.0%	0.5%	0.2%	0.0%	63.6%	0.0%	13.6%	0.2%
DANNON	Raspberry - La Crème	-4	11.4%	5.3%	0.3%	0.2%	0.1%	65.5%	0.0%	17.2%	0.2%
DANNON	Blueberries 'n Cream - Light & Fit, Carb & Sugar Control	-3	Contains Artificial Sweetener								
DANNON	Blueberry - Light & Fit Nonfat	-3	Contains Artificial Sweetener								
FAGE (Greek)	Total Classic	-3	33.0%	15.5%	1.0%	0.5%	0.1%	15.0%	0.0%	35.0%	0.2%
FAGE (Greek)	Total 0%	+4	0.0%	0.0%	0.0%	0.0%	0.0%	31.6%	0.0%	68.4%	0.3%
FAGE (Greek)	Total 2%	+2	9.8%	4.6%	0.3%	0.1%	0.0%	22.2%	0.0%	63.0%	0.2%
FAGE (Greek)	Total Light	-1	22.0%	10.3%	0.7%	0.3%	0.1%	20.8%	0.0%	45.8%	0.3%
FAGE (Greek)	Total with Strawberry	-4	25.5%	12.0%	0.8%	0.4%	0.1%	35.5%	0.0%	25.8%	0.1%
FAGE (Greek)	Total with Honey	-5	16.5%	7.8%	0.5%	0.3%	0.0%	58.3%	0.0%	16.7%	0.1%
HORIZON ORGANIC	Plain - Fat Free	-3	0.0%	0.0%	0.0%	0.0%	0.0%	78.6%	0.0%	21.4%	0.3%
HORIZON ORGANIC	Blueberry - Fruit on the Bottom - Fat Free	-1	0.0%	0.0%	0.0%	0.0%	0.0%	76.5%	2.9%	20.6%	0.3%
HORIZON ORGANIC	Blueberry Blended - Lowfat	-1	3.4%	1.6%	0.1%	0.1%	0.0%	71.8%	5.1%	17.9%	0.3%
HORIZON ORGANIC	Whole Milk	-2	14.9%	7.0%	0.5%	0.2%	0.1%	45.2%	0.0%	32.3%	0.5%
HORIZON ORGANIC	Baby Yogurt	-4	7.9%	3.7%	0.2%	0.1%	0.0%	72.0%	0.0%	16.0%	0.3%
HORIZON ORGANIC	Blueberry - Kids Lowfat Tubes	-4	4.4%	2.1%	0.1%	0.1%	0.0%	80.0%	0.0%	13.3%	0.3%
HORIZON ORGANIC	Soaring Strawberry Yo-Yo's Organic Lowfat	-2	2.6%	1.2%	0.1%	0.0%	0.0%	76.0%	4.0%	16.0%	0.3%
NANCY'S	Plain Lowfat	-1	6.6%	3.1%	0.2%	0.1%	0.1%	53.3%	0.0%	36.7%	0.6%
NANCY'S	Blueberry Lowfat	-1	4.1%	1.9%	0.1%	0.1%	0.0%	66.7%	2.5%	24.7%	0.4%
NANCY'S	Plain Nonfat	0	0.0%	0.0%	0.0%	0.0%	0.1%	58.6%	0.0%	41.4%	0.6%
NANCY'S	Blueberry Fruit on Top Nonfat	-1	0.0%	0.0%	0.5%	0.2%	0.0%	71.8%	2.6%	25.6%	0.4%
NANCY'S	Organic Whole Milk	-3	15.8%	7.4%	0.5%	0.2%	0.1%	44.0%	0.0%	32.0%	0.5%
NANCY'S	Plain Organic Lowfat	-1	6.6%	3.1%	0.2%	0.1%	0.1%	53.3%	0.0%	36.7%	0.6%

YOGURT		Score	SFA	MUFA	LA	ALA	Chol	NFC	Fiber	Protein	Na
NANCY'S	Blueberry - Organic Fruit on Top Nonfat	-1	0.0%	0.0%	0.0%	0.0%	0.0%	71.1%	2.6%	26.3%	0.4%
REDWOOD HILL FARM	Blueberry - Goat Milk	-1	6.4%	3.0%	0.2%	0.1%	0.0%	67.7%	6.5%	16.1%	0.3%
REDWOOD HILL FARM	Plain - Goat Milk	-1	13.8%	6.5%	0.4%	0.2%	0.1%	46.5%	4.7%	27.9%	0.2%
SILK	Blueberry - Live! - Soy	-3	3.8%	1.8%	0.1%	0.1%	0.0%	80.0%	2.9%	11.4%	0.1%
SILK	Vanilla - Live! - Soy	-3	6.4%	3.0%	0.2%	0.1%	0.0%	73.2%	2.4%	14.6%	0.1%
STONYFIELD	Blueberry - All Natural Fat Free	0	0.0%	0.0%	0.0%	0.0%	0.0%	75.0%	6.3%	18.8%	0.3%
STONYFIELD	Blueberry - Light - All Natural Fat Free	+1	0.0%	0.0%	0.0%	0.0%	0.0%	73.5%	8.8%	17.6%	0.3%
STONYFIELD	Plain - All Natural Fat Free	+4	0.0%	0.0%	0.0%	0.0%	0.0%	54.5%	9.1%	36.4%	0.5%
STONYFIELD	Blueberry - Organic Lowfat	0	3.0%	1.4%	0.1%	0.1%	0.0%	70.8%	6.2%	18.5%	0.3%
STONYFIELD	Plain - Organic Lowfat	+3	4.6%	2.2%	0.1%	0.1%	0.0%	51.2%	9.3%	32.6%	0.5%
STONYFIELD	Wild Blueberry - Organic Whole Milk	-2	11.3%	5.3%	0.3%	0.2%	0.1%	62.9%	5.7%	14.3%	0.2%
STONYFIELD	Plain - Organic Whole Milk	+1	17.5%	8.2%	0.5%	0.3%	0.1%	38.2%	8.8%	26.5%	0.4%
STONYFIELD	Yo Baby Blueberry	0	12.0%	5.6%	0.4%	0.2%	0.0%	54.5%	9.1%	18.2%	0.3%
STONYFIELD	Yo Baby Plus Mixed Berry - Fruit & Cereal	0	9.8%	4.6%	0.3%	0.2%	0.0%	59.6%	8.5%	17.0%	0.2%
STONYFIELD	Banana - Yo Baby Drinkable	-2	11.8%	5.6%	0.4%	0.2%	0.0%	61.5%	5.1%	15.4%	0.2%
STONYFIELD	Raspberry - Yo Kids	0	2.5%	1.2%	0.1%	0.0%	0.0%	73.1%	7.7%	15.4%	0.3%
WALLABY ORGANIC	Blueberry - Lowfat	-3	4.6%	2.2%	0.1%	0.1%	0.0%	73.2%	0.0%	19.7%	0.2%
WALLABY ORGANIC	Plain - Lowfat	-2	8.9%	4.2%	0.3%	0.1%	0.1%	53.7%	0.0%	32.8%	0.4%
WALLABY ORGANIC	Strawberry - Nonfat	-3	0.0%	0.0%	0.0%	0.0%	0.0%	79.4%	0.0%	20.6%	0.3%
WALLABY ORGANIC	Plain - Nonfat	0	0.0%	0.0%	0.0%	0.0%	0.0%	61.3%	0.0%	38.7%	0.5%
WEIGHT WATCHERS	Blueberry	+4	1.4%	0.7%	0.0%	0.0%	0.0%	59.6%	12.8%	25.5%	0.5%
WOODSTOCK WATER BUFFALO	Plain	-5	33.0%	15.5%	1.0%	0.5%	0.1%	25.0%	0.0%	25.0%	0.3%
WOODSTOCK WATER BUFFALO	Plain - Low Fat	+8	7.6%	3.6%	0.2%	0.1%	0.0%	34.6%	19.2%	34.6%	0.3%
WOODSTOCK WATER BUFFALO	Blueberry	-5	17.5%	8.2%	0.5%	0.3%	0.1%	58.8%	0.0%	14.7%	0.2%
WOODSTOCK WATER BUFFALO	Vermont Honey	-5	18.9%	8.9%	0.6%	0.3%	0.1%	57.1%	0.0%	14.3%	0.2%

YOGURT		Score	SFA	MUFA	LA	ALA	Chol	NFC	Fiber	Protein	Na
YOPLAIT	Mountain Blueberry - Original	-4	2.5%	1.2%	0.1%	0.1%	0.0%	83.5%	0.0%	12.7%	0.2%
YOPLAIT	Blueberry Mist - Whips	-4	5.1%	2.4%	0.2%	0.1%	0.0%	76.9%	0.0%	15.4%	0.2%
YOPLAIT	Strawberry Banana - Healthy Heart	-4	2.4%	1.1%	0.1%	0.0%	0.0%	84.3%	0.0%	12.0%	0.2%
YOPLAIT	Blueberries 'N Cream Thick & Creamy Custard Style	-4	5.4%	2.6%	0.2%	0.1%	0.0%	75.3%	0.0%	16.5%	0.2%
YOPLAIT	Mixed Berry Light Thick & Creamy Custard Style	-3	Contains Artificial Sweetener								
YOPLAIT	Raspberry Crème Carb Monitor	-3	Contains Artificial Sweetener								
YOPLAIT	Strawberry Yoplait Kids	-1	5.5%	2.6%	0.2%	0.1%	0.0%	66.7%	4.2%	20.8%	0.3%
YOPLAIT	Blueberry Patch Light Fat Free	-3	Contains Artificial Sweetener								

Fats and Oils

The NQI rates 17 fats and oils based on *overall* nutritional quality. Scores range from -10 (toxic) to +10 (exceptional) reflecting the dramatic variation in molecular contents and predicted metabolic and health consequences of different oils.

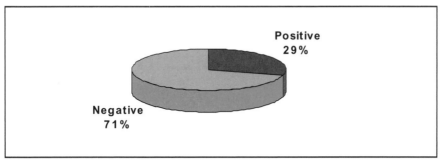

Figure 4: Fats and Oils. Five of seventeen oils (29%) evaluated by the NQI receive favorable ratings.

Because **unsaturated** fats tend to have better health properties than **saturated** fats, oil labeling claims often focus attention on their high unsaturated fat content. In fact, the FDA allows "heart healthy" labeling claims on virtually *any* oil containing >80% unsaturated fats. However, **there are several different subtypes of unsaturated fats, each with distinct health properties.** Importantly, most U.S. oils contain massive amounts of omega-6 fats and little or no omega-3 fats. These high omega-6 to omega-3 ratios promote a variety of metabolic disturbances and may predispose to the Big 7 U.S. epidemic diseases (see Parts 2 and 3). Like omega-3 fats, monounsaturated fats have favorable metabolic and health properties. Failure to distinguish between these different subtypes of unsaturated fats allows unhealthy oils to masquerade as beneficial. **Despite health claims to the contrary, most available oils are low quality foods.**

The NQI easily distinguishes between high and low quality oils. Highly rated oils contain no trans fats and have low concentrations of saturated fats, high concentrations of monounsaturated fats, and low omega-6 to omega-3 ratios. As part of a healthy diet, regular consumption of these high quality oils will optimize your metabolism and reduce your risk of developing the Big 7 epidemic U.S. diseases.

NQI SUPERIOR SELECTIONS

TOP 5 OUTSTANDING OILS

+9	Extra Virgin Olive Oil
+8	Canola Oil
+7	*High-Oleic** Safflower Oil
+6	Olive oil (non-virgin)
+5	Flaxseed Oil**

Author's Notes:

- *Unlike conventional safflower oil which consists of nearly 80% omega-6 linoleic acid, high oleic safflower oil consists of predominantly monounsaturated oleic acid. This modification dramatically improves the nutritional composition of the high-oleic variety.*

- **Because high temperatures may damage flaxseed oil, it is not suitable for cooking. For best results, flaxseed oil should be added to uncooked items (i.e. salad dressings) or after cooking. Better yet, after cooking add **ground** flaxseed, a rich source of omega-3 ALA, fiber, **and** protein.*

FATS & OILS	Score	SFA	MUFA	LA	ALA	AOX
Canola	+8	8.0%	60.0%	24.0%	8.0%	1.0
Coconut	-10	94.0%	6.0%	0.0%	0.0%	1.0
Corn	-9	14.0%	25.0%	60.0%	1.0%	1.0
Cottonseed	-10	27.0%	19.0%	54.0%	0.0%	1.0
Flaxseed	+5	10.0%	20.0%	14.0%	56.0%	2.0
Olive - extra virgin	+9	15.0%	74.0%	10.0%	1.0%	4.0
Olive	+6	15.0%	74.0%	10.0%	1.0%	1.0
Palm	-8	50.0%	40.0%	10.0%	0.0%	1.0
Palm kernel	-10	86.0%	12.0%	2.0%	0.0%	1.0
Peanut	-4	18.0%	50.0%	32.0%	0.0%	0.0
Rice bran	-3	20.0%	42.0%	36.0%	2.0%	2.0
Safflower	-10	7.0%	15.0%	78.0%	0.0%	1.0
Safflower - high oleic	+7	6.0%	79.0%	15.0%	0.0%	1.0
Sesame	-5	15.0%	42.0%	43.0%	0.0%	1.0
Soybean	-3	15.0%	25.0%	53.0%	7.0%	2.0
Sunflower	-10	10.0%	20.0%	70.0%	0.0%	1.0
Sunflower - high oleic	-2	10.0%	50.0%	40.0%	0.0%	1.0

Finfish

The NQI rates 29 fish based on *overall* nutritional quality. Scores range from **-10** (toxic) to **+10** (exceptional) reflecting the dramatic variation in molecular contents and predicted metabolic and health consequences of different fish.

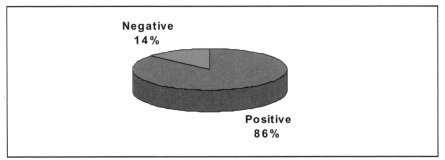

Figure 5: Finfish. Twenty-five of twenty-nine fish (86%) evaluated by the NQI receive favorable ratings.

Finfish have perhaps the best overall health impact of *any* food group and regular fish consumption is strongly linked to reduced risk of the Big 7 epidemic U.S. diseases. However, ***not all fish have equivalent metabolic health properties***. In fact, regular consumption of a few types may have serious adverse health consequences.

Fish are a concentrated source of protein. However, different species naturally contain radically different concentrations of long-chain omega-3 fatty acids and toxins (PCBs and mercury). Additionally, agribusiness practices can profoundly alter the contents of fish in the same species. For example, farm raised Atlantic salmon contain much greater quantities of PCBs and up to fifteen times as much omega-6 arachidonic acid as wild salmon.

The NQI easily distinguishes between high and low quality finfish. In light of widespread U.S. deficiency of omega-3 EPA and DHA, it is crucially important to identify and consume high omega-3, low mercury and PCB fish. As part of a healthy diet, regular consumption of high quality fish will optimize your metabolism and reduce your risk of developing the Big 7 epidemic U.S. diseases.

NQI SUPERIOR SELECTIONS

TOP 15 FANTASTIC FINFISH

+10	Salmon Chinook/king (wild)
+10	Salmon Pink/humpback (wild)
+10	Salmon Sockeye/red (wild)
+10	Salmon Coho/silver (wild)
+10	Whitefish
+10	Ocean perch
+9	Herring
+9	Mackerel
+8	Haddock
+7	Flounder
+7	Cod
+6	Perch
+6	Snapper
+6	Trout
+6	*Canned light* Tuna

Author's Note:

- Though controversial, women of childbearing years should probably avoid all fish with mercury content above 0.30 ppm (see table p.74), and should restrict intake of fish with between 0.10 ppm to 0.30 ppm to one serving per week (This includes canned light tuna).

- If budgetary concerns or geographic location limit your access to high quality fish, purified, omega-3 EPA and DHA-rich fish oil or cod liver oil can provide a viable alternative. All three samples listed below score off the charts on the NQI. Talk to a qualified and informed health care provider before taking these or any supplements.

FINFISH	Score	SFA	MUFA	LA	ArA	ALA	EPA/DHA	Chol	Protein	Na	TOX
Catfish - wild	+4	3.9%	4.5%	0.5%	0.8%	0.4%	2.0%	0.3%	87.6%	0.2%	4.0
Catfish - farmed	+3	7.9%	16.1%	3.9%	0.4%	0.4%	1.2%	0.2%	69.8%	0.2%	3.0
Cod	+7	0.7%	0.5%	0.1%	0.1%	0.0%	1.0%	0.2%	97.4%	0.3%	1.6
Flounder	+7	1.4%	1.2%	0.0%	0.2%	0.0%	1.0%	0.2%	95.8%	0.4%	1.8
Grouper	-2	1.2%	1.0%	0.1%	0.2%	0.0%	1.2%	0.2%	96.2%	0.3%	11.0
Haddock	+8	0.7%	0.6%	0.0%	0.1%	0.0%	1.0%	0.3%	97.3%	0.3%	0.6
Halibut	+4	1.4%	3.3%	0.1%	0.6%	0.3%	1.6%	0.1%	92.4%	0.2%	4.6
Halibut - cold water	+5	9.2%	31.8%	0.5%	0.2%	0.2%	3.5%	0.2%	54.5%	0.3%	4.6
Herring	+9	8.0%	14.6%	0.5%	0.2%	0.4%	6.1%	0.2%	70.0%	0.4%	0.8
Mackerel	+9	9.7%	14.2%	0.6%	0.5%	0.4%	6.6%	0.2%	67.9%	0.3%	1.4
Mackerel, King	-5	1.7%	3.5%	0.2%	0.0%	0.0%	1.4%	0.2%	93.0%	0.7%	14.6
Ocean perch	+10	1.2%	3.1%	0.1%	0.0%	0.3%	1.5%	0.2%	93.5%	0.4%	0.2
Orange roughy	-4	0.1%	1.4%	0.2%	0.1%	0.0%	0.1%	0.4%	97.7%	0.4%	10.8
Perch	+6	0.9%	0.8%	0.1%	0.3%	0.1%	1.3%	0.4%	96.2%	0.3%	2.8
Salmon, Atlantic - farmed	+1	7.3%	13.0%	2.0%	3.9%	0.3%	6.4%	0.2%	66.9%	0.2%	6.8
Salmon, Chinook/king	+10	10.4%	14.8%	0.4%	0.5%	0.3%	6.6%	0.2%	66.9%	0.2%	0.2
Salmon, Coho/silver - wild	+10	4.7%	8.0%	0.8%	0.5%	0.6%	4.1%	0.2%	81.2%	0.2%	0.2
Salmon, Coho/silver - farmed	+5	6.4%	11.8%	1.2%	0.3%	0.3%	4.3%	0.2%	75.5%	0.2%	5.0
Salmon, Pink/humpback	+10	2.5%	4.1%	0.2%	0.3%	0.2%	4.4%	0.2%	88.0%	0.3%	0.2
Salmon, Sockeye/red	+10	5.2%	14.4%	1.3%	0.3%	0.3%	4.1%	0.2%	74.2%	0.2%	0.2
Sea Bass	+2	2.6%	2.1%	0.1%	0.0%	0.0%	3.0%	0.2%	92.0%	0.3%	7.6
Snapper	+6	1.3%	1.2%	0.1%	0.2%	0.0%	1.4%	0.2%	95.5%	0.3%	3.8

FINFISH	Score	SFA	MUFA	LA	ArA	ALA	EPA/DHA	Chol	Protein	Na	TOX
Swordfish	-10	4.7%	6.6%	0.1%	0.3%	0.8%	2.7%	0.2%	84.6%	0.4%	26.2
Tilapia - farmed	+5	2.7%	2.3%	0.7%	0.1%	0.1%	0.4%	0.2%	93.5%	0.2%	1.3
Trout	+6	4.3%	12.3%	0.7%	0.7%	0.6%	2.8%	0.2%	78.4%	0.2%	4.0
Tuna, Skipjack	+5	1.4%	0.8%	0.1%	0.1%	0.0%	1.1%	0.2%	96.2%	0.2%	4.1
Tuna, Yellowfin	+4	1.0%	0.6%	0.0%	0.1%	0.0%	0.9%	0.2%	97.1%	0.2%	5.1
Tuna, Albacore - canned "white" in water	+4	3.0%	3.0%	0.2%	0.2%	0.3%	3.3%	0.2%	89.9%	1.4%	6.5
Tuna, Skipjack or Yellowfin - canned "light" in water	+6	0.9%	0.6%	0.0%	0.1%	0.0%	1.0%	0.1%	97.2%	1.3%	2.4
Whitefish	+9	3.8%	8.3%	1.1%	0.9%	0.8%	5.2%	0.3%	79.6%	0.2%	1.4
Fish Oil, Salmon	+10	23.7%	34.6%	1.8%	0.8%	1.3%	37.2%	0.6%	0.0%	0.0%	0.2
Fish Oil, Herring	+10	23.3%	62.0%	1.3%	0.3%	0.8%	11.5%	0.8%	0.0%	0.0%	0.2
Fish Oil, Cod Liver	+10	25.0%	50.9%	1.0%	1.0%	1.0%	19.7%	0.6%	0.0%	0.0%	0.2

Shellfish

The NQI rates 13 crustaceans and mollusks based on *overall* nutritional quality. On a scale of -10 (toxic) to +10 (exceptional), scores range from -4 to +10 reflecting the dramatic variation in molecular contents and predicted metabolic and health consequences of different shellfish.

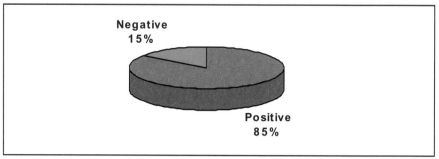

Figure 6: Shellfish. Eleven of thirteen shellfish (85%) evaluated by the NQI receive favorable ratings.

Like finfish, regular shellfish consumption is likely to have a variety of health benefits. However, not all shellfish have equivalent metabolic and health properties. In fact, regular consumption of certain types may have serious adverse health consequences. For instance, while all shellfish are an excellent source of protein, concentrations of both mercury and omega-3 fats can vary 30-fold or more among different varieties!

The NQI easily distinguishes between high and low quality shellfish.
Top rated crustaceans and mollusks contain high concentrations of protein and long-chain omega-3 fats and low concentrations of mercury and PCBs. In fact, certain low-toxin shellfish contain higher concentrations of omega-3 fats than many finfish. As part of a healthy diet, regular consumption of high quality shellfish will optimize your metabolism and reduce your risk of developing the Big 7 epidemic U.S. diseases.

NQI SUPERIOR SELECTIONS

TOP 11 SHELLFISH

+10	Oyster
+10	Shrimp
+9	Squid (Calamari)
+9	Crab (Dungeness)
+8	Crab (Blue)
+7	Mussel
+7	Crayfish
+6	Scallop
+6	Clam
+5	Octopus
+5	Spiny (Rock) Lobster

SHELLFISH		Score	SFA	MUFA	LA	ArA	ALA	EPA/DHA	Chol	NFC	Fiber	Protein	Na	TOX
CRUSTACEANS	Crab, blue	+8	1.2%	1.0%	0.1%	0.3%	0.0%	1.7%	0.4%	0.2%	0.0%	95.2%	1.5%	1.2
CRUSTACEANS	Crab, dungeness	+9	0.7%	0.9%	0.0%	0.0%	0.0%	1.6%	0.3%	3.9%	0.0%	92.5%	1.6%	1.2
CRUSTACEANS	Crab, imitation/surimi	-4	0.5%	0.7%	0.2%	0.0%	0.0%	0.1%	0.1%	63.1%	2.2%	33.2%	3.7%	0.8
CRUSTACEANS	Crayfish/crawfish	+7	1.0%	1.0%	0.3%	0.3%	0.2%	0.9%	0.7%	0.0%	0.0%	95.7%	0.4%	0.8
CRUSTACEANS	Lobster, Atlantic Maine	-1	0.9%	1.3%	0.0%	0.0%	0.0%	0.0%	0.5%	2.5%	0.0%	94.8%	1.5%	6.2
CRUSTACEANS	Lobster, Rock/spiny	+5	1.0%	1.1%	0.1%	0.6%	0.0%	1.5%	0.3%	10.1%	0.0%	85.3%	0.7%	1.8
CRUSTACEANS	Shrimp	+10	1.5%	1.1%	0.1%	0.4%	0.1%	2.1%	0.7%	4.0%	0.0%	90.0%	0.7%	0.2
MOLLUSKS	Clam	+6	0.6%	0.5%	0.1%	0.3%	0.0%	0.9%	0.2%	16.3%	0.0%	81.1%	0.4%	0.2
MOLLUSKS	Mussel	+7	2.5%	3.0%	0.1%	0.4%	0.1%	2.6%	0.2%	21.6%	0.0%	69.6%	1.7%	1.4
MOLLUSKS	Octopus	+5	1.3%	0.9%	0.1%	0.2%	0.0%	0.9%	0.3%	12.4%	0.0%	84.0%	1.3%	0.6
MOLLUSKS	Oyster	+10	4.4%	2.3%	0.3%	0.4%	0.3%	4.3%	0.4%	30.6%	0.0%	57.0%	1.6%	0.2
MOLLUSKS	Scallop	+6	0.4%	0.2%	0.0%	0.1%	0.0%	1.0%	0.2%	12.1%	0.0%	86.0%	0.8%	1.0
MOLLUSKS	Squid/calamari	+9	1.8%	0.5%	0.0%	0.0%	0.0%	2.5%	1.2%	15.5%	0.0%	78.4%	0.2%	1.4

Animal Meats

The NQI rates 40 animal meats based on *overall* nutritional quality. On a scale of -10 (toxic) to +10 (exceptional), scores range from -5 to +6 reflecting the dramatic variation in molecular contents and predicted metabolic and health consequences of different meats.

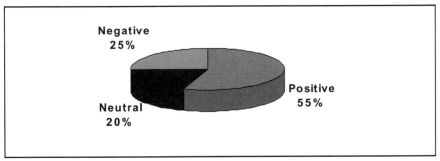

Figure 7: Animal meats. Twenty-two out of forty meats (55%) evaluated by the NQI receive favorable ratings.

All meats are concentrated sources of protein. However, recent changes in agribusiness practices have radically altered the *fat* content of most U.S. meats. For example, the corn-fed cattle that currently provide over 95% of beef consumed in the U.S., contain much more saturated fats, and less monounsaturated and omega-3 fats than the wild meats consumed by our ancestors. Similar agribusiness practices have increased the saturated fat content and omega-6 to omega-3 ratios of poultry, pork, and other meats. However, high quality meats *are* available, you just need to know how to identify them. Because modern feeding practices reduce fat quality, lean meats are a viable option. Alternatively, meats from grass-fed animals naturally contain less saturated fat, more monounsaturated fat, and lower omega-6 to omega-3 ratios.

The NQI easily distinguishes between high and low quality meats. Top rated meats contain high concentrations of protein and monounsaturated fats, as well as low omega-6 to omega-3 ratios. As part of a healthy diet, regular consumption of high quality meats will optimize your metabolism and reduce your risk of developing the Big 7 epidemic U.S. diseases.

NQI SUPERIOR SELECTIONS

TOP 10 CHOICE CUTS

+6	Chicken Breast/Light Meat*
+6	Turkey Breast/Light Meat*
+5	Pork Tenderloin
+4	Chicken Leg/Dark Meat*
+4	Grass-fed Ground Beef
+4	Bison – Top Sirloin
+4	Bison – Ribeye
+4	Elk
+4	Venison/deer
+3	Grass-fed Beef Tenderloin

*=skinless

Author's Notes:

1) Bacon, sausages, hot dogs and other processed meats typically contain nitrates which are converted to cancer-causing nitrosamines. Similarly, red meat consumption is linked to an increased risk of cancer. It is not known whether this association is due to the presence of heme iron, omega-6 arachidonic acid, or other cancer-promoting substances.

2) Cooking methods can alter the nutritional quality of meats, fish, and shellfish. Specifically, overcooking (essentially burning) these high protein foods creates cancer-promoting heterocyclic amines (HCAs). Therefore, meats are ideally cooked at moderate temperatures to avoid charring.

POULTRY		Score	SFA	MUFA	LA	ArA	ALA	EPA/DHA	Chol	Protein	Na
Chicken	Light meat, breast	+6	1.4%	1.2%	0.7%	0.2%	0.0%	0.1%	0.2%	96.1%	0.3%
Chicken	Dark meat, leg & thigh	+4	4.7%	5.7%	3.5%	0.4%	0.2%	0.2%	0.3%	85.0%	0.4%
Chicken	Whole, meat & skin	+1	13.3%	19.3%	8.9%	0.2%	0.4%	0.1%	0.2%	57.5%	0.2%
Chicken	Cornish hen, whole	0	12.9%	20.5%	8.2%	0.5%	0.4%	0.1%	0.3%	57.1%	0.2%
Turkey	Breast	+6	0.8%	0.4%	0.4%	0.1%	0.0%	0.0%	0.2%	97.9%	0.2%
Turkey	Light meat	+5	2.0%	1.1%	1.1%	0.3%	0.0%	0.1%	0.3%	95.1%	0.3%
Turkey	Dark meat, with skin	+3	5.9%	6.4%	4.4%	0.4%	0.2%	0.1%	0.2%	82.3%	0.3%
Duck	Wild, with skin	+2	16.1%	21.7%	5.9%	0.0%	0.5%	0.0%	0.2%	55.5%	0.2%
Duck	Domestic, with skin	-2	27.2%	38.5%	9.7%	0.0%	0.8%	0.0%	0.3%	23.7%	0.1%
Ostrich	Domestic, tenderloin	+1	4.6%	4.9%	1.9%	0.9%	0.2%	0.0%	0.3%	87.2%	0.3%

BEEF/ VEAL		Score	SFA	MUFA	LA	ArA	ALA	EPA/DHA	Chol	NFC	Protein	Na
BEEF	Frankfurter	-5	27.5%	33.6%	2.4%	0.1%	0.4%	0.0%	0.2%	9.5%	26.4%	2.7%
BEEF	Ground beef - 20% fat	-1	22.4%	25.6%	1.2%	0.1%	0.2%	0.0%	0.2%	0.0%	50.2%	0.2%
BEEF	Ground beef - 15% fat	0	18.6%	20.8%	1.1%	0.1%	0.2%	0.0%	0.3%	0.0%	59.0%	0.2%
BEEF	Ground beef - 10% fat	+1	14.1%	15.1%	0.9%	0.1%	0.2%	0.0%	0.2%	0.0%	69.4%	0.2%
BEEF	Chuck pot roast	0	21.2%	22.5%	1.3%	0.1%	0.6%	0.0%	0.2%	0.0%	54.1%	0.2%
BEEF	Shortribs	-3	32.9%	34.2%	1.7%	0.0%	1.0%	0.0%	0.2%	0.0%	30.0%	0.1%
BEEF	London Broil, top round steak	+3	11.1%	12.2%	0.7%	0.1%	0.3%	0.0%	0.3%	0.0%	75.5%	0.2%
BEEF	Steak, Porterhouse	0	22.4%	25.0%	1.3%	0.1%	0.6%	0.0%	0.2%	0.0%	50.3%	0.1%
BEEF	Steak, tenderloin	0	20.4%	21.6%	1.2%	0.1%	0.6%	0.0%	0.2%	0.0%	55.9%	0.1%
BEEF	Ground beef - grass-fed	+4	5.1%	4.7%	1.4%	0.5%	0.7%	0.4%	0.2%	0.0%	87.0%	0.2%
BEEF	Tenderloin - grass-fed	+3	7.1%	6.4%	1.1%	0.4%	0.5%	0.4%	0.2%	0.0%	83.9%	0.2%
VEAL	Ground	+1	11.1%	10.2%	1.4%	0.3%	0.2%	0.0%	0.3%	0.0%	76.6%	0.3%
VEAL	Top round	+3	5.0%	4.7%	0.8%	0.2%	0.1%	0.0%	0.3%	0.0%	88.9%	0.3%
VEAL	Loin, chop or steak	0	14.4%	13.1%	1.7%	0.3%	0.2%	0.0%	0.3%	0.0%	70.0%	0.3%

PORK	Score	SFA	MUFA	LA	ArA	ALA	Chol	NFC	Protein	Na
Bacon	-5	28.8%	38.6%	8.3%	0.2%	0.4%	0.2%	1.3%	22.3%	1.6%
Canadian bacon	0	7.8%	11.1%	1.9%	0.2%	0.3%	0.3%	5.9%	72.8%	5.0%
Ham, lean	0	7.0%	9.5%	1.9%	0.3%	0.2%	0.2%	0.2%	80.8%	5.5%
Ground pork	-1	21.8%	26.2%	4.6%	0.2%	0.2%	0.2%	0.0%	46.8%	0.2%
Pork Frankfurter	-3	25.0%	31.2%	5.6%	0.1%	0.4%	0.3%	0.5%	36.7%	2.3%
Ribs, spareribs	-1	23.2%	26.5%	5.1%	0.2%	0.2%	0.2%	0.0%	44.4%	0.2%
Roasts or chops	+1	15.0%	19.3%	3.8%	0.3%	0.3%	0.3%	0.0%	61.0%	0.2%
Roasts or chops, lean	+5	8.1%	10.6%	2.0%	0.3%	0.1%	0.2%	0.0%	78.7%	0.2%
Tenderloin, lean	+5	4.9%	6.4%	1.2%	0.2%	0.0%	0.3%	0.0%	87.0%	0.2%

LAMB & GAME	Score	SFA	MUFA	LA	ArA	ALA	EPA/DHA	Chol	Protein	Na
Lamb, ground	-2	26.6%	25.1%	3.6%	0.2%	1.1%	0.0%	0.2%	43.3%	0.2%
Lamb, leg	0	19.5%	18.6%	2.7%	0.2%	0.8%	0.0%	0.3%	58.1%	0.2%
Lamb, stew or kabob, lean	+3	7.6%	8.6%	1.5%	0.2%	0.3%	0.0%	0.2%	81.6%	0.3%
Bison/Buffalo, topsirloin, lean	+4	3.7%	4.2%	0.9%	0.4%	0.0%	0.2%	0.2%	90.3%	0.2%
Bison/Buffalo, ribeye, lean	+4	3.7%	4.1%	0.8%	0.4%	0.0%	0.2%	0.3%	90.6%	0.2%
Elk	+4	2.2%	1.5%	0.7%	0.4%	0.2%	0.2%	0.2%	94.8%	0.2%
Venison/Deer	+4	3.8%	2.7%	1.2%	0.4%	0.3%	0.2%	0.3%	91.3%	0.2%

EGGS

The NQI rates 4 varieties of eggs based on *overall* nutritional quality. On a scale of -10 (toxic) to +10 (exceptional), scores range from -2 to +3 reflecting the considerable variation in molecular contents and predicted metabolic and health consequences of different eggs.

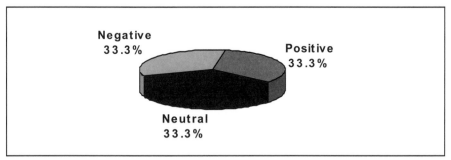

Figure 8: Eggs. One out of the three (33%) available U.S. types of eggs receives a favorable rating.

Like animal meats, modern agribusiness practices have radically altered the fat content of U.S. eggs. Specifically, typical corn-fed hens produce eggs with higher concentrations of omega-6 fats and a tiny fraction of omega-3 fats as their naturally raised peers. For example, conventional U.S. eggs contain twice as much omega-6 linoleic acid and less than one-fifth as much omega-3 ALA, EPA, and DHA as free-range Greek eggs.

The NQI easily distinguishes between high and low quality eggs. Highly rated eggs contain high concentrations of protein and low omega-6 to omega-3 ratios. The only readily available U.S. eggs meeting these criteria are flax-fed eggs. As part of a healthy diet, regular consumption of these high quality eggs will optimize your metabolism and reduce your risk of developing the Big 7 epidemic U.S. diseases.

NQI SUPERIOR SELECTIONS

TOP RATED EGG

+3	Flax-fed eggs

Author's Note: *Many people restrict their consumption of eggs due to the belief that "all cholesterol is bad." However, as explained in Parts 2 and 3, unlike* **blood** *(or serum) cholesterol, there is little convincing evidence linking* **dietary** *cholesterol to any disease. In fact, roughly two-thirds of Americans halt production of cholesterol when* **dietary** *cholesterol is increased. The other one-third responds with elevations of both "bad cholesterol" (LDL) and "good cholesterol" (HDL) levels. Because egg intake results in little change in LDL to HDL ratios and may actually reduce the atherogenicity of LDL particles by increasing their size and buoyancy, consumption of high quality eggs may actually reduce the risk of cardiovascular disease. For a thorough discussion of the major determinants of* **blood** *cholesterol see Part 3: Diet and Cholesterol Metabolism, pages 121-131.*

EGGS	Score	SFA	MUFA	LA	ArA	ALA	EPA/DHA	Chol	NFC	Protein
Standard - USDA	-2	14.1%	17.3%	5.2%	0.6%	0.1%	0.2%	1.9%	3.5%	57.1%
Fish-meal fed	0	13.2%	15.5%	9.7%	0.6%	0.6%	1.0%	1.9%	3.5%	54.0%
Flax-fed	+3	13.7%	15.8%	6.6%	0.4%	3.3%	0.8%	1.9%	3.5%	53.9%
Greek - free-range	+2	14.7%	20.6%	2.3%	0.8%	1.0%	1.1%	1.9%	3.5%	54.2%

Fruits

The NQI rates 36 fruits based on *overall* nutritional quality. On a scale of -10 (toxic) to +10 (exceptional), scores range from -3 to +10 reflecting the dramatic variation in molecular contents and predicted metabolic and health consequences of different fruits.

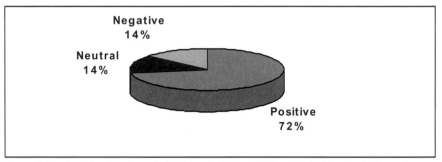

Figure 9: Fruits. Twenty-six out of thirty-six fruits (72%) evaluated by the NQI receive favorable ratings.

As a category, fruits have a variety of beneficial health attributes and replacement of processed foods with fruits is likely to reduce your risk of the Big 7 epidemic U.S. diseases. However, **not all fruits have equivalent metabolic and health properties.** In fact, habitual consumption of some fruits may actually have adverse metabolic and health consequences.

Different fruits contain radically different amounts of fiber, protein, antioxidants, monounsaturated fats, sugars, and other important components. For example, non-fiber carbohydrates (sugar equivalents) range from less than 8% to over 90% of water-free weight of different fruits! Similarly, fiber and antioxidant contents vary up to 15-fold and 35-fold, respectively. Comparable variations exist for protein, monounsaturated fats, and other beneficial components.

The NQI easily distinguishes between high and low quality fruits. The highest rated fruits contain significant quantities of antioxidants, fiber, and other beneficial components, as well as low non-fiber carbohydrate to fiber ratios. As part of a healthy diet, regular consumption of high quality fruits will optimize your metabolism and reduce your risk of developing the Big 7 epidemic U.S. diseases.

NQI SUPERIOR SELECTIONS

TOP RATED FRUITS

+10	Blackberry
+10	Raspberry
+10	Cranberry
+10	Avocado
+10	Olive (black or green)
+10	Strawberry
+9	Lemon*
+8	Lime*
+6	Blueberry
+5	Cherry (tart)
+5	Orange
+5	Plum
+5	Pear

* includes pulp

FRUIT		Score	SFA	MUFA	LA	ALA	NFC	Fiber	Protein	Na	AOX
BERRIES, CHERRIES & GRAPES	Blackberry	+10	0.1%	0.4%	1.6%	0.8%	38.0%	46.7%	12.3%	0.0%	4.1
BERRIES, CHERRIES & GRAPES	Blueberry	+6	0.2%	0.3%	0.6%	0.4%	78.3%	15.5%	4.8%	0.0%	4.2
BERRIES, CHERRIES & GRAPES	Cherry, sour	+5	0.5%	0.6%	0.3%	0.3%	78.8%	11.9%	7.5%	0.0%	4.0
BERRIES, CHERRIES & GRAPES	Cherry, sweet	+2	0.2%	0.3%	0.2%	0.2%	80.8%	12.2%	6.2%	0.0%	1.7
BERRIES, CHERRIES & GRAPES	Cranberry	+10	0.1%	0.1%	0.3%	0.2%	60.0%	36.3%	3.1%	0.0%	7.3
BERRIES, CHERRIES & GRAPES	Grape, green	-2	0.5%	0.6%	0.3%	0.1%	90.3%	5.1%	3.7%	0.0%	0.6
BERRIES, CHERRIES & GRAPES	Grape, red	-1	0.5%	0.6%	0.3%	0.1%	90.3%	5.1%	3.7%	0.0%	1.6
BERRIES, CHERRIES & GRAPES	Raisin	-3	0.1%	0.1%	0.0%	0.0%	91.6%	4.5%	3.7%	0.1%	0.6
BERRIES, CHERRIES & GRAPES	Raspberry	+10	0.1%	0.5%	1.8%	0.9%	40.0%	47.8%	8.8%	0.0%	3.5
BERRIES, CHERRIES & GRAPES	Strawberry	+10	0.2%	0.5%	1.1%	0.8%	66.4%	23.4%	7.8%	0.0%	4.0
CITRUS	Grapefruit	+2	0.2%	0.1%	0.2%	0.1%	79.7%	12.6%	7.2%	0.0%	1.4
CITRUS	Lemon	+9	0.4%	0.1%	0.6%	0.2%	61.7%	26.5%	10.4%	0.0%	1.0
CITRUS	Lime	+8	0.4%	0.4%	0.3%	0.2%	68.3%	24.7%	6.2%	0.0%	1.0
CITRUS	Orange	+5	0.1%	0.2%	0.1%	0.1%	73.3%	18.8%	7.4%	0.0%	1.4
CITRUS	Tangerine	+1	0.3%	0.4%	0.3%	0.1%	80.6%	12.6%	5.7%	0.0%	0.6
COMMON	Apple (with skin)	+4	0.2%	0.0%	0.3%	0.1%	80.6%	16.9%	1.8%	0.0%	2.1
COMMON	Apricot	+4	0.2%	1.3%	0.6%	0.0%	71.3%	15.6%	10.9%	0.0%	1.0
COMMON	Banana	0	0.5%	0.1%	0.2%	0.1%	83.8%	10.8%	4.5%	0.0%	0.3
COMMON	Cantaloupe	0	0.6%	0.0%	0.4%	0.5%	79.4%	9.8%	9.2%	0.2%	0.3
COMMON	Date	0	0.0%	0.0%	0.0%	0.0%	86.4%	10.3%	3.2%	0.0%	0.4
COMMON	Fig	+2	0.3%	0.3%	0.7%	0.0%	80.6%	14.4%	3.7%	0.0%	0.5
COMMON	Honeydew	-2	0.4%	0.0%	0.3%	0.3%	85.2%	8.2%	5.5%	1.8%	0.3
COMMON	Kiwi	+4	0.2%	0.3%	1.5%	0.3%	72.2%	18.6%	7.1%	0.0%	0.6
COMMON	Mango	0	0.4%	0.6%	0.1%	0.2%	85.7%	10.2%	2.9%	0.0%	0.6
COMMON	Nectarine	+3	0.2%	0.7%	0.9%	0.0%	74.7%	14.4%	9.0%	0.0%	0.6
COMMON	Peach	+3	0.2%	0.6%	0.8%	0.0%	75.7%	14.1%	8.6%	0.0%	1.6
COMMON	Pear	+5	0.0%	0.2%	0.2%	0.0%	77.7%	19.5%	2.4%	0.0%	1.1
COMMON	Pineapple	0	0.1%	0.1%	0.2%	0.1%	84.8%	10.6%	4.1%	0.0%	0.6

FRUIT		Score	SFA	MUFA	LA	ALA	NFC	Fiber	Protein	Na	AOA
COMMON	Plum	+5	0.1%	1.1%	0.4%	0.0%	81.3%	11.4%	5.7%	0.0%	5.0
COMMON	Pomegranate	+1	0.2%	0.3%	0.3%	0.0%	90.7%	3.3%	5.2%	0.0%	5.0
COMMON	Prune	+1	0.1%	0.1%	0.1%	0.0%	85.7%	10.7%	3.3%	0.0%	1.3
COMMON	Watermelon	-2	0.2%	0.4%	0.6%	0.0%	86.5%	4.9%	7.4%	0.0%	0.2
FRUIT - Other	Avocado	+10	8.8%	40.3%	6.9%	0.5%	7.4%	28.0%	8.2%	0.0%	0.7
FRUIT - Other	Avocado, Florida	+10	10.2%	28.7%	8.2%	0.5%	11.6%	29.2%	11.6%	0.0%	0.7
FRUIT - Other	Olive, black	+10	8.2%	45.6%	4.9%	0.4%	17.7%	18.5%	4.9%	5.0%	4.0
FRUIT - Other	Olive, green	+10	10.4%	58.0%	6.2%	0.5%	2.8%	16.9%	5.3%	8.0%	3.0

Vegetables

The NQI rates 38 vegetables based on *overall* nutritional quality. On a scale of -10 (toxic) to +10 (exceptional), scores range from -1 to +10 reflecting the considerable variation in molecular contents and predicted metabolic and health consequences of different vegetables.

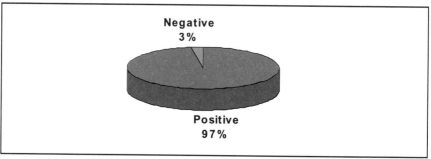

Figure 10: Vegetables. Thirty-seven out of thirty-eight vegetables (97%) evaluated by the NQI receive favorable ratings.

Like fruits, vegetables have a variety of beneficial health properties, and replacement of processed foods with vegetables is likely to reduce your risk of the Big 7 epidemic U.S. diseases. In fact, twenty-four of thirty-eight vegetables (63%) receive the maximum score of +10. These high scores reflect their high concentrations of fiber and relatively high contents of antioxidants, protein, and other beneficial components. However, ***not all vegetables have equivalent metabolic and health properties.***   Seven of thirty-eight vegetables (18%) receive a score of +2 or below, reflecting only moderately beneficial or even neutral metabolic and health properties. In general, these lower scores reflect higher concentrations of non-fiber carbohydrates (sugar equivalents) and minimal antioxidant and fiber content.

The NQI easily distinguishes between high and low quality vegetables. The highest rated vegetables contain significant quantities of antioxidants, fiber, and other beneficial components, as well as low non-fiber carbohydrate to fiber ratios. As part of a healthy diet, regular consumption of high quality vegetables will optimize your metabolism and reduce your risk of developing the Big 7 epidemic U.S. diseases.

NQI SUPERIOR SELECTIONS
TOP 24 VEGETABLES

+10	Eggplant
+10	Artichoke
+10	Collards
+10	Romaine lettuce
+10	Asparagus
+10	Spinach
+10	Looseleaf lettuce
+10	Broccoli
+10	Radish
+10	Alfalfa sprouts
+10	Jalapeno pepper
+10	Okra
+10	Cauliflower
+10	Brussel sprouts
+10	Green bean
+10	Celery
+10	Arugula
+10	Cabbage
+10	Iceberg lettuce
+10	Green onion (scallion)
+10	Pea
+10	Summer squash
+10	Red Cabbage
+10	Beet

Authors Notes
- *Although the raw scores of some vegetables are considerably higher, final scores are capped at +10. They are listed above in descending order.*
- *Eggplant and artichoke receive among the highest scores of all NQI-rated foods! High ratings reflect their exceptionally high concentrations of fiber, protein, and antioxidants.*
- *The +10 score of iceberg lettuce reflects its surprisingly high content of fiber, omega-3 ALA, and antioxidants.*

www.theNQI.com

VEGETABLES	Score	SFA	MUFA	LA	ALA	NFC	Fiber	Protein	Na	AOX
Alfalfa sprouts	+10	0.8%	0.7%	2.8%	2.1%	15.4%	30.1%	48.1%	0.1%	0.5
Artichoke	+10	0.3%	0.0%	0.3%	0.1%	36.8%	38.9%	23.6%	0.7%	7.2
Arugula	+10	1.3%	0.7%	1.9%	2.5%	30.7%	24.0%	38.7%	0.4%	2.0
Asparagus	+10	0.6%	0.0%	0.6%	0.0%	28.8%	34.0%	35.7%	0.0%	4.1
Beet	+10	0.2%	0.3%	0.5%	0.0%	59.9%	24.8%	14.3%	0.7%	2.3
Broccoli	+10	0.6%	0.3%	0.4%	1.5%	26.4%	35.4%	35.2%	0.3%	1.7
Brussel sprouts	+10	0.5%	0.2%	0.4%	0.8%	41.1%	30.2%	26.9%	0.2%	2.0
Cabbage	+10	0.5%	0.2%	0.2%	0.0%	46.2%	35.0%	17.9%	0.3%	1.6
Cabbage, red	+10	0.2%	0.1%	0.4%	0.5%	59.1%	23.6%	16.0%	0.3%	2.5
Carrot	+8	0.3%	0.1%	1.1%	0.0%	63.5%	26.2%	8.7%	0.6%	1.1
Cauliflower	+10	0.4%	0.2%	0.1%	0.5%	38.0%	33.9%	26.9%	0.4%	0.9
Celery	+10	1.1%	0.8%	2.1%	0.0%	36.0%	42.0%	18.1%	2.1%	1.2
Collards	+10	0.7%	0.4%	1.0%	1.3%	24.8%	42.8%	29.1%	0.2%	2.5
Corn	+2	0.8%	1.5%	2.3%	0.1%	70.0%	11.6%	13.8%	0.1%	0.3
Cucumber	+2	0.8%	0.1%	0.6%	0.1%	71.8%	11.5%	14.9%	0.0%	0.3
Eggplant	+10	0.5%	0.2%	0.9%	0.2%	33.6%	49.7%	14.8%	0.0%	3.1
Green (or yellow) bean	+10	0.3%	0.1%	0.3%	0.4%	41.3%	37.6%	20.1%	0.1%	0.5
Kale	+8	0.7%	0.4%	1.0%	1.3%	58.2%	14.5%	24.0%	0.3%	2.5
Leek	+2	0.3%	0.0%	0.4%	0.6%	77.9%	11.3%	9.5%	0.1%	1.1
Lettuce, iceberg	+10	0.5%	0.2%	0.5%	1.3%	44.6%	30.2%	22.7%	0.3%	1.1
Lettuce, looseleaf	+10	0.8%	0.2%	0.9%	2.3%	31.9%	37.9%	25.9%	0.2%	3.1
Lettuce, romaine	+10	0.8%	0.3%	1.0%	2.4%	25.2%	44.4%	26.0%	0.2%	1.9
Mushroom	+8	0.7%	0.0%	2.1%	0.0%	43.9%	15.2%	47.1%	0.1%	1.5
Mushroom, portobello	+9	0.3%	0.0%	1.0%	0.0%	46.5%	19.5%	32.6%	0.1%	1.5
Okra	+10	0.3%	0.2%	0.3%	0.0%	42.1%	35.2%	22.0%	0.1%	1.0

VEGETABLES	Score	SFA	MUFA	LA	ALA	NFC	Fiber	Protein	Na	AOX
Onion	+4	0.4%	0.1%	0.1%	0.0%	72.7%	16.2%	10.5%	0.0%	1.1
Onion, scallion/green onion	+10	0.3%	0.3%	0.8%	0.0%	51.0%	28.0%	19.7%	0.2%	1.1
Pea	+10	0.4%	0.2%	0.8%	0.2%	46.4%	25.3%	26.9%	0.0%	0.2
Pepper, bell (green, red, yellow)	+8	0.7%	0.1%	1.2%	0.5%	60.4%	23.1%	14.0%	0.0%	1.1
Pepper, jalapeno	+10	0.8%	0.4%	4.0%	0.2%	40.5%	36.5%	17.6%	0.0%	2.5
Potato, red (with skin)	+1	0.2%	0.0%	0.2%	0.1%	79.4%	9.5%	10.6%	0.0%	0.6
Potato, white (with skin)	+2	0.1%	0.0%	0.2%	0.1%	76.2%	13.7%	9.6%	0.0%	0.6
Pumpkin	-1	0.7%	0.2%	0.0%	0.0%	79.3%	6.6%	13.2%	0.0%	0.4
Radish	+10	0.8%	0.4%	0.4%	0.7%	43.1%	38.3%	16.3%	0.9%	2.2
Spinach	+10	0.9%	0.1%	0.4%	2.1%	21.2%	32.7%	42.5%	1.2%	2.6
Squash, summer	+10	0.9%	0.3%	0.7%	1.2%	47.8%	23.4%	25.7%	0.0%	0.5
Squash, winter	+4	0.5%	0.2%	0.4%	0.6%	73.1%	15.5%	9.8%	0.0%	0.5
Sweet potato (with skin)	+2	0.1%	0.0%	0.1%	0.0%	78.8%	13.8%	7.2%	0.3%	0.4
Tomato	+8	0.6%	0.6%	1.6%	0.1%	55.1%	24.3%	17.8%	0.1%	0.7

Nuts and Seeds

The NQI rates 13 nuts and seeds based on *overall* nutritional quality. On a scale of **-10** (toxic) to **+10** (exceptional), scores range from **-6** to **+10** reflecting the dramatic variation in molecular contents and predicted metabolic and health consequences of different nuts and seeds.

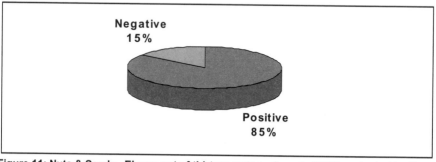

Figure 11: Nuts & Seeds. Eleven out of thirteen nuts and seeds (85%) evaluated by the NQI receive favorable ratings.

Like fruits and vegetables, nuts and seeds have a variety of beneficial health attributes, and replacement of other snack foods with nuts and seeds is likely to reduce your risk of the Big 7 epidemic U.S. diseases. However, ***not all nuts and seeds have equivalent metabolic and health properties and regular consumption of a few may even have adverse health consequences.*** For instance, the respective concentrations of fiber, monounsaturated fats, omega-6 fats, and omega-3 fats vary more than 8-fold, 30-fold, 25-fold, and 100-fold among different nuts and seeds. The two nuts receiving negative scores reflect high concentrations of saturated fats and unbalanced omega-6 to omega-3 ratios, as well as low contents of fiber, protein, monounsaturated fats, and antioxidants.

The NQI easily distinguishes between high and low quality nuts and seeds. The highest quality nuts and seeds contain significant quantities of monounsaturated fats, fiber, protein, and other beneficial components, as well as low omega-6 to omega-3 ratios. As part of a healthy diet, regular consumption of high quality nuts and seeds will optimize your metabolism and reduce your risk of developing the Big 7 epidemic U.S. diseases.

NQI SUPERIOR SELECTIONS

TOP 6 NUTS & SEEDS

+10	Flaxseed
+10	Hazelnut
+10	Macadamia
+9	Almond
+8	Pecan
+6	Pistachio

Author's Notes: *These ratings reflect the nutritional compositions of **raw** nuts and seeds. Processing reduces the nutritional quality of nuts in several ways:*

- *Roasting destroys many of the antioxidants.*
- *The addition of omega-6 rich vegetable and seed oils reduces the overall fat quality.*
- *The addition of salt significantly reduces overall nutritional quality.*

NUTS	Score	SFA	MUFA	LA	ALA	NFC	Fiber	Protein	Na	AOX
Almond	+9	4.3%	36.0%	13.7%	0.0%	8.9%	13.2%	23.8%	0.0%	0.5
Cashew	+1	9.9%	29.6%	8.3%	0.2%	32.2%	3.3%	16.6%	0.0%	0.2
Coconut	-6	59.3%	2.8%	0.7%	0.0%	12.4%	18.0%	6.7%	0.0%	1.0
Hazelnut	+10	5.0%	50.9%	8.7%	0.1%	7.8%	10.8%	16.7%	0.0%	1.0
Macadamia	+10	12.8%	62.5%	1.4%	0.2%	5.5%	9.1%	8.4%	0.0%	0.2
Peanut	+5	7.7%	27.5%	17.5%	0.0%	8.6%	9.6%	29.1%	0.0%	0.3
Pecan	+8	6.7%	44.5%	22.5%	1.1%	4.6%	10.5%	10.0%	0.0%	1.9
Pine nut	-2	5.8%	22.4%	39.6%	0.2%	11.2%	4.4%	16.3%	0.0%	0.1
Pistachio	+6	6.0%	25.7%	14.5%	0.3%	19.5%	11.3%	22.7%	0.0%	0.8
Walnut	+4	6.7%	9.8%	41.8%	10.0%	7.7%	7.3%	16.7%	0.0%	1.4

SEEDS	Score	SFA	MUFA	LA	ALA	NFC	Fiber	Protein	Na	AOX
Flaxseed	+10	4.2%	8.6%	6.8%	26.2%	1.8%	31.4%	21.0%	0.0%	1.0
Sesame	+4	7.8%	21.2%	24.1%	0.4%	13.1%	13.3%	20.0%	0.0%	0.5
Sunflower	+1	5.8%	10.6%	36.7%	0.1%	9.3%	11.8%	25.6%	0.0%	0.5

Legumes

The NQI rates 13 legumes based on *overall* nutritional quality. On a scale of -10 (toxic) to +10 (exceptional), scores range from +4 to +10 reflecting significant variation in molecular contents and predicted metabolic and health consequences of different legumes.

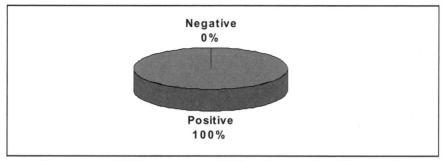

Figure 12: Legumes. All thirteen legumes (100%) evaluated by the NQI receive favorable ratings.

Like other unprocessed plant-based foods, legumes have a variety of beneficial health attributes, and replacement of processed foods with legumes is likely to reduce your risk of the Big 7 epidemic U.S. diseases. In fact, all thirteen legumes rated by the NQI receive a score of at least +4. These high scores reflect their high fiber and protein contents, and relatively high contents of antioxidants and other beneficial components. Despite these high scores, ***not all legumes have equivalent metabolic and health properties.*** In general, lower scores reflect higher concentrations of non-fiber carbohydrates (sugar equivalents) and modest antioxidant and fiber contents.

The NQI easily identifies the highest quality legumes. The highest rated legumes contain significant quantities of fiber, protein, antioxidants, and other beneficial components, as well as low non-fiber carbohydrate to fiber ratios. As part of a healthy diet, regular consumption of high quality legumes will optimize your metabolism and reduce your risk of developing the Big 7 epidemic U.S. diseases.

NQI SUPERIOR SELECTIONS

TOP 5 LEGUMES

+10	Lentil
+10	Kidney bean
+10	Split pea
+10	Fava bean
+10	Great Northern bean

LEGUMES	Score	SFA	MUFA	LA	ALA	NFC	Fiber	Protein	AOX
Black bean	+7	0.4%	0.1%	0.4%	0.3%	55.4%	17.9%	25.4%	0.9
Chickpea/garbanzo	+8	0.7%	1.6%	3.1%	0.1%	51.1%	20.6%	22.8%	1.0
Cowpea, blackeye	+4	0.4%	0.1%	0.4%	0.2%	58.5%	12.5%	27.8%	0.5
Edamame/soybean	+7	3.4%	5.2%	11.7%	1.6%	24.5%	10.9%	42.8%	1.0
Fava bean	+10	0.3%	0.4%	0.7%	0.1%	38.9%	29.2%	30.5%	0.5
Great Northern bean	+10	0.4%	0.1%	0.3%	0.3%	49.5%	23.7%	25.7%	1.0
Kidney bean	+10	0.1%	0.1%	0.2%	0.3%	41.7%	29.6%	28.0%	1.6
Lentil	+10	0.2%	0.2%	0.5%	0.1%	34.1%	35.2%	29.7%	1.0
Lima bean	+8	0.2%	0.1%	0.3%	0.1%	52.0%	22.3%	25.1%	0.0
Navy bean	+7	0.2%	0.2%	0.4%	0.6%	57.1%	18.2%	23.4%	0.3
Pinto bean	+8	0.3%	0.3%	0.2%	0.3%	55.5%	18.3%	25.2%	1.4
Split pea	+10	0.2%	0.3%	0.5%	0.1%	40.6%	29.7%	28.6%	1.0
White bean	+7	0.3%	0.1%	0.2%	0.2%	53.5%	18.0%	27.7%	1.0

For more information or to download NQI Ratings
for additional food categories as they become available
please visit us at www.theNQI.com